Vascular Disruptive Agents for the Treatment of Cancer

Tim Meyer
Editor

Vascular Disruptive Agents for the Treatment of Cancer

Springer

Editor
Tim Meyer
Senior Lecturer in Medical Oncology
UCL Cancer Institute
Paul O'Gorman Building
University College London
72 Huntley Street
London
WC1E 6BT
t.meyer@ucl.ac.uk

ISBN 978-1-4419-6608-7 e-ISBN 978-1-4419-6609-4
DOI 10.1007/978-1-4419-6609-4
Springer New York Dordrecht Heidelberg London

Library of Congress Control Number: 2010934905

Printed on acid-free paper

Springer is part of Springer Science+Business Media (www.springer.com)

Contents

Development of Vascular Disrupting Agents 1
Graeme J. Dougherty and David J. Chaplin

Part I Pre-Clinical Development

The Discovery and Characterisation of Tumour Endothelial Markers 31
Dario Neri and Roy Bicknell

The Use of Animal Models in the Assessment of Tumour Vascular Disrupting Agents (VDAs) 49
R. Barbara Pedley and Gillian M. Tozer

Combination Therapy with Chemotherapy and VDAs 77
Givlia Taraboletti, Katiuscia Bonezzi, and Raffaella Giavazzi

Lessons from Animal Imaging in Preclinical Models 95
Lesley D. McPhail and Simon P. Robinson

Combining Antiangiogenic Drugs with Vascular Disrupting Agents Rationale and Mechanisms of Action 117
Yuval Shaked, Paul Nathan, Laura G.M. Daenen, and Robert S. Kerbel

Part II Imaging in the Development of Vascular Disruptive Agents

MRI to Assess Vascular Disruptive Agents 137
Martin Zweifel and Anwar R. Padhani

Contrast Ultrasound in Imaging Tumor Angiogenesis 165
Grzegorz Korpanty and Rolf A. Brekken

Part III Clinical Development

The Clinical Development of Tubulin Binding Vascular Disrupting Agents 183
Martin Zweifel and Gordon Rustin

ASA404 (DMXAA): New Concepts in Tumour Vascular Targeting Therapy 217
Bruce C. Baguley

Vascular Disruptive Agents in Combination with Radiotherapy 231
Henry C. Mandeville and Peter J. Hoskin

Index 251

Contributors

Bruce C. Baguley
Auckland Cancer Society Research Centre, The University of Auckland, Auckland, New Zealand
b.baguley@auckland.ac.nz

Roy Bicknell
Cancer Research UK Angiogenesis Group, Institute for Biomedical Research, College of Medicine and Dentistry, University of Birmingham, Birmingham, B15 2TT, UK

Katiuscia Bonezzi
Mario Negri Institute for Pharmacological Research, c/o Parco Scientifico Technologico Kilometro Rosso Via Stezzano, 87, 24126 Bergamo, Italy

Rolf A. Brekken
Division of Surgical Oncology, Departments of Surgery and Pharmacology, The Hamon Center for Therapeutic Oncology Research, UT Southwestern Medical Center, 6000 Harry Hines Blvd, Dallas, TX 75390-8593, USA
rolf.brekken@utsouthwestern.edu

David J. Chaplin
OXiGENE Inc., Magdalen Centre, 1 Robert Robinson Road, Oxford, OX44GA, UK

Laura G.M. Daenen
Division of Molecular and Cellular Biology Research, Sunnybrook Health, Sciences Centre, 2075 Bayview Avenue, Toronto, ON, M4N 3M5, Canada

Graeme J. Dougherty
Department of Radiation Oncology, University of Arizona, 1501 North Campbell Avenue, Tucson, AZ 85724, USA
gdougherty@azcc.arizona.edu

Raffaella Giavazzi
Mario Negri Institute for Pharmacological Research,
via Giuseppe La Masa 19, 20156, Milano, Italy
raffaella.giavazzi@marionegri.it

Peter J. Hoskin
Marie Curie Research Wing, Mount Vernon Hospital, Northwood, UK
peterhoskin@nhs.net

Robert S. Kerbel
Division of Molecular and Cellular Biology Research, Sunnybrook Health, Sciences Centre, 2075 Bayview Avenue, Toronto, ON M4N 3M5, Canada and Department of Medical Biophysics, University of Toronto,
S-217,2075 Bayview Avenue, Toronto, ON M4N 3M5, Canada
Robert.kerbel@sri.utoronto.ca

Grzegorz Korpanty
Department of Medical Oncology, Mater Misericordiae University Hospital, Eccles St, Dublin 7, Ireland

Henry C. Mandeville
Marie Curie Research Wing, Mount Vernon Hospital, Northwood, UK

Lesley D. McPhail
Cancer Research Technology, The Beatson Institute for Cancer Research, Garscube Estate, Switchback Road, Bearsden, Glasgow, G61 1BD, UK
lmcphail@cancertechnology.com

Paul Nathan
Department of Medical Oncology, Mount Vernon Cancer Centre, Northwood, Middlesex, UK

Dario Neri
Department of Chemistry and Applied Biosciences, ETH Zurich,
Wolfgang-Pauli-Str. 10, CH-8093 Zurich, Switzerland
dario.neri@pharma.ethz.ch

Anwar R. Padhani
Paul Strickland Scanner Centre, Mount Vernon Cancer Centre,
Rickmansworth Road,
Northwood, Middlesex, HA6 2RN, UK

R. Barbara Pedley
UCL Cancer Institute, Paul O'Gorman Building,
University College London, 72 Huntley St, London, WC1E 6BT

Simon P. Robinson
Cancer Research UK Clinical Magnetic Resonance Research Group,
The Institute of Cancer Research, Sutton, Surrey, SM2 5NG, UK

Gordon Rustin
Department of Oncology, Mount Vernon Cancer Centre , Northwood, Middlesex, HA6 2RN, UK

Yuval Shaked
Department of Molecular Pharmacology, Rappaport Faculty of Medicine, Technion – Israel Institute of Technology, Haifa, 31096, Israel

Giulia Taraboletti
Mario Negri Institute for Pharmacological Research, c/o Parco Scientifico Technologico Kilometro Rosso Via Stezzano, 87, 24126 Bergamo, Italy

Gillian M. Tozer
Academic Unit of Surgical Oncology, School of Medicine & Biomedical Sciences, University of Scheffield, Beech Hill Road, Sheffield S10 2RX, UK

Martin Zweifel
Department of Oncology, Mount Vernon Cancer Centre, Rickmansworth Road, Northwood, Middlesex, HA6 2RN, UK

Development of Vascular Disrupting Agents

Graeme J. Dougherty and David J. Chaplin

Abstract The majority of the cancer therapies in use today target the malignant cell population. In broad terms, specificity is achieved by exploiting intrinsic differences between normal cells and tumor cells with respect to various key processes including proliferative activity, DNA repair and responsiveness to apoptotic stimuli. Although progress continues to be made, it remains the case that chemotherapy alone is rarely curative. Thus, in recent years increased interest has focused on alternative strategies that instead target various normal cell types upon which the survival and growth of a tumor depends. In this chapter we explore the historical events that lead to development of vascular disrupting therapies and discuss the major approaches currently employed to selectively destroy the neovasculature of solid tumors.

1 Introduction

For largely historical reasons, the majority of the cancer therapies in use today directly target the malignant cell population. Specificity is achieved by exploiting intrinsic differences between normal cells and tumor cells with respect to various key processes including proliferative activity, DNA repair, responsiveness to apoptotic stimuli and so on. While new tumor-directed therapies targeting novel pathways continue to be developed, it remains the case that chemotherapy alone is rarely curative. Thus, in recent years increased interest has focused on alternative strategies that instead target various normal cell types upon which the survival and growth of a tumor depends (Lorusso and Ruegg 2008; Mbeunkui and Johann 2009). Although a number of such approaches have been explored (Anton and Glod 2009; Dickens and Jubinsky 2009; Hanna et al. 2009; Kiaris et al. 2008; Ma and Adjei 2009; Zhang 2008), perhaps the most dramatic progress has been made in the area of vascular-directed therapies (Heath and Bicknell 2009).

G.J. Dougherty (✉)
Department of Radiation Oncology, University of Arizona,
1501 North Campbell Avenue, Tucson, AZ 85724, USA
e-mail: gdougherty@azcc.arizona.edu

T. Meyer (ed.), *Vascular Disruptive Agents for the Treatment of Cancer*,
DOI 10.1007/978-1-4419-6609-4_1, © Springer Science+Business Media, LLC 2010

As is the case for normal tissues, the growth of a tumor requires the provision of adequate levels of oxygen and nutrients and the removal of waste products generated in the course of metabolic activity (Cao 2009). Since the vascular system plays an essential role in each of these processes (Nikitenko 2009), it follows that approaches that compromise blood flow may provide therapeutic benefit (Siemann and Horsman 2009).

Tumors generally arise from a single cell that has undergone a number of genetic events that allow escape from the normal growth control mechanisms that operate within a tissue. Initially, the growing tumor receives sufficient oxygen and nutrients simply by diffusion from nearby blood vessels. However, as the mass increases in size, a point is quickly reached whereby consumption by cells closer to a vessel prevents more distant cells from receiving sufficient oxygen and nutrients to maintain viability, restricting further expansion and resulting in a tumor remaining localized (Fig. 1) (Bertout et al. 2008). For a tumor to continue to grow and ultimately metastasize to distant tissue sites, it is necessary that it trigger the production of new blood vessels (Fig. 1) (Bertout et al. 2008). This process, which is known as angiogenesis, is controlled by a large number of soluble mediators released by tumor cells and/or various tumor-associated normal cell types including macrophages and fibroblasts (Bertout et al. 2008). Working together in a hierarchical fashion, these so called "angiogenic factors" trigger the proliferation of endothelial cells in nearby vessels and coordinate the complex series of cell–cell and cell–matrix interactions that ultimately give rise to new tumor-associated blood vessels. Unlike in normal tissues, the aberrant and/or disregulated nature of the angiogenic process that occurs within tumors generates a structurally and functionally abnormal vasculature that is often described as "chaotic" (Cao 2009).

As understanding of the molecular events involved in the regulation of angiogenesis has increased, the possibility that the process might serve as a target for the development of novel cancer therapies, has gained support. Two distinct but potentially complimentary strategies have emerged. By far the greatest effort has focused on so-called "anti-angiogenic therapies." As first advocated by the late Professor M. Judah Folkman (Klagsbrun and Moses 2008), the goal of such treatments is to inhibit

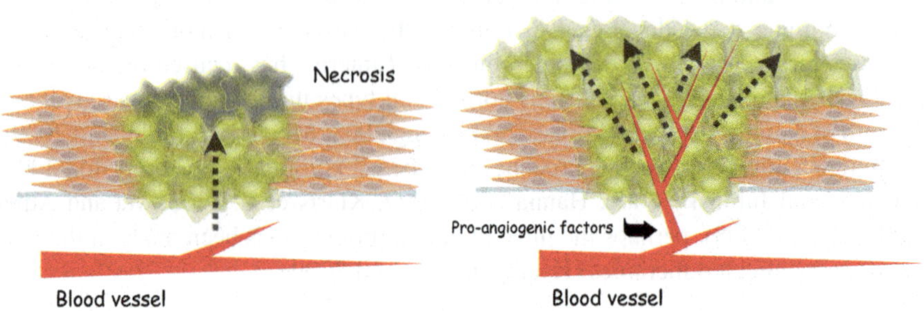

Fig. 1 Requirement for angiogenesis in tumor progression. As oxygen is consumed as it diffuses through tissue, cells more than ~150 μm from the nearest blood vessel receive insufficient supply to maintain their viability. Thus, in order for a tumor to continue to grow, it must induce the formation of new blood vessels. Tumors that fail to do so do not progress and remain localized

the angiogenic process so as to prevent the *formation* of new blood vessels (Ribatti 2009). Approaches targeting the pro-angiogenic cytokine vascular endothelial cell growth factor (VEGF) have shown the most promise (Fig. 2). Bevacizumab (Avastin), a humanized antibody directed against VEGF, was the first rationally-designed anti-angiogenic agent to be granted approval by the FDA, initially as a first line treatment for metastatic colorectal cancer in combination with fluorouracil-based chemotherapy (Rhee and Hoff 2005; Chase 2008; Grothey and Ellis 2008; Ribatti 2009). A number of small molecule tyrosine kinase inhibitors that block the signal transduction events induced upon the interaction of VEGF with its cognate receptor have also been developed (Wakelee and Schiller 2005; Baka et al. 2006). Examples include SU11248 (Sunitinib), BAY-43-9006 (Sorafenib/Nexavar) and ZD6474 (Zactima) (Fig. 2).

Although anti-angiogenic therapies are clearly of benefit in certain advanced malignancies, there are potential drawbacks with this approach that may limit its usefulness in other settings. Most importantly, while it is evident anti-angiogenic therapies not only prevent the formation of new blood vessels, but can induce the regression or normalization of the tumor-associated neovasculature (Heath and Bicknell 2009; Fukumura and Jain 2007; Huang and Chen 2008), the agents may need to be administered continuously over an extended period of time in order to produce a durable response. Indeed, there is evidence from both human and animal studies to suggest that vessels rapidly regrow once therapy is stopped (Mancuso et al. 2006). More worryingly, it has long been appreciated that since most anti-angiogenic agents including bevacizumab target a single pathway (e.g. VEGF), other angiogenic factors may simply take over in the presence of a specific inhibitor (Kuhn et al. 2006; Ruegg

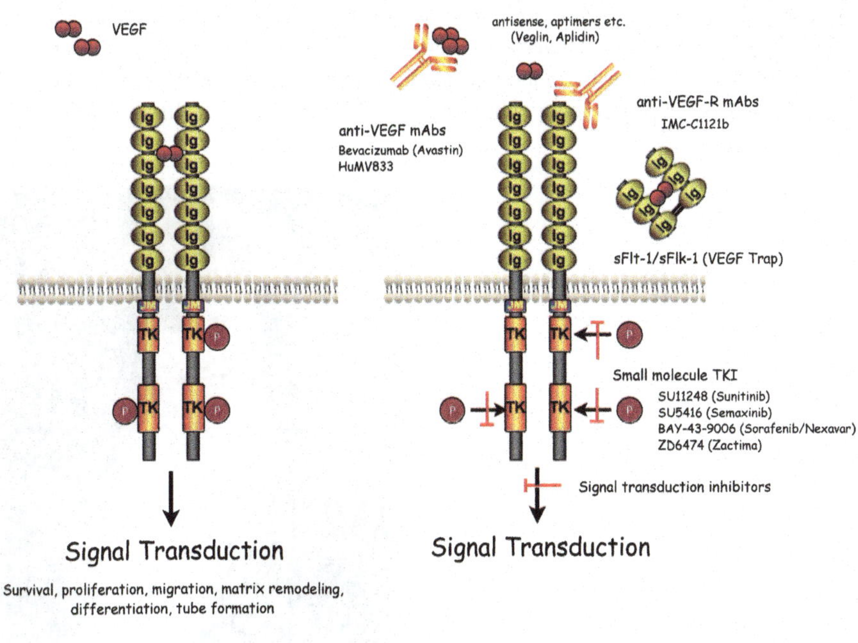

Fig. 2 Anti-angiogenic therapies targeting the VEGF pathway

and Mutter 2007). Indeed, the results of some mouse experiments suggest that angiogenic inhibitors targeting the VEGF pathway may trigger an adaptive response within a tumor and/or the host that may inadvertently result in enhanced invasiveness and metastatic potential (Paez-Ribes et al. 2009; Ebos et al. 2009). Such findings may be highly relevant with respect to several ongoing studies in which anti-angiogenic agents are being evaluated in an adjuvant and/or neoadjuvant setting in patients with earlier stage disease. In this regard, it may be telling that a recently completed Phase III study (NSABP C-08) in which patients with stage II or III colorectal cancer were assigned to receive FOLFOX chemotherapy with or without bevacizumab following surgery failed to demonstrate improved disease free survival in the arm receiving anti-angiogenic therapy (Wolmark et al. 2009).

It is for these and other reasons that efforts have been made to explore alternative vascular targeting strategies that involve not simply preventing angiogenesis but rather specifically disrupting the existing abnormal vasculature that is found within a tumor so as to prevent the delivery of the oxygen and nutrients required to maintain tumor cell viability (Siemann and Horsman 2009). Originally championed by the late Professor Juliana Denekamp (Fig. 3) (Denekamp 1982, 1984, 1990, 1991, 1993; Denekamp et al. 1983, 1998), this approach has gained acceptance in recent years with the development of several small molecule Vascular Disrupting Agents (VDAs) that have been shown to induce vascular shutdown and anti-tumor responses at well tolerated doses in the clinic (Cai 2007; LoRusso et al. 2008; Rehman and Rustin 2008; Siemann et al. 2009).

Vascular disrupting strategies offer a number of advantages over approaches that directly target tumor cells. With conventional chemotherapeutic agents, eradication of even a small tumor mass with a volume of around 1 cm^3 requires that an effective dose of the drug in question be delivered to each of up to 10^9 cells. Poor and/or intermittent perfusion resulting from the abnormal nature of tumor vasculature, high interstitial pressure and other physiologic considerations conspire to make this a challenging

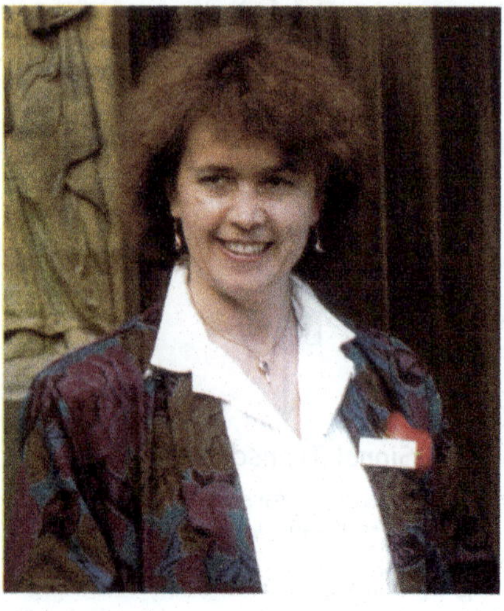

Fig. 3 Professor Juliana Denekamp (1943–2001)

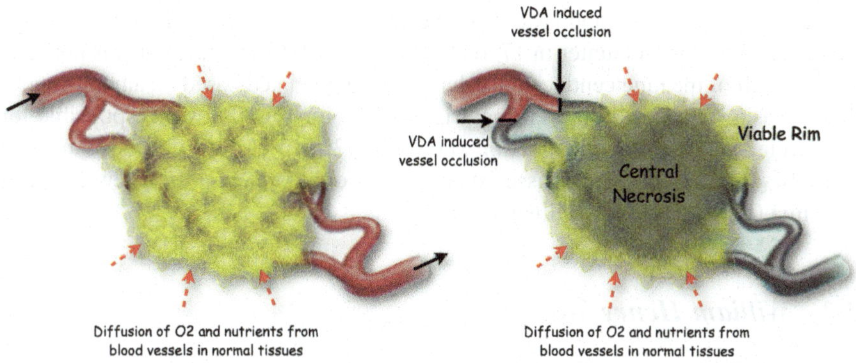

Fig. 4 Anti-tumor activity of vascular disrupting agents (VDAs). Vessel occlusion resulting from the selective action of VDAs on tumor-associated endothelial cells blocks blood flow and prevents the delivery of required oxygen and nutrients to a tumor mass. Not only are tumor cells in the direct vicinity of the point of damage killed but also all downstream cells supplied by that vessel. Thus VDAs typically produce massive necrosis particularly within central regions of a treated tumor. Cells around the periphery survive as they receive sufficient oxygen and nutrients to maintain viability by diffusion from vessels in surrounding normal tissues. In the absence of additional treatment, cells in this so called "viable rim" can repopulate necrotic regions allowing tumor growth to resume

objective. In contrast, for VDAs, the cells being targeted (i.e. endothelial cells lining tumor-associated blood vessels) are in direct contact with the circulation and thus easily accessible to intravenously administered agents. Moreover, it is not even necessary to kill endothelial cells in order to mediate an effect, as any change in their shape or function, even if temporary, which interferes with blood flow, may be effective. Most importantly, as blood vessels are effectively pipelines through which oxygen and nutrients are carried to, and the toxic waste products of metabolism removed from, a tumor mass it follows that damage at any one point that obstructs blood flow will result in the death not only of cells in the direct vicinity of the point of damage but also all downstream cells supplied by that vessel segment (Fig. 4). Thus even limited damage to the tumor vasculature may result in the death of many thousands of tumor cells if blood flow is shutdown for an adequate period of time.

2 Early Studies Supporting the Development of Vascular Disrupting Cancer Therapies

2.1 Testicular Torsion

The discovery that transient disruption of vascular function can cause rapid tissue death came from studies involving various normal tissues. For example, testicular torsion, in which the spermatic cord carrying the blood supply to a testicle becomes twisted, reducing or abolishing blood flow and leading, if untreated, to atrophy or loss of the affected testicle, was first described in the medical literature by the London surgeon John Hunter in 1776 (Noske et al. 1998). However, it was not until the later half of the nineteenth century that it was appreciated based on animal studies that it was a reduction in blood flow triggered by torsion that was responsible for the resultant hemorrhagic infarction (Follin 1852; Miflet 1879). It is of interest from these studies that gross tissue damage was only evident after a few hours of ischemia (Enderlen 1896; Hellner 1933).

2.2 *William Henry Woglom*

By the mid 1800s there were occasional apocryphal reports that tumors too sometimes regressed if their blood supply was compromised as a result of torsion of the vascular pedicle or thrombosis of a major feeding vessel (Walshe 1844). However, the therapeutic potential of vascular disrupting strategies seems to have remained largely unrealized until a seminal paper from William Henry Woglom, published in 1923 (Woglom 1923). It is obvious from comments made in this publication, that Woglam understood not only the causal relationship between vessel thrombosis and tumor regression, but more importantly, the unique opportunity that this relationship presented with respect to the development of novel therapies. Clearly, he also appreciated the challenge, when he noted that "the problem of treatment would be to find some agent capable of thrombosing the vessels of a tumor and no others." Most perceptively, he also outlined a potential problem with vascular disrupting therapies when he stated that "even though all the vessels of a tumor could be thrombosed, there would often remain single cells or small groups of cells invading the surrounding tissue and supported, not by the blood-vessels of the neoplasm from which they escaped, but by the fluids imbibed from the normal tissues about them." As discussed below, it is precisely such a mechanism that is believed to explain the characteristic persistence of a so-called "viable rim" around the periphery of a tumor after treatment with a VDA.

2.3 *Tumor Clamping Studies*

As indicated above, Juliana Denekamp and her colleagues at the CRC Gray Laboratory in the UK played an instrumental role in advancing the concept of vascular disrupting therapy and in providing an experimental basis for the rational development of effective small molecule therapeutics. Of key importance were a series of studies in which ischemia was induced by applying D-shaped metal clamps across the base of transplantable subcutaneous murine tumors (Denekamp et al. 1983). As one would expect from the studies on vessel torsion described above, the extent of tumor cell death was directly proportional to the duration of clamping. Temperature was also important with a much reduced rate of cell death observed for a given period of ischemia if tumors were allowed to cool during treatment (Chaplin and Horsman 1994b). Generally speaking, if tumors were maintained at

37°C greater than 99% of cells were killed if blood flow was interrupted for 2 h (Chaplin and Horsman 1994a, b). However, up to 15 h of vessel occlusion was necessary if the subsequent regrowth of treated tumors was to be prevented (Denekamp et al. 1983). In contrast, studies with C3H mammary tumors indicated that a 6 h period of ischemia was sufficient to cure three of seven treated tumors maintained at 37°C (Chaplin and Horsman 1994a, b). Similar results were also obtained using the CaNT tumor model (Parkins et al. 1994). Together with the work on testicular torsion, these studies demonstrate the potent impact of ischemia on tumor cell survival and suggest that shutting off the blood supply to a tumor for just a few hours may be sufficient to cause extensive cell death and necrosis.

2.4 Coley's Toxins

There have been reports dating back to at least the beginning of the eighteenth century suggesting a causal relationship between infection, particularly bacterial infection, and cancer regression (Hoption Cann et al. 2002). Over the years, various attempts have been made to develop treatments that exploit this relationship. Among the best known early proponents of such an strategy was the New York surgeon Dr. William B. Coley (Hoption Cann et al. 2003). His interest was apparently triggered by his frustration over the poor prognosis of sarcoma patients in his care. In reviewing the associated medical records he became aware of the case of an apparently terminal patient who staged a remarkable recovery after suffering two episodes of erysipelas, associated with infection with the bacterium *Streptococcus pyogenes* (McCarthy 2006). Although this relationship had been noted by others (Busch 1866; Gresser 1987), Coley was among the first to deliberately inoculate cancer patients with bacterial preparations in an effort to induce a therapeutic response (Coley 1891). "Coley's Toxins," a mixture of killed *S. pyogenes* and *Serratia marcescens* (Coley 1914), has been evaluated in numerous clinical trials and although the results were at best mixed, the occasional response served to stimulate interest in this area. Subsequent analysis of the active components in Coley's Toxins suggested a key role for lipopolysaccharide (LPS) (Shear et al. 1943). Importantly from the perspective of vascular disruption, early studies in mice demonstrated that purified LPS can induce the collapse of tumor capillaries producing a pattern of hemorrhagic necrosis, particularly within central regions of a tumor, characteristic of that seen subsequently with small molecule VDAs (Shear 1944; Algire et al. 1952). Similar results were obtained with other non-specific bacterial immunostimulants including *Corynebacterium parvum* and bacillus Calmette-Guérin (BCG).

An important step in the understanding of the mechanisms involved in this effect came with the finding that LPS and can induce the production of various pro-inflammatory cytokines including one that is now known as tumor necrosis factor-alpha (TNF-α) (Carswell et al. 1975; Flick and Gifford 1986). As its name suggests, TNF-α can, in the absence of other factors, induce the collapse of tumor vessels triggering a necrotic response (Carswell et al. 1975; Flick and Gifford 1986). Although

TNF-α is clearly pleiotropic and has both positive and negative effects on endothelial cells (Pober 1987; Balkwill 1989), this finding served to validate vasculature as a target in cancer therapy. It is unfortunate that the systemic toxicity of TNF-α prevents its use as a vascular disrupting agent (Hundsberger et al. 2008). It should also be remembered that bacteria and their products can potentially affect the viability and function of endothelial cells through other mechanisms. For example, it has recently been shown that platelets activated by bacterial endotoxin, induced endothelial cells to produce reactive oxygen species that triggered apoptotic death through a caspase 8- and caspase 9-dependent process (Kuckleburg et al. 2008). Findings such as this help explain the endothelial damage associated with infection with certain bacterial species including *Haemophilus somnus* (Kuckleburg et al. 2008). Whether such bacteria have therapeutic potential in the treatment of cancer remains largely unexplored.

3 Vascular Disrupting Therapies Employing High Molecular Weight Agents

The physical obstacles that contrive to limit the efficacy of antibodies, peptides and other large high molecular weight reagents in cancer treatment are far less important in the context of vascular targeted anti-angiogenic and vascular disrupting therapies as the cells being targeted (i.e. endothelial cells) are in direct contact with the circulation and are thus readily accessible to intravenously administered agents (Thorpe et al. 2003). The possibility that limited damage to the vasculature may produce a large downstream effect is an additional benefit.

A number of determinants differentially expressed on the surface of tumor-associated vascular endothelial cells have been identified (Folkman 1999; Thorpe and Ran 2002; Enback and Laakkonen 2007) and in some cases antibodies or other molecules directed against these structures have been shown to express vascular disrupting activity of sufficient magnitude to impact on tumor grown in experimental systems (Thorpe 2004).

3.1 Engineered Ligands

Ligands that interact with receptors that are induced or activated at sites of active angiogenesis can be engineered so as induce endothelial cell death or other changes upon binding. Examples include a fusion between the pro-angiogenic cytokine VEGF and the toxin gelonin, which acts as a potent inhibitor of protein synthesis ($VEGF_{121}$/rGel) (Veenendaal et al. 2002). Studies have shown that the purified homodimeric fusion protein selectively killed proliferating endothelial cells that overexpress the VEGF receptor Flk-1/KDR with an IC50 in the low nM range. Non-dividing endothelial cells were relatively resistant. In a prostate tumor model, $VEGF_{121}$/rGel caused thrombotic damage to tumor vessels, induced hemorrhagic necrosis and reduced tumor volume (Veenendaal et al. 2002). The growth of MDA-MB-231 breast tumor metastases in SCID mice was similarly inhibited by treatment with $VEGF_{121}$/rGel (Ran et al. 2005b). As one might expect, the lung colonies that did grow in treated animals tended to be smaller and their vascularity was substantially reduced relative to controls (Ran et al. 2005b). The growth of orthotopic human bladder cancer xenografts was also inhibited by this treatment (Mohamedali et al. 2005).

3.2 Antibody-Based Approaches

Encouraging results have been obtained using a number of antibodies and antibody fragments directed against proteins or other molecules that are upregulated or differentially expressed on tumor-associated blood vessels (Pasqualini and Arap 2002). Targets include receptors that bind various angiogenic factors, adhesion proteins that mediate the cell–cell and cell–matrix interactions involved in the formation of new blood vessels and lectins and other molecules induced in response to the plethora of pro-inflammatory cytokines and other stimuli produced within the tumor microenvironment (Thorpe 2004).

While antibody binding alone could potentially cause vessel occlusion as the result, for example, of complement activation, most strategies that have been explored so far have utilized immunoconjugates of one type or another. L19, a humanized scFv antibody fragment specific for the oncofetal ED-B domain of fibronectin fused to the extracellular domain of tissue factor can trigger clotting and block nutritive blood flow after being bound by immature and/or proliferating endothelial cells. The same antibody fragment has also been used with some success to target radioisotopes (Demartis et al. 2001) and various cytokines including TNF-α (Borsi et al. 2003; Balza et al. 2006), IFN-γ (Borsi et al. 2003), IL-12 (Gafner et al. 2006) and IL-15 and GM-CSF (Kaspar et al. 2007) to the tumor vasculature. Tissue factor can also produce vessel occlusion, tumor necrosis and tumor growth delay if localized to tumor vasculature using an antibody to the adhesion protein VCAM-1 (Ran et al. 1998; Dienst et al. 2005).

Recently, much interest in the area of antibody-mediated vascular disrupting therapy has focused on the targeting potential of anionic phospholipids. Although normally found only on the internal (i.e. cytoplasmic) surface of the plasma membrane, negatively charged phospholipids, including most notably phosphatidylserine (PS), are exposed on the outer surface of injured, activated and apoptotic cells. Unexpectedly, PS is also present on the luminal surface on a large proportion of apparently viable endothelial cells in tumor vessels (Ran et al. 2002). While the precise signals responsible for this effect remain to be determined, inflammatory cytokines, thrombin, acidity and periods of hypoxia and reoxygenation all trigger the surface expression of PS on endothelial cells in vitro (Ran and Thorpe 2002). Injury induced by exposure to reactive oxygen intermediates may be key (Ran and Thorpe 2002). Systemic administration of a monoclonal antibody designated 3G4 that specifically binds to surface-expressed PS in the presence of the plasma protein beta-2-glycoprotein 1 (Luster et al. 2006), produced extensive vascular damage and a resultant reduction in vascular density and functional vascular volume in a number of murine tumor models (Ran et al. 2005a). Evidence suggests that monocyte-mediated antibody-dependent cytotoxic mechanisms may be involved in this effect (Ran et al. 2005a). While tumor growth was substantially reduced, normal tissues were unaffected (Ran et al. 2005a). Additional inhibition of tumor growth was obtained when anti-PS antibodies were combined with conventional cytotoxic agents including docetaxel (Huang et al. 2005) and gemcitabine (Beck et al. 2006). Radiation therapy also enhanced the vascular disrupting and anti-tumor activity of anti-PS antibodies (He et al. 2007). In this later case, there is evidence that exposure to radiation increases the expression of PS on the surface of endothelial cells in tumor vessels, which in turn improves the efficiency of antibody-dependent cell-mediated cytotoxicity (He et al. 2007).

The therapeutic potential of bavituximab, a chimeric version of the anti-PS monoclonal antibody 2aG4, is currently being investigated in three Phase II trials. Two are focused on advanced breast cancer and employ bavituximab in combination with docetaxel or paclitaxel and carboplatin respectively. In the third, bavituximab is being evaluated in combination with paclitaxel and carboplatin for the treatment of advanced non-small cell lung cancers. A Phase I trial of bavituximab monotherapy is also currently underway.

3.3 *Gene Therapy*

While there are significant practical and regulatory obstacles to the commercial development of molecular approaches to cancer treatment, the exquisite targeting specificity that can be achieved through the use of such techniques has served to stimulate interest in this potentially important area (Edelstein et al. 2004).

A key factor that has limited the more widespread adoption of molecular therapies designed to target the malignant cell population is the relatively poor transduction efficiencies that can be achieved using currently available viral and non-viral vectors (Kouraklis 1999; Kesmodel and Spitz 2003; Dass and Choong 2006; Arnberg 2009). It is partly for this reason that vascular directed gene therapy approaches are so attractive, as there are grounds to believe that even modest damage to tumor vasculature may cause the death of substantial numbers of tumor cells if the gene being expressed results in vessel occlusion thereby preventing the delivery of essential oxygen and/or nutrients to the tumor site (Dougherty et al. 2004; Liu and Deisseroth 2006). Thus, in contrast to other forms of cancer gene therapy it does not seem entirely unreasonable to expect that dramatic anti-tumor effects may be produced even if the therapeutic gene in question is expressed only transiently in subset of endothelial cells in a tumor-associated vessel (Dougherty et al. 2004).

Among the genes that might prove useful in the context of vascular disrupting molecular therapies are those encoding the bacterial toxins *Pseudomonas* exotoxin A and diphtheria toxin, both of which posses potent ADP ribosyltransferase activity and can thus kill endothelial and other cell types by attacking elongation factor 2 and inhibiting protein synthesis. Genes that encode enzymes that activate various prodrugs or which sensitize endothelial cells to the cytotoxic effects of ionizing radiation and/or chemotherapeutic agents all have their supporters. Genes that activate complement or induce coagulation are also attractive. Rather more speculatively, the results of studies employing small molecule tubulin-deploymerizing agents, as described below, suggest that some thought might be given to the therapeutic potential of genes that can alter the shape and/or adhesive properties of endothelial cells.

Finally, we have advocated a functional targeting strategy that employs genes that are activated to produce an effect (i.e. endothelial cell death) only when triggered by signals that are uniquely present within the tumor microenvironment. One example of this approach involves a chimeric protein in which the extracellular domain of the VEGF receptor Flk-1/KDR is fused in frame to the cytoplasmic death domain of the pro-apoptotic protein Fas (Carpenito et al. 2002; Dougherty and Dougherty 2009). Rather than triggering the growth promoting signals that are normally transduced when Flk-1/KDR binds the angiogenic cytokine VEGF, the chimeric Flk-1/Fas protein instead triggers apoptotic cell death when expressed in endothelial cells (Carpenito et al. 2002). Since the induction of apoptosis requires oligomerization of the chimeric receptor (Carpenito et al. 2002), death only occurs at sites where VEGF is present at a reasonably high level. This ensures that endothelial cells within the tumor microenvironment are selectively killed even if the therapeutic gene is widely expressed.

Endothelial cells can be readily transduced with viral and non-viral vectors both in vitro and in vivo (Nabel et al. 1991; Baker et al. 2005). Differential transduction of endothelial cells lining tumor-associated vessels is more challenging but is necessary if normal tissue damage is to be avoided (Baker et al. 2005). Approaches in which peptides are incorporated into viral receptors in order to redirect or restrict infection to cells expressing a particular differentially expressed counter-receptor have proven effective in endothelial cell targeting (Krasnykh et al. 1998; Cowan et al. 2003; Nicklin et al. 2004; White et al. 2004; Parker et al. 2005; Hajitou et al. 2006; Work et al. 2006; White et al. 2008). Although cell surface structures involved in angiogenesis or induced on endothelial cells in response to signals produced within the tumor microenvironment can be targeted, recently developed phage display techniques allow the identification of defined peptides that bind specifically to tumor-associated endothelial cells without any knowledge of the nature of the structures with which they interact (Nicklin et al. 2004).

Additional control of therapeutic genes in order to ensure that they act only on endothelial cells in tumor vessels can be achieved by placing their expression under the control of an appropriate promoter and/or enhancer element. Sequences upstream of a number of endothelial cell-specific genes have been cloned and several tested for their ability to drive gene expression within tumor-associated endothelial cells (Graulich et al. 1999; Jager et al. 1999; Nicklin et al. 2001; Dancer et al. 2003; De Palma et al. 2003; Greenberger et al. 2004; Work et al. 2004; Dong and Nor 2009; Hodish et al. 2009). The results so far have been encouraging. Screening strategies that permit the isolation of entirely synthetic regulatory elements that possess a desired level of specificity and activity have also proven fruitful in the context of endothelial cell targeting and are likely to grow in importance (Dai et al. 2004).

4 Small Molecule Vascular Disrupting Agents

4.1 Metals and Metalloids

The induction of a massive necrotic response within a few hours of drug administration is a defining feature of agents that mediate their anti-tumor effects via vascular damage. Various metals and metalloids that have been used in cancer therapy over the years produce such an effect and in some cases this activity has been attributed to induced changes in blood flow. Thus early studies on lead colloids noted not only the rapid regression of large tumor masses (Fitzwilliams 1927) but related this activity to the thrombosis of tumor vessels (Mottram 1923; Wood 1926). Certain arsenic compounds, too, appear to induce both vascular damage and rapid tumor necrosis although such effects are generally only observed when these compounds are used at, or close to, their maximum tolerated dose (MTD) (Leiter et al. 1952). Of the compounds tested, trivalent arsenicals were among the most effective. More recent animal studies have confirmed that arsenic trioxide, which is employed primarily in the treatment of promyelocytic leukemia, has dramatic effects on blood flow in a number of solid tumor models (Lew et al. 1999; Griffin et al. 2003). It may be relevant in connection with the studies on colchicine described below, that arsenic trioxide has been shown to inhibit GTP-induced polymerization of monomeric tubulin and microtubule formation (Li and Broome 1999). Given their mechanism of action (Lew et al. 1999; Griffin et al. 2003) further rational development of these compounds as vascular disrupting agents may be warranted.

4.2 Flavonoids/Xanthenones

Several investigators have demonstrated that the flavonoid Flavone Acetic Acid (FAA) can reduce tumor blood flow and trigger hemorrhagic necrosis in animal tumor models. The proposed mechanism of action has been attributed to the ability of FAA to trigger the local production of TNF-α by tumor-associated macrophages and/or other tumor-associated host cell types (Baguley 2001). Although a number of trials were initiated, the absence of convincing responses when used as a monotherapy ultimately caused clinical development to be discontinued. While there may be other reasons, the lack of an obvious effect of FAA in the clinic was attributed to the fact that, unlike the situation in rodents, the compound was a only a weak inducer of TNF-α by human cells (Philpott et al. 2001). However, we are now aware that because of the "viable rim effect" VDAs are unlikely to be very effective when used as a monotherapy and in the absence of tumor blood flow data it may have been premature to list this agent as an ineffective VDA in the clinic.

These studies nevertheless served to stimulate interest in finding structurally related compounds that retain activity in humans (Aitken et al. 1998; Pinto et al. 2005).

The most promising agent identified to date is 5,6-dimethylxanthenone 4-acetic acid (DMXAA) (Philpott et al. 1997, 2001; Baguley 2003). DMXAA performed well in certain animal models (Seshadri et al. 2007) both as a single agent and in combination with other treatments and has demonstrated evidence of blood flow reduction in the clinic (Zhou et al. 2002; Baguley and Wilson 2002; Baguley 2003; McKeage 2008; Rehman and Rustin 2008). Acquired by Antisoma, the compound has recently been licensed to Novartis AG and is now referred to as ASA404. In Phase II studies, ASA404 was evaluated in combination with conventional chemotherapy in the treatment of lung, prostate and ovarian cancers (McKeage et al. 2008, 2009). Phase III trials in lung cancer are currently underway and a breast cancer trial is planned (Rehman and Rustin 2008).

4.3 N-Cadherin Antagonists

Adhesive interactions between endothelial cells play an essential role in maintaining the functional integrity of blood vessels (Blaschuk and Rowlands 2000; Vestweber et al. 2009; Gavard 2009; London et al. 2009). The cell surface structures that mediate such interactions are thus obvious targets for therapy (Blaschuk and Rowlands 2000; Lu et al. 2009; Alghisi et al. 2009). In this regard, a cyclic peptide termed ADH-1 or Exherin that blocks the homotypic binding of N-cadherin molecules has been shown to trigger blood flow reductions and hemorrhage within animal tumors (Kelland 2007; Li et al. 2007; Mariotti et al. 2007). Phase Ib/II and Phase II trials of ADH-1 monotherapy have already been completed and combination studies are ongoing (Perotti et al. 2009).

4.4 Colchicine

Colchicine is an tricyclic alkaloid originally extracted from the Autumn crocus (Meadow saffron) *Colchicum autumnale*. While *Colchicum* preparations have been employed since at least Roman times as a treatment for gout, the use of colchicine as an anti-cancer agent has a more recent history. Among the key early studies were those of Eric and Margaret Boyland at the Chester Beatty Research Institute in London. Working with both transplantable and spontaneous chemically-induced tumors they demonstrated that intraperitoneal injection of colchicine could induce hemorrhagic necrosis similar to that produced by bacterial extracts (Boyland and Boyland 1937, 1940). They noted, however, that such effects only occurred at, or very close to, MTD.

Further work on the mechanism of action of colchicine on tumor tissue was carried out by Ludford (Ludford 1948). These important studies provided clear evidence that the anti-tumor activity of colchicine could be attributed mostly to vascular damage that preferentially affected newly formed tumor vessels. Again, it was noted that these effects only occurred at doses that resulted in the death of significant numbers of treated animals (Ludford 1948).

Concerns over the low therapeutic index of colchicine, did not, at least initially, discourage its evaluation in the treatment of human tumors. In a study carried out by Seed et al. published in 1940 (Seed et al. 1940) two of four patients with large advanced carcinomas that received high doses of colchicine exhibited evidence of "rapid (tumor) degeneration" that occurred within a few days of treatment. Emphasizing the systemic toxicity of the doses of colchicine used in this study, the other two patients could not be evaluated as they died from the effects of colchicine poisoning! Interestingly, in the two patients that did survive, tumor control was only temporary, presumably because malignant cells surviving toward the periphery of the tumor mass rapidly repopulated necrotic regions re-establishing tumor growth. It is now appreciated that this presentation is typical of that seen with newer less toxic VDAs (Chaplin and Hill 2002; Davis et al. 2002; West and Price 2004; Gaya and Rustin 2005; Chaplin et al. 2006; Pilat and Lorusso 2006).

Other more recently discovered tubulin depolymerizing agents used in cancer therapy including podophyllotoxin (Leiter et al. 1950) and the vinca alkaloids vinblastine and vincristine (Baguley et al. 1991; Hill et al. 1994) also disrupt tumor vasculature and induce rapid hemorrhagic necrosis but as with colchicine do so only at doses near MTD.

4.5 Novel Vascular Disrupting Tubulin Depolymerizing Agents

The encouraging results obtained with colchicine and related compounds motivated the search for novel tubulin depolymerizing agents that have vascular disrupting activity at doses well below MTD. These studies were facilitated by the development of a simple perfusion assay involving intravenous injection of the fluorochrome Hoechst 33342 that permitted the effect of drug treatment on tumor blood flow to be rapidly and quantitatively determined (Chaplin et al. 1987). Although most compounds possessed anti-vascular activity only when administered at near toxic doses, several agents were identified that had dramatic effects on tumor blood flow at doses as low as 1/10th MTD (Chaplin et al. 1996; Dark et al. 1997).

One of the first agents identified in this way, was the soluble phosphate prodrug of combretastatin A4 (CA4P), a compound isolated initially from the bark of the South African "bushwillow" *Combretum caffrum* by Pettit and colleagues in the early 1980s (Dark et al. 1997; Pettit et al. 1989; el-Zayat et al. 1993).

The active moiety CA4, released upon dephosphorylation of CA4P, binds rapidly to β-tubulin, at or near the site recognized by colchicine (kd = 0.4 ± 0.06 μM). It can competitively inhibit colchicine binding with a Ki of 0.14 μM and shares with colchicine the ability to prevent tubulin polymerization. Where it differs from colchicine is with respect to dissociation rate. While colchicine dissociates from tubulin with a half-life of approximately 405 min at 37°C, CA4 has a half-life of only 3.6 min. It is this characteristic of CA4 that in part explains the absence of the toxicities commonly associated with tubulin-directed anti-mitotic agents when the compound is administered in vivo.

Similar functional screening approaches have been used by other groups to identify additional agents that can disrupt tumor blood flow and induce a necrotic response. Of those that have progressed furthest in human trials, most, including ZD6126 (Angiogene), MN029/Denibulin (Medicinova), AVE8062E (Sanofi Aventis), NPI-2358 (Nereus) and BNC-105 (Bionomics) also bind to and disrupt tubulin (Hinnen and Eskens 2007; Cai 2007; Lippert, 2007). A number of other tubulin-binding agents that were originally identified on the basis of their anti-mitotic activity have subsequently been tested for vascular effects. Examples include MPC6827 (Azixa, a brain-penetrating anti-mitotic from Myriad), ABT751 (Abott, an oral anti-mitotic), LP261 (an oral anti-mitotic from Locus), CYT997 (Cytopia) and EPC2407 (Epicept). Although it is not unexpected that certain of these agents will, like vinblastine, vincristine and colchicine, possess tumor-selective VDA activity, it remains to be determined whether the doses required to achieve such effects are sufficiently below MTD so as to permit them to be used in this manner.

The question of specificity is obviously key to the success of VDAs. When administered in vivo, VDAs appear to cause the immature endothelial cells lining the structurally abnormal blood vessels that supply a growing tumor mass to round up and detach from the basement membrane (Blakey et al. 2002b). Intravascular coagulation is subsequently induced resulting in vessel blockage and the slowing or cessation of nutritive blood flow (Blakey et al. 2002b). Without adequate oxygen and nutrients, cells soon die and a massive necrotic response results particularly within central regions of a treated tumor mass (Blakey et al. 2002b). In part, the selective destruction of tumor vasculature can be attributed to the reliance of endothelial cells in newly formed or immature vessels on a tubulin cytoskeleton for the maintenance of their elongated shape, while in more mature non-proliferating endothelial cells this function is largely supplanted by actin (Gotlieb 1990; Galbraith et al. 2001; Lee and Gotlieb 2005). CA4P has also been demonstrated to disrupt adhesive interactions between endothelial cells mediated by the vascular endothelial (VE)-cadherin/β-catenin complex (Vincent et al. 2005). The presence of smooth muscle cells, a characteristic feature of normal tissue vasculature, inhibits this disruption (Vincent et al. 2005). The targeting of recently formed endothelial cells in immature or abnormal vessels which lack a full complement of smooth muscle or pericyte support is thus believed to be responsible in large part for the specificity of tubulin binding VDAs.

It has been suggested that an early consequence of endothelial cell shape change is an increase in vascular permeability. Clearly, if rapid changes in endothelial cell morphology and detachment do occur in vivo, exposure of the basement membrane and a physical narrowing of the vessel lumen will contribute to the reduction in capillary blood flow, increasing vascular resistance as well as inducing hemorrhage and coagulation. The sensitivity of the immature tumor vasculature to CA4P probably relates to not only structural differences between newly formed and mature endothelial cells and the absence or presence of support cells but also to characteristics of the tumor microcirculation such as high interstitial fluid pressure, pro-coagulant status, vessel tortuosity and heterogeneous blood flow distribution.

Pharmacokinetic considerations are also likely to be important. Thus, in contrast to established cytotoxic agents such as vinblastine or colchicine that bind to and destabilize tubulin, or microtubule-stabilizing cytotoxins such as paclitaxel and docetaxel, the depolymerizing activity of VDAs is rapidly reversible (Blakey et al. 2002b; Chaplin and Hill 2002). As the compounds also have a relatively short plasma elimination half-life following intravenous administration (Blakey et al. 2002a; Dowlati et al. 2002; Beerepoot et al. 2006), effects on the shape and adhesive properties of immature tubulin-dependent endothelial cells are achieved without the toxicities commonly associated with the use of tubulin-directed anti-mitotic drugs (Beerepoot et al. 2006; LoRusso et al. 2008).

Although almost all the focus on the development of VDAs has centered on solid tumor indications, CA4P has recently been shown to elicit significant anti-tumor activity against orthotopically implanted leukemia when used as a single agent (Petit et al. 2008). This activity is believed to result from the ability of CA4P to alter the adherence and attachment of leukemic cells which exist in treatment resistant stromal niches (Petit et al. 2008). It is probable that, as with the effects on immature endothelial cells, alterations in both cell shape and adhesion molecule expression and/or function trigger this release. These results offer the possibility that tubulin binding VDAs may have a role in the treatment of chemotherapy resistant leukemias (Petit et al. 2008; Fang et al. 2008; Xu et al. 2008; Billard et al. 2008).

5 Combining VDAs with Other Therapies

As Woglom predicted almost 100 years ago (Woglom 1923), a characteristic of VDA therapy, is the persistence around the periphery of a treated tumor of a layer of viable cells that survive because they obtain the oxygen and nutrients necessary to remain viable, by diffusion from unaffected mature vessels present in surrounding non-malignant tissues (Chaplin and Hill 2002; Davis et al. 2002). In the absence of further treatment, this so called "viable rim" can serve as a reservoir from which malignant cells can invade and repopulate the necrotic central regions of a treated tumor (Chaplin and Hill 2002; Davis et al. 2002). It is for this reason that VDAs are generally most effective when used in combination with conventional cytotoxic agents or radiation therapy that kill the comparatively well-oxygenated and mitotically active cells remaining within the viable rim (Thorpe 2004; Siemann et al. 2004; Siemann and Horsman 2004; Siemann and Shi 2004).

As repopulation of the necrotic regions produced within a tumor as a result of VDA treatment is dependent upon revascularization, it follows that combining small molecule VDA approaches with anti-angiogenic therapies may provide another way of slowing or preventing tumor regrowth. VEGF, upregulated in response to hypoxic stimuli, is a key regulator of revascularization following vascular shutdown (Ferrario et al. 2000) and therapies that target this particular pro-angiogenic pathway have proven effective when used in conjunction with VDAs in pre-clinical studies (Siemann and Shi 2004; Shi and Siemann 2005; Siemann and Shi 2008). This strategy has now moved into clinical testing.

VDA treatment also appears to stimulate the release of circulating endothelial cell progenitor cells (CEPs) from the bone marrow and their recruitment to the tumor (Shaked et al. 2006). It has been suggested that such cells may contribute to both new vessel formation and the rapid "recanulisation" of recently blocked sections of vessels following VDA treatment (Shaked et al. 2006). Interestingly, recent evidence suggests that anti-angiogenic therapies and approaches that target local angiogenic responses can inhibit the VDA-induced release of CEPs (Shaked et al. 2006).

6 Clinical Experience with VDAs

Small molecule VDAs first entered clinical testing over 10 years ago and three agents are now in Phase III clinical trials. Table 1 lists the current clinical status of small molecule VDAs. As the clinical experience with VDAs has been the subject of several recent reviews (Siemann et al. 2009; Chaplin et al. 2006; Siemann and Chaplin 2007) and is covered in another chapter in this book, only a brief summary of findings will be discussed here. The main finding from Phase I studies are that these agents are able to induce blood flow reductions in a range of solid tumors. Surprisingly given their mode of action which, in the absence of a cytotoxic component, spares a viable rim of tumor cells, a number of objective tumor responses were seen when these agents were administered as monotherapy. However, Phase II studies have focused on combinations with conventional cytotoxic/antiproliferative chemotherapy with a particular focus on platinum and taxane based treatment regimes. These combinations have been well tolerated, as would be expected from their non overlapping toxicity profiles. Encouraging signs of anti-tumor activity in these trials have led to the initiation of ongoing Phase III trials in lung, sarcoma and anaplastic thyroid.

As discussed above the potential of combining VDAs with anti-angiogenic treatments is receiving increased attention. The encouraging preclinical data obtained to date has led to the completion of a Phase I trial using CA4P in combination with bevacizumab. This trial demonstrates that the combination is well tolerated and in turn has led to an ongoing Phase II trial in Stage IIIb/IV NSCLC where CA4P is added to the approved treatment of bevacizumab with carboplatin and paclitaxel.

One of the most common side effects seen in the clinic, certainly with VDAs which act through depolymerization of tubulin, is transient hypertension (Rustin et al. 2003; Zweifel et al. 2009). Microtubules help resist constriction of smooth muscle cells and thus their depolymerization may make vessels more sensitive to vasoconstriction. The use of anti-hypertensives such as nitrates and calcium channel blockers has been shown to eliminate the blood pressure effects of VDAs both in animals and in patients (Gould et al. 2007; Zweifel et al. 2009). The importance of this finding is that if left uncontrolled acute hypertensive episodes can, in the presence of underlying cardiovascular disease, lead to cardiac toxicity (LoRusso

Table 1 Small molecule VDAs in active clinical development

Compound	Mechanism	Current clinical development status	Tumor blood reductions established in clinic	Company
CA4P (fosbretabulin) (Zybrestat)	Tubulin depolymerising agent	Phase II and III	Yes	OXiGENE Inc.
DMXAA (AS1404)	TNF induction	Phase III	Yes	Novartis/Antisoma
AVE8062 (AC7700)	Tubulin depolymerising Agent	Phase III	Yes	Sanofi-Aventis
CYT 997	Tubulin depolymerising agent	Phase II	Yes	Cytopia
NPI 2358	Tubulin depolymerising Agent	Phase II	Yes	Nereus
MPC-6827 (Azixa)	Tubulin deolymerising Agent	Phase II	Yes	Myriad
ZD6126	Tubulin depolymerising agent	Phase I Trials Completed	Yes	Angiogene Pharmaceuticals Ltd
MN 029 (Denebulin)	Tubulin depolymerising Agent	Phase I Trials completed	Yes	Medicinova
OXi4503	Tubulin depolymerising Agent	Phase I Trials ongoing	Studies ongoing	OXiGENE Inc.
BNC-105	Tubulin depolymerising Agent	Phase I Trials ongoing	Studies ongoing	Bionomics
EPC-2407	Tubulin depolymerising Agent	Phase I Trials ongoing	Studies ongoing	Epicept

et al. 2008; Cooney et al. 2004; van Heeckeren et al. 2006). Active monitoring and management of hypertension should be an ongoing part of clinical application of VDAs. It is possible that routine prophylaxis with a calcium channel blocker could become part of the treatment for some patients receiving VDAs. It should be noted that hypertension is short lived (i.e. lasting for just a few hours after drug administration) so control measures should only be required for a short period of time.

7 Concluding Remarks

The appeal of vascular directed anticancer therapy lies not only in the recognition of the critical function of the vasculature in tumor growth and spread but also in the realization that by attacking a component distinct from that targeted by cytotoxic agents there exists great potential for complementary therapeutic activity. Rapid developments in recent years have now resulted in the identification of a number of promising investigational drugs. Tubulin depolymerizing VDAs are the most widely studied subset of a group of compounds that induce hemorrhagic necrosis in tumors. Preclinical evidence has demonstrated not only that VDA treatment leads to extensive tumor necrosis but that application of these agents in combination with radiotherapy and anticancer drugs, as well as anti-angiogenic therapies, can lead to markedly enhanced tumor responses. These concepts are now being actively explored in the clinic in late stage trials.

References

Aitken RA, Bibby MC, Bielefeldt F, Double JA, Laws AL, Mathieu AL, Ritchie RB, Wilson DW (1998) Synthesis and antitumour activity of new derivatives of flavone-8-acetic acid (FAA). Part 3: 2-Heteroaryl derivatives. Arch Pharm (Weinheim) 331:405–411

Alghisi GC, Ponsonnet L, Ruegg C (2009) The integrin antagonist cilengitide activates alphaVbeta3, disrupts VE-cadherin localization at cell junctions and enhances permeability in endothelial cells. PLoS One 4:e4449

Algire GH, Legallais FY, Anderson BF (1952) Vascular reactions of normal and malignant tissues in vivo. V. Role of hypotension in the action of bacterial polysaccharide on tumors. J Natl Cancer Inst 12:1279–1295

Anton K, Glod J (2009) Targeting the tumor stroma in cancer therapy. Curr Pharm Biotechnol 10:185–191

Arnberg N (2009) Adenovirus receptors: implications for tropism, treatment and targeting. Rev Med Virol 19:165–178

Baguley BC (2001) Small-molecule cytokine inducers causing tumor necrosis. Curr Opin Investig Drugs 2:967–975

Baguley BC (2003) Antivascular therapy of cancer: DMXAA. Lancet Oncol 4:141–148

Baguley BC, Wilson WR (2002) Potential of DMXAA combination therapy for solid tumors. Expert Rev Anticancer Ther 2:593–603

Baguley BC, Holdaway KM, Thomsen LL, Zhuang L, Zwi LJ (1991) Inhibition of growth of colon 38 adenocarcinoma by vinblastine and colchicine: evidence for a vascular mechanism. Eur J Cancer 27:482–487

Baka S, Clamp AR, Jayson GC (2006) A review of the latest clinical compounds to inhibit VEGF in pathological angiogenesis. Expert Opin Ther Targets 10:867–876

Baker AH, Kritz A, Work LM, Nicklin SA (2005) Cell-selective viral gene delivery vectors for the vasculature. Exp Physiol 90:27–31

Balkwill FR (1989) Tumour necrosis factor. Br Med Bull 45:389–400

Balza E, Mortara L, Sassi F, Monteghirfo S, Carnemolla B, Castellani P, Neri D, Accolla RS, Zardi L, Borsi L (2006) Targeted delivery of tumor necrosis factor-alpha to tumor vessels induces a therapeutic T cell-mediated immune response that protects the host against syngeneic tumors of different histologic origin. Clin Cancer Res 12:2575–2582

Beck AW, Luster TA, Miller AF, Holloway SE, Conner CR, Barnett CC, Thorpe PE, Fleming JB, Brekken RA (2006) Combination of a monoclonal anti-phosphatidylserine antibody with gemcitabine strongly inhibits the growth and metastasis of orthotopic pancreatic tumors in mice. Int J Cancer 118:2639–2643

Beerepoot LV, Radema SA, Witteveen EO, Thomas T, Wheeler C, Kempin S, Voest EE (2006) Phase I clinical evaluation of weekly administration of the novel vascular-targeting agent, ZD6126, in patients with solid tumors. J Clin Oncol 24:1491–1498

Bertout JA, Patel SA, Simon MC (2008) The impact of O_2 availability on human cancer. Nat Rev Cancer 8:967–975

Billard C, Menasria F, Quiney C, Faussat AM, Finet JP, Combes S, Kolb JP (2008) 4-arylcoumarin analogues of combretastatins stimulate apoptosis of leukemic cells from chronic lymphocytic leukemia patients. Exp Hematol 36:1625–1633

Blakey DC, Ashton SE, Westwood FR, Walker M, Ryan AJ (2002a) ZD6126: a novel small molecule vascular targeting agent. Int J Radiat Oncol Biol Phys 54:1497–1502

Blakey DC, Westwood FR, Walker M, Hughes GD, Davis PD, Ashton SE, Ryan AJ (2002b) Antitumor activity of the novel vascular targeting agent ZD6126 in a panel of tumor models. Clin Cancer Res 8:1974–1983

Blaschuk OW, Rowlands TM (2000) Cadherins as modulators of angiogenesis and the structural integrity of blood vessels. Cancer Metastasis Rev 19:1–5

Borsi L, Balza E, Carnemolla B, Sassi F, Castellani P, Berndt A, Kosmehl H, Biro A, Siri A, Orecchia P, Grassi J, Neri D, Zardi L (2003) Selective targeted delivery of TNFalpha to tumor blood vessels. Blood 102:4384–4392

Boyland E, Boyland ME (1937) Studies in tissue metabolism: the action of colchicine and B. typhosus extract. Biochem J 31:454–460

Boyland E, Boyland ME (1940) Studies in tissue metabolism: the action of colchicine on transplanted, induced and spontaneous mouse tumours. Biochem J 34:280–284

Busch W (1866) Einfluβ von erysipel. Beliner Klin Wschr 3:245–246

Cai SX (2007) Small molecule vascular disrupting agents: potential new drugs for cancer treatment. Recent Pat Anticancer Drug Discov 2:79–101

Cao Y (2009) Tumor angiogenesis and molecular targets for therapy. Front Biosci 14:3962–3973

Carpenito C, Davis PD, Dougherty ST, Dougherty GJ (2002) Exploiting the differential production of angiogenic factors within the tumor microenvironment in the design of a novel vascular-targeted gene therapy-based approach to the treatment of cancer. Int J Radiat Oncol Biol Phys 54:1473–1478

Carswell EA, Old LJ, Kassel RL, Green S, Fiore N, Williamson B (1975) An endotoxin-induced serum factor that causes necrosis of tumors. Proc Natl Acad Sci U S A 72:3666–3670

Chaplin DJ, Hill SA (2002) The development of combretastatin A4 phosphate as a vascular targeting agent. Int J Radiat Oncol Biol Phys 54:1491–1496

Chaplin DJ, Horsman MR (1994a) The effect of artificially induced ischemia on tumour cell survival. Adv Exp Med Biol 345:437–443

Chaplin DJ, Horsman MR (1994b) The influence of tumour temperature on ischemia-induced cell death: potential implications for the evaluation of vascular mediated therapies. Radiother Oncol 30:59–65

Chaplin DJ, Olive PL, Durand RE (1987) Intermittent blood flow in a murine tumor: radiobiological effects. Cancer Res 47:597–601
Chaplin DJ, Pettit GR, Parkins CS, Hill SA (1996) Antivascular approaches to solid tumour therapy: evaluation of tubulin binding agents. Br J Cancer Suppl 27:S86–S88
Chaplin DJ, Horsman MR, Siemann DW (2006) Current development status of small-molecule vascular disrupting agents. Curr Opin Investig Drugs 7:522–528
Chase JL (2008) Clinical use of anti-vascular endothelial growth factor monoclonal antibodies in metastatic colorectal cancer. Pharmacotherapy 28:23S–30S
Coley WB (1891) Contribution to the knowledge of sarcoma. Ann Surg 14:199–220
Coley WB (1914) The treatment of malignant tumors by repeated inoculations of erysipelas and *Bacillus prodigiosus*. Brussels: M. Weissenbruch
Cooney MM, Radivoyevitch T, Dowlati A, Overmoyer B, Levitan N, Robertson K, Levine SL, DeCaro K, Buchter C, Taylor A, Stambler BS, Remick SC (2004) Cardiovascular safety profile of combretastatin a4 phosphate in a single-dose phase I study in patients with advanced cancer. Clin Cancer Res 10:96–100
Cowan PJ, Shinkel TA, Fisicaro N, Godwin JW, Bernabeu C, Almendro N, Rius C, Lonie AJ, Nottle MB, Wigley PL, Paizis K, Pearse MJ, d'Apice AJ (2003) Targeting gene expression to endothelium in transgenic animals: a comparison of the human ICAM-2, PECAM-1 and endoglin promoters. Xenotransplantation 10:223–231
Dai C, McAninch RE, Sutton RE (2004) Identification of synthetic endothelial cell-specific promoters by use of a high-throughput screen. J Virol 78:6209–6221
Dancer A, Julien S, Bouillot S, Pointu H, Vernet M, Huber P (2003) Expression of thymidine kinase driven by an endothelial-specific promoter inhibits tumor growth of Lewis lung carcinoma cells in transgenic mice. Gene Ther 10:1170–1178
Dark GG, Hill SA, Prise VE, Tozer GM, Pettit GR, Chaplin DJ (1997) Combretastatin A-4, an agent that displays potent and selective toxicity toward tumor vasculature. Cancer Res 57:1829–1834
Dass CR, Choong PF (2006) Selective gene delivery for cancer therapy using cationic liposomes: in vivo proof of applicability. J Control Release 113:155–163
Davis PD, Dougherty GJ, Blakey DC, Galbraith SM, Tozer GM, Holder AL, Naylor MA, Nolan J, Stratford MR, Chaplin DJ, Hill SA (2002) ZD6126: a novel vascular-targeting agent that causes selective destruction of tumor vasculature. Cancer Res 62:7247–7253
De Palma M, Venneri MA, Naldini L (2003) In vivo targeting of tumor endothelial cells by systemic delivery of lentiviral vectors. Hum Gene Ther 14:1193–1206
Demartis S, Tarli L, Borsi L, Zardi L, Neri D (2001) Selective targeting of tumour neovasculature by a radiohalogenated human antibody fragment specific for the ED-B domain of fibronectin. Eur J Nucl Med 28:534–539
Denekamp J (1982) Endothelial cell proliferation as a novel approach to targeting tumour therapy. Br J Cancer 45:136–139
Denekamp J (1984) Vascular endothelium as the vulnerable element in tumours. Acta Radiol Oncol 23:217–225
Denekamp J (1990) Vascular attack as a therapeutic strategy for cancer. Cancer Metastasis Rev 9:267–282
Denekamp J (1991) The current status of targeting tumour vasculature as a means of cancer therapy: an overview. Int J Radiat Biol 60:401–408
Denekamp J (1993) Review article: angiogenesis, neovascular proliferation and vascular pathophysiology as targets for cancer therapy. Br J Radiol 66:181–196
Denekamp J, Hill SA, Hobson B (1983) Vascular occlusion and tumour cell death. Eur J Cancer Clin Oncol 19:271–275
Denekamp J, Dasu A, Waites A (1998) Vasculature and microenvironmental gradients: the missing links in novel approaches to cancer therapy? Adv Enzyme Regul 38:281–299
Dickens DS, Jubinsky PT (2009) Therapeutic strategies for targeting mononuclear phagocytes in cancer. J Pediatr Hematol Oncol 31:14–17

Dienst A, Grunow A, Unruh M, Rabausch B, Nor JE, Fries JW, Gottstein C (2005) Specific occlusion of murine and human tumor vasculature by VCAM-1-targeted recombinant fusion proteins. J Natl Cancer Inst 97:733–747

Dong Z, Nor JE (2009) Transcriptional targeting of tumor endothelial cells for gene therapy. Adv Drug Deliv Rev 61:542–552

Dougherty GJ, Dougherty ST (2009) Exploiting the tumor microenvironment in the development of targeted cancer gene therapy. Cancer Gene Ther 16:279–290

Dougherty GJ, Davis PD, Dougherty ST (2004) Vascular-targeted cancer gene therapy. Expert Opin Biol Ther 4:1911–1920

Dowlati A, Robertson K, Cooney M, Petros WP, Stratford M, Jesberger J, Rafie N, Overmoyer B, Makkar V, Stambler B, Taylor A, Waas J, Lewin JS, McCrae KR, Remick SC (2002) A phase I pharmacokinetic and translational study of the novel vascular targeting agent combretastatin a-4 phosphate on a single-dose intravenous schedule in patients with advanced cancer. Cancer Res 62:3408–3416

Ebos JM, Lee CR, Cruz-Munoz W, Bjarnason GA, Christensen JG, Kerbel RS (2009) Accelerated metastasis after short-term treatment with a potent inhibitor of tumor angiogenesis. Cancer Cell 15:232–239

Edelstein ML, Abedi MR, Wixon J, Edelstein RM (2004) Gene therapy clinical trials worldwide 1989–2004-an overview. J Gene Med 6:597–602

el-Zayat AA, Degen D, Drabek S, Clark GM, Pettit GR, Von Hoff DD (1993) In vitro evaluation of the antineoplastic activity of combretastatin A-4, a natural product from *Combretum caffrum* (arid shrub). Anticancer Drugs 4:19–25

Enback J, Laakkonen P (2007) Tumour-homing peptides: tools for targeting, imaging and destruction. Biochem Soc Trans 35:780–783

Enderlen E (1896) Klinische und experimentelle Studien zur Frage der Torsion des Hodens. Dtsch Z Chir 43:177

Fang L, Shen L, Fang Y, Hu Y, He Q, Yang B (2008) MZ3 can induce G2/M-phase arrest and apoptosis in human leukemia cells. J Cancer Res Clin Oncol 134:1337–1345

Ferrario A, von Tiehl KF, Rucker N, Schwarz MA, Gill PS, Gomer CJ (2000) Antiangiogenic treatment enhances photodynamic therapy responsiveness in a mouse mammary carcinoma. Cancer Res 60:4066–4069

Fitzwilliams DCL (1927) The treatment of carcinoma by lead colloids. Br Med J 1:822

Flick DA, Gifford GE (1986) Production of tumor necrosis factor in unprimed mice: mechanism of endotoxin-mediated tumor necrosis. Immunobiology 171:320–328

Folkman J (1999) Angiogenic zip code. Nat Biotechnol 17:749

Follin F (1852) De la cryptorchidie chez l'homme Mem Soc Biol

Fukumura D, Jain RK (2007) Tumor microvasculature and microenvironment: targets for anti-angiogenesis and normalization. Microvasc Res 74:72–84

Gafner V, Trachsel E, Neri D (2006) An engineered antibody-interleukin-12 fusion protein with enhanced tumor vascular targeting properties. Int J Cancer 119:2205–2212

Galbraith SM, Chaplin DJ, Lee F, Stratford MR, Locke RJ, Vojnovic B, Tozer GM (2001) Effects of combretastatin A4 phosphate on endothelial cell morphology in vitro and relationship to tumour vascular targeting activity in vivo. Anticancer Res 21:93–102

Gavard J (2009) Breaking the VE-cadherin bonds. FEBS Lett 583:1–6

Gaya AM, Rustin GJ (2005) Vascular disrupting agents: a new class of drug in cancer therapy. Clin Oncol (R Coll Radiol) 17:277–290

Gotlieb AI (1990) The endothelial cytoskeleton: organization in normal and regenerating endothelium. Toxicol Pathol 18:603–617

Gould S, Westwood FR, Curwen JO, Ashton SE, Roberts DW, Lovick SC, Ryan AJ (2007) Effect of pretreatment with atenolol and nifedipine on ZD6126-induced cardiac toxicity in rats. J Natl Cancer Inst 99:1724–1728

Graulich W, Nettelbeck DM, Fischer D, Kissel T, Muller R (1999) Cell type specificity of the human endoglin promoter. Gene 227:55–62

Greenberger S, Shaish A, Varda-Bloom N, Levanon K, Breitbart E, Goldberg I, Barshack I, Hodish I, Yaacov N, Bangio L, Goncharov T, Wallach D, Harats D (2004) Transcription-controlled gene therapy against tumor angiogenesis. J Clin Invest 113:1017–1024

Gresser I (1987) A. Chekhov, M.D., and Coley's toxins. N Engl J Med 317:457

Griffin RJ, Monzen H, Williams BW, Park H, Lee SH, Song CW (2003) Arsenic trioxide induces selective tumour vascular damage via oxidative stress and increases thermosensitivity of tumours. Int J Hyperthermia 19:575–589

Grothey A, Ellis LM (2008) Targeting angiogenesis driven by vascular endothelial growth factors using antibody-based therapies. Cancer J 14:170–177

Hajitou A, Pasqualini R, Arap W (2006) Vascular targeting: recent advances and therapeutic perspectives. Trends Cardiovasc Med 16:80–88

Hanna E, Quick J, Libutti SK (2009) The tumour microenvironment: a novel target for cancer therapy. Oral Dis 15:8–17

He J, Luster TA, Thorpe PE (2007) Radiation-enhanced vascular targeting of human lung cancers in mice with a monoclonal antibody that binds anionic phospholipids. Clin Cancer Res 13:5211–5218

Heath VL, Bicknell R (2009) Anticancer strategies involving the vasculature. Nat Rev Clin Oncol 6:395–404

Hellner H (1933) Die örtlichen Kreislaufstörungen des Hodens. Bruns Beitr Klin Chir 158:225

Hill SA, Lonergan SJ, Denekamp J, Chaplin DJ (1994) The effect of vinca alkaloids on tumour blood flow. Adv Exp Med Biol 345:417–422

Hinnen P, Eskens FA (2007) Vascular disrupting agents in clinical development. Br J Cancer 96:1159–1165

Hodish I, Tal R, Shaish A, Varda-Bloom N, Greenberger S, Rauchwerger A, Breitbart E, Bangio L, Ben-Shushan D, Pfeffer R, Feder B, Waitsman A, Barshack I, Goldberg I, Mazaki-Tovi S, Peled M, Harats D (2009) Systemic administration of radiation-potentiated anti-angiogenic gene therapy against primary and metastatic cancer based on transcriptionally controlled HSV-TK. Cancer Biol Ther 8:424–432

Hoption Cann SA, van Netten JP, van Netten C, Glover DW (2002) Spontaneous regression: a hidden treasure buried in time. Med Hypotheses 58:115–119

Hoption Cann SA, van Netten JP, van Netten C (2003) Dr William Coley and tumour regression: a place in history or in the future. Postgrad Med J 79:672–680

Huang G, Chen L (2008) Tumor vasculature and microenvironment normalization: a possible mechanism of antiangiogenesis therapy. Cancer Biother Radiopharm 23:661–667

Huang X, Bennett M, Thorpe PE (2005) A monoclonal antibody that binds anionic phospholipids on tumor blood vessels enhances the antitumor effect of docetaxel on human breast tumors in mice. Cancer Res 65:4408–4416

Hundsberger H, Verin A, Wiesner C, Pfluger M, Dulebo A, Schutt W, Lasters I, Mannel DN, Wendel A, Lucas R (2008) TNF: a moonlighting protein at the interface between cancer and infection. Front Biosci 13:5374–5386

Jager U, Zhao Y, Porter CD (1999) Endothelial cell-specific transcriptional targeting from a hybrid long terminal repeat retrovirus vector containing human prepro-endothelin-1 promoter sequences. J Virol 73:9702–9709

Lippert JW, III (2007) Vascular disrupting agents. Bioorg Med Chem 15:605–615

Kaspar M, Trachsel E, Neri D (2007) The antibody-mediated targeted delivery of interleukin-15 and GM-CSF to the tumor neovasculature inhibits tumor growth and metastasis. Cancer Res 67:4940–4948

Kelland L (2007) Drug evaluation: ADH-1, an N-cadherin antagonist targeting cancer vascularization. Curr Opin Mol Ther 9:86–91

Kesmodel SB, Spitz FR (2003) Gene therapy for cancer and metastatic disease. Expert Rev Mol Med 5:1–18

Kiaris H, Trimis G, Papavassiliou AG (2008) Regulation of tumor-stromal fibroblast interactions: implications in anticancer therapy. Curr Med Chem 15:3062–3067

Klagsbrun M, Moses MA (2008) Obituary: M. Judah Folkman (1933–2008). Nature 451:781
Kouraklis G (1999) Progress in cancer gene therapy. Acta Oncol 38:675–683
Krasnykh V, Dmitriev I, Mikheeva G, Miller CR, Belousova N, Curiel DT (1998) Characterization of an adenovirus vector containing a heterologous peptide epitope in the HI loop of the fiber knob. J Virol 72:1844–1852
Kuckleburg CJ, Tiwari R, Czuprynski CJ (2008) Endothelial cell apoptosis induced by bacteria-activated platelets requires caspase-8 and -9 and generation of reactive oxygen species. Thromb Haemost 99:363–372
Kuhn H, Konrad J, Holtz S, Salameh A, Gessner C, Hammerschmidt S, Wirtz H (2006) Enhanced expression of VEGF following bFGF inhibition in non-small cell lung cancer cell lines. Lung Cancer 54:149–153
Lee JS, Gotlieb AI (2005) Microtubules regulate aortic endothelial cell actin microfilament reorganization in intact and repairing monolayers. Histol Histopathol 20:455–465
Leiter J, Downing V, Hartwell JL, Shear MJ (1950) Damage induced in sarcoma 37 with podophyllin, podophyllotoxin alpha-peltatin, beta-peltatin, and quercetin. J Natl Cancer Inst 10:1273–1293
Leiter J, Downing V, Hartwell JL, Shear MJ (1952) Damage induced in sarcoma 37 with chemical agents. II. Trivalent and pentavalent arsenicals. J Natl Cancer Inst 13:365–378
Lew YS, Brown SL, Griffin RJ, Song CW, Kim JH (1999) Arsenic trioxide causes selective necrosis in solid murine tumors by vascular shutdown. Cancer Res 59:6033–6037
Li YM, Broome JD (1999) Arsenic targets tubulins to induce apoptosis in myeloid leukemia cells. Cancer Res 59:776–780
Li H, Price DK, Figg WD (2007) ADH1, an N-cadherin inhibitor, evaluated in preclinical models of angiogenesis and androgen-independent prostate cancer. Anticancer Drugs 18:563–568
Liu Y, Deisseroth A (2006) Tumor vascular targeting therapy with viral vectors. Blood 107:3027–3033
London NR, Whitehead KJ, Li DY (2009) Endogenous endothelial cell signaling systems maintain vascular stability. Angiogenesis 12:149–158
Lorusso G, Ruegg C (2008) The tumor microenvironment and its contribution to tumor evolution toward metastasis. Histochem Cell Biol 130:1091–1103
LoRusso PM, Gadgeel SM, Wozniak A, Barge AJ, Jones HK, DelProposto ZS, DeLuca PA, Evelhoch JL, Boerner SA, Wheeler C (2008) Phase I clinical evaluation of ZD6126, a novel vascular-targeting agent, in patients with solid tumors. Invest New Drugs 26:159–167
Lu L, Payvandi F, Wu L, Zhang LH, Hariri RJ, Man HW, Chen RS, Muller GW, Hughes CC, Stirling DI, Schafer PH, Bartlett JB (2009) The anti-cancer drug lenalidomide inhibits angiogenesis and metastasis via multiple inhibitory effects on endothelial cell function in normoxic and hypoxic conditions. Microvasc Res 77:78–86
Ludford RJ (1948) Factors determining the action of colchicine on tumour growth. Br J Cancer 2:75–86
Luster TA, He J, Huang X, Maiti SN, Schroit AJ, de Groot PG, Thorpe PE (2006) Plasma protein beta-2-glycoprotein 1 mediates interaction between the anti-tumor monoclonal antibody 3G4 and anionic phospholipids on endothelial cells. J Biol Chem 281:29863–29871
Ma WW, Adjei AA (2009) Novel agents on the horizon for cancer therapy. CA Cancer J Clin 59:111–137
Mancuso MR, Davis R, Norberg SM, O'Brien S, Sennino B, Nakahara T, Yao VJ, Inai T, Brooks P, Freimark B, Shalinsky DR, Hu-Lowe DD, McDonald DM (2006) Rapid vascular regrowth in tumors after reversal of VEGF inhibition. J Clin Invest 116:2610–2621
Mariotti A, Perotti A, Sessa C, Ruegg C (2007) N-cadherin as a therapeutic target in cancer. Expert Opin Investig Drugs 16:451–465
Mbeunkui F, Johann DJJ (2009) Cancer and the tumor microenvironment: a review of an essential relationship. Cancer Chemother Pharmacol 63:571–582
McCarthy EF (2006) The toxins of William B. Coley and the treatment of bone and soft-tissue sarcomas. Iowa Orthop J 26:154–158
McKeage MJ (2008) The potential of DMXAA (ASA404) in combination with docetaxel in advanced prostate cancer. Expert Opin Investig Drugs 17:23–29

McKeage MJ, Von Pawel J, Reck M, Jameson MB, Rosenthal MA, Sullivan R, Gibbs D, Mainwaring PN, Serke M, Lafitte JJ, Chouaid C, Freitag L, Quoix E (2008) Randomised phase II study of ASA404 combined with carboplatin and paclitaxel in previously untreated advanced non-small cell lung cancer. Br J Cancer 99:2006–2012

McKeage MJ, Reck M, Jameson MB, Rosenthal MA, Gibbs D, Mainwaring PN, Freitag L, Sullivan R, Von Pawel J (2009) Phase II study of ASA404 (vadimezan, 5,6-dimethylxanthenone-4-acetic acid/DMXAA) 1800 mg/m(2) combined with carboplatin and paclitaxel in previously untreated advanced non-small cell lung cancer. Lung Cancer 65:192–197

Miflet J (1879) Über die pathologischen Veränderungen des Hodens, welche durch Störungen der lokalen Blutzirkulation veranlaßt werden Arch Klin Chir 24:399

Mohamedali KA, Kedar D, Sweeney P, Kamat A, Davis DW, Eve BY, Huang S, Thorpe PE, Dinney CP, Rosenblum MG (2005) The vascular-targeting fusion toxin VEGF121/rGel inhibits the growth of orthotopic human bladder carcinoma tumors. Neoplasia 7:912–920

Mottram JC (1923) Observations on the combined action of colloidal lead and radiation on tumours. Br Med J 1:132–133

Nabel EG, Plautz G, Nabel GJ (1991) Gene transfer into vascular cells. J Am Coll Cardiol 17:189B–194B

Nicklin SA, Reynolds PN, Brosnan MJ, White SJ, Curiel DT, Dominiczak AF, Baker AH (2001) Analysis of cell-specific promoters for viral gene therapy targeted at the vascular endothelium. Hypertension 38:65–70

Nicklin SA, White SJ, Nicol CG, Von Seggern DJ, Baker AH (2004) In vitro and in vivo characterisation of endothelial cell selective adenoviral vectors. J Gene Med 6:300–308

Nikitenko LL (2009) Vascular endothelium in cancer. Cell Tissue Res 335:223–240

Noske HD, Kraus SW, Altinkilic BM, Weidner W (1998) Historical milestones regarding torsion of the scrotal organs. J Urol 159:13–16

Paez-Ribes M, Allen E, Hudock J, Takeda T, Okuyama H, Vinals F, Inoue M, Bergers G, Hanahan D, Casanovas O (2009) Antiangiogenic therapy elicits malignant progression of tumors to increased local invasion and distant metastasis. Cancer Cell 15:220–231

Parker AL, Fisher KD, Oupicky D, Read ML, Nicklin SA, Baker AH, Seymour LW (2005) Enhanced gene transfer activity of peptide-targeted gene-delivery vectors. J Drug Target 13:39–51

Parkins CS, Hill SA, Lonergan SJ, Horsman MR, Chadwick JA, Chaplin DJ (1994) Ischaemia induced cell death in tumors: importance of temperature and pH. Int J Radiat Oncol Biol Phys 29:499–503

Pasqualini R, Arap W (2002) Translation of vascular diversity into targeted therapeutics. Ann Hematol 81 Suppl 2:S66–S67

Perotti A, Sessa C, Mancuso A, Noberasco C, Cresta S, Locatelli A, Carcangiu ML, Passera K, Braghetti A, Scaramuzza D, Zanaboni F, Fasolo A, Capri G, Miani M, Peters WP, Gianni L (2009) Clinical and pharmacological phase I evaluation of Exherin (ADH-1), a selective anti-N-cadherin peptide in patients with N-cadherin-expressing solid tumours. Ann Oncol 20:741–745

Petit I, Karajannis MA, Vincent L, Young L, Butler J, Hooper AT, Shido K, Steller H, Chaplin DJ, Feldman E, Rafii S (2008) The microtubule-targeting agent CA4P regresses leukemic xenografts by disrupting interaction with vascular cells and mitochondrial-dependent cell death. Blood 111:1951–1961

Pettit GR, Singh SB, Hamel E, Lin CM, Alberts DS, Garcia-Kendall D (1989) Isolation and structure of the strong cell growth and tubulin inhibitor combretastatin A-4. Experientia 45:209–211

Philpott M, Joseph WR, Crosier KE, Baguley BC, Ching LM (1997) Production of tumour necrosis factor-alpha by cultured human peripheral blood leucocytes in response to the anti-tumour agent 5,6-dimethylxanthenone-4-acetic acid (NSC 640488). Br J Cancer 76:1586–1591

Philpott M, Ching LM, Baguley BC (2001) The antitumour agent 5,6-dimethylxanthenone-4-acetic acid acts in vitro on human mononuclear cells as a co-stimulator with other inducers of tumour necrosis factor. Eur J Cancer 37:1930–1937

Pilat MJ, Lorusso PM (2006) Vascular disrupting agents. J Cell Biochem 99:1021–1039

Pinto MM, Sousa ME, Nascimento MS (2005) Xanthone derivatives: new insights in biological activities. Curr Med Chem 12:2517–2538

Pober JS (1987) Effects of tumour necrosis factor and related cytokines on vascular endothelial cells. Ciba Found Symp 131:170–184

Ran S, Thorpe PE (2002) Phosphatidylserine is a marker of tumor vasculature and a potential target for cancer imaging and therapy. Int J Radiat Oncol Biol Phys 54:1479–1484

Ran S, Gao B, Duffy S, Watkins L, Rote N, Thorpe PE (1998) Infarction of solid Hodgkin's tumors in mice by antibody-directed targeting of tissue factor to tumor vasculature. Cancer Res 58:4646–4653

Ran S, Downes A, Thorpe PE (2002) Increased exposure of anionic phospholipids on the surface of tumor blood vessels. Cancer Res 62:6132–6140

Ran S, He J, Huang X, Soares M, Scothorn D, Thorpe PE (2005a) Antitumor effects of a monoclonal antibody that binds anionic phospholipids on the surface of tumor blood vessels in mice. Clin Cancer Res 11:1551–1562

Ran S, Mohamedali KA, Luster TA, Thorpe PE, Rosenblum MG (2005b) The vascular-ablative agent VEGF(121)/rGel inhibits pulmonary metastases of MDA-MB-231 breast tumors. Neoplasia 7:486–496

Rehman F, Rustin G (2008) ASA404: update on drug development. Expert Opin Investig Drugs 17:1547–1551

Rhee J, Hoff PM (2005) Angiogenesis inhibitors in the treatment of cancer. Expert Opin Pharmacother 6:1701–1711

Ribatti D (2009) The discovery of antiangiogenic molecules: a historical review. Curr Pharm Des 15:345–352

Ruegg C, Mutter N (2007) Anti-angiogenic therapies in cancer: achievements and open questions. Bull Cancer 94:753–762

Rustin GJ, Galbraith SM, Anderson H, Stratford M, Folkes LK, Sena L, Gumbrell L, Price PM (2003) Phase I clinical trial of weekly combretastatin A4 phosphate: clinical and pharmacokinetic results. J Clin Oncol 21:2815–2822

Seed L, Slaughter DP, Limarzi LR (1940) Effect of colchicine on human carcinoma. Surgery 7:696–709

Seshadri M, Spernyak JA, Maiery PG, Cheney RT, Mazurchuk R, Bellnier DA (2007) Visualizing the acute effects of vascular-targeted therapy in vivo using intravital microscopy and magnetic resonance imaging: correlation with endothelial apoptosis, cytokine induction, and treatment outcome. Neoplasia 9:128–135

Shaked Y, Ciarrocchi A, Franco M, Lee CR, Man S, Cheung AM, Hicklin DJ, Chaplin D, Foster FS, Benezra R, Kerbel RS (2006) Therapy-induced acute recruitment of circulating endothelial progenitor cells to tumors. Science 313:1785–1787

Shear MJ (1944) Chemical treatment of tumors. IX. Reactions of mice with primary subcutaneous tumors to injection of a hemorrhage-producing bacterial polysaccharide. J Natl Cancer Inst 4:461–476

Shear MJ, Turner FC, Perrault A (1943) Chemical treatment of tumors. Isolation of haemorrhage-producing fractions fromSerratia marcescens (*Bacillus prodrigiosus*) culture filtrate (*Bacillus prodrigiosus*) culture filtrate J Natl Cancer Inst 4:81–97

Shi W, Siemann DW (2005) Targeting the tumor vasculature: enhancing antitumor efficacy through combination treatment with ZD6126 and ZD6474. In Vivo 19:1045–1050

Siemann DW, Chaplin DJ (2007) An update on the clinical development of drugs to disable tumor vasculature. Expert Opin Drug Discov 2:1–11

Siemann DW, Horsman MR (2004) Targeting the tumor vasculature: a strategy to improve radiation therapy. Expert Rev Anticancer Ther 4:321–327

Siemann DW, Horsman MR (2009) Vascular targeted therapies in oncology. Cell Tissue Res 335:241–248

Siemann DW, Shi W (2004) Efficacy of combined antiangiogenic and vascular disrupting agents in treatment of solid tumors. Int J Radiat Oncol Biol Phys 60:1233–1240

Siemann DW, Shi W (2008) Dual targeting of tumor vasculature: combining Avastin and vascular disrupting agents (CA4P or OXi4503). Anticancer Res 28:2027–2031

Siemann DW, Chaplin DJ, Horsman MR (2004) Vascular-targeting therapies for treatment of malignant disease. Cancer 100:2491–2499

Siemann DW, Chaplin DJ, Walicke PA (2009) A review and update of the current status of the vasculature-disabling agent combretastatin-A4 phosphate (CA4P). Expert Opin Investig Drugs 18:189–197

Thorpe PE (2004) Vascular targeting agents as cancer therapeutics. Clin Cancer Res 10:415–427

Thorpe PE, Ran S (2002) Mapping zip codes in human vasculature. Pharmacogenomics J 2:205–206

Thorpe PE, Chaplin DJ, Blakey DC (2003) The first international conference on vascular targeting: meeting overview. Cancer Res 63:1144–1147

van Heeckeren WJ, Bhakta S, Ortiz J, Duerk J, Cooney MM, Dowlati A, McCrae K, Remick SC (2006) Promise of new vascular-disrupting agents balanced with cardiac toxicity: is it time for oncologists to get to know their cardiologists? J Clin Oncol 24:1485–1488

Veenendaal LM, Jin H, Ran S, Cheung L, Navone N, Marks JW, Waltenberger J, Thorpe P, Rosenblum MG (2002) In vitro and in vivo studies of a VEGF121/rGelonin chimeric fusion toxin targeting the neovasculature of solid tumors. Proc Natl Acad Sci U S A 99:7866–7871

Vestweber D, Winderlich M, Cagna G, Nottebaum AF (2009) Cell adhesion dynamics at endothelial junctions: VE-cadherin as a major player. Trends Cell Biol 19:8–15

Vincent L, Kermani P, Young LM, Cheng J, Zhang F, Shido K, Lam G, Bompais-Vincent H, Zhu Z, Hicklin DJ, Bohlen P, Chaplin DJ, May C, Rafii S (2005) Combretastatin A4 phosphate induces rapid regression of tumor neovessels and growth through interference with vascular endothelial-cadherin signaling. J Clin Invest 115:2992–3006

Wakelee HA, Schiller JH (2005) Targeting angiogenesis with vascular endothelial growth factor receptor small-molecule inhibitors: novel agents with potential in lung cancer. Clin Lung Cancer 7 Suppl 1:S31–S38

Walshe WW (1844) The Anatomy, Physiology, Pathology and Treatment of Cancer, William D. Ticknor & Co: Boston.

West CM, Price P (2004) Combretastatin A4 phosphate. Anticancer Drugs 15:179–187

White SJ, Nicklin SA, Buning H, Brosnan MJ, Leike K, Papadakis ED, Hallek M, Baker AH (2004) Targeted gene delivery to vascular tissue in vivo by tropism-modified adeno-associated virus vectors. Circulation 109:513–519

White K, Buning H, Kritz A, Janicki H, McVey J, Perabo L, Murphy G, Odenthal M, Work LM, Hallek M, Nicklin SA, Baker AH (2008) Engineering adeno-associated virus 2 vectors for targeted gene delivery to atherosclerotic lesions. Gene Ther 15:443–451

Woglom WH (1923) A critique of tumour resistance. J Cancer Res 7:283–311

Wolmark N, Yothers G, O'Connell MJ, Sharif S, Atkins JN, Seay TE, Feherenbacher L, O'Reilly S, Allegra CJ (2009) A phase III trial comparing mFOLFOX6 to mFOLFOX6 plus bevacizumab in stage II or III carcinoma of the colon: results of NSABP Protocol C-08. J Clin Oncol 27:15s. (abstr LBA4)

Wood FC (1926) Use of colloidal lead in the treatment of cancer. J Am Med Assoc 87:717–722

Work LM, Ritchie N, Nicklin SA, Reynolds PN, Baker AH (2004) Dual targeting of gene delivery by genetic modification of adenovirus serotype 5 fibers and cell-selective transcriptional control. Gene Ther 11:1296–1300

Work LM, Buning H, Hunt E, Nicklin SA, Denby L, Britton N, Leike K, Odenthal M, Drebber U, Hallek M, Baker AH (2006) Vascular bed-targeted in vivo gene delivery using tropism-modified adeno-associated viruses. Mol Ther 13:683–693

Xu D, Fang L, Zhu Q, Hu Y, He Q, Yang B (2008) Antimultidrug-resistant effect and mechanism of a novel CA-4 analogue MZ3 on leukemia cells. Pharmazie 63:528–533

Zhang B (2008) Targeting the stroma by T cells to limit tumor growth. Cancer Res 68:9570–9573

Zhou S, Kestell P, Baguley BC, Paxton JW (2002) 5,6-dimethylxanthenone-acetic acid (DMXAA): a new biological response modifier for cancer therapy. Invest New Drugs 20:281–295

Zweifel M, Jayson G, Reed N, Osborne R, Hassan B, Shreeves G, Poupard L, Walicke PA, Balkissoon J, Chaplin D, Rustin G (2009) Combretastatin A-4 phosphate (CA4P) carboplatin and paclitaxel in patients with platinum-resistant ovarian cancer: final phase II trial results. J Clin Oncol 27:15s. (suppl; abstr 5502)

Part I
Pre-Clinical Development

The Discovery and Characterisation of Tumour Endothelial Markers

Dario Neri and Roy Bicknell

Abstract One avenue towards the development of more selective anti-cancer drugs consists in the targeted delivery of bioactive molecules (drugs, cytokines, procoagulant factors, photosensitizers, radionuclides, etc.) to the tumor environment by means of binding molecules (e.g., human antibodies) specific to tumor-associated markers. In this context, the targeted delivery of therapeutic agents to newly-formed blood vessels ("vascular targeting") is particularly attractive, because of the dependence of tumors on new blood vessels to sustain growth and invasion, and because of the accessibility of neo-vascular structures for therapeutic agents injected intravenously.

This chapter reviews modern methodologies for the discovery of vascular tumor markers for pharmacodelivery applications and outlines the key properties of some of the best characterized targets.

1 Vascular Tumor Targeting: Concepts and Definitions

One avenue towards the development of more selective anti-cancer drugs consists in the targeted delivery of bioactive molecules (drugs, cytokines, procoagulant factors, photosensitizers, radionuclides, etc.) to the tumor environment by means of binding molecules (e.g., human antibodies) specific to tumor-associated markers. In this context, the targeted delivery of therapeutic agents to newly-formed blood vessels ("vascular targeting") is particularly attractive, because the formation of new vascular structures is a rare event in the adult and because tumors rely on new blood vessels to sustain growth and invasion. Neo-vascular structures are readily

D. Neri (✉)
Department of Chemistry and Applied Biosciences, ETH Zurich,
Wolfgang-Pauli-Str. 10, CH-8093 Zurich, Switzerland
e-mail: dario.neri@pharma.ethz.ch

T. Meyer (ed.), *Vascular Disruptive Agents for the Treatment of Cancer*,
DOI 10.1007/978-1-4419-6609-4_2, © Springer Science+Business Media, LLC 2010

accessible for therapeutic agents that are injected intravenously, thus facilitating their preferential localization at the tumor site.

In this chapter, we will restrict the definition of vascular tumor targeting to pharmacodelivery applications based on ligands capable of selective recognition of markers expressed at sites of tumor angiogenesis. This therapeutic area is different from the development and use of vascular disrupting agents such as combretastatins, where small organic molecules are used to destabilize the cytoskeleton of tumor endothelial cells (Chaplin et al. 2006). Similarly, vascular tumor targeting is clearly distinct (both conceptually and in terms of experimental methodologies) from the inhibition of angiogenesis, as achieved by the blockade of soluble growth factors such as VEGF-A by means of the monoclonal antibody bevacizumab (Ferrara 2004). While the inhibition of angiogenesis aims at preventing the growth of new blood vessels, vascular tumor targeting delivers therapeutic agents to tumor blood vessels that already exist.

Tumors rely on an over-exhuberant growth of blood vessels for the supply of oxygen and nutrients (Folkman 1990). The selective destruction or occlusion of tumor blood vessels (e.g., by the antibody-mediated targeted delivery of toxins or of pro-coagulant factors) interrupts the blood supply to the neoplastic tissue, thus causing a cascade of tumor cell death (Denekamp 1990; Burrows and Thorpe 1993; Huang et al. 1997). More recently, other vascular tumor targeting strategies have been considered, which still rely on the selective localization of antibody derivatives on tumor blood vessels but which manifest an anti-cancer activity without direct damage to the tumor cells (Neri and Bicknell 2005). For example, antibody–cytokine fusion proteins ("immunocytokines") which accumulate on the sub-endothelial extracellular matrix at tumor sites can promote the proliferation and activation of immune cells (e.g., NK cells), which infiltrate the neoplastic mass and which directly kill tumor cells (e.g., Carnemolla et al. 2002; Halin et al. 2002). Alternatively, radiolabeled antibodies or antibody–photosensitizer conjugates may be used to deliver diffusible toxic moieties to the surroundings of tumor blood vessels (e.g., electrons or reactive oxygen species) (Berndorff et al. 2005; Tijink et al. 2006; Birchler et al. 1999; Fabbrini et al. 2006).

Several types of vascular tumor targeting agents have begun clinical testing, as we will see in the following chapters (Jennewein et al. 2008; Soares et al. 2008; Corti et al. 2008; Bieker et al. 2009; Carnemolla et al. 2002; Mårlind et al. 2008; Sauer et al. 2009; Brack et al. 2006).

2 Methodologies for the Discovery of Vascular Tumor Targets

Vascular tumor targeting applications crucially rely on good-quality markers of angiogenesis, which are expressed at sites of tumor angiogenesis, which display a restricted pattern of expression in normal tissues and which can be drugged with antibody derivatives.

Historically, the first markers of angiogenesis were discovered as a result of extensive immunohistochemical profiling of certain monoclonal antibodies.

For example, the discovery by limited proteolysis experiments that tumor fibronectin may contain an alternatively-spliced extra-domain not present in plasma fibronectin ("EDB"; Zardi et al. 1987) was followed by the observation that antibodies specific to EDB-containing fibronectin preferentially stain blood vessels in many cancer types, but do not stain normal tissues (exception made for the endometrium in the proliferating phase, some vessels in the ovaries and placenta) (Carnemolla et al. 1989, 1996; Castellani et al. 1994, 2002; Neri et al. 1997; Birchler et al. 2003; Driemel et al. 2007; Schliemann et al. 2009; Sauer et al. 2009).

Similarly, immunization of rodents with tumor-derived complex antigen mixtures have led to the discovery of markers (e.g., endoglin, endosialin, prostate-specific membrane antigen), which were found to be over-expressed at sites of tumor angiogenesis (Rettig et al. 1992; Nanus et al. 2003; Dallas et al. 2008). Antibody phage libraries may be panned directly on endothelial cells in culture (Mutuberria et al. 2004), on tissue sections followed by laser capture microdisection and recovery of phage (Ruan et al. 2006) or directly in vivo. For example, the latter was used to isolate phage that homes to the breast vasculature. The target was later shown to be aminopeptidase P (Essler and Ruoslahti 2002).

The search for tumor endothelial cell markers has initially been tackled using subtractive cDNA analysis methodologies (Wyder et al. 2000). Subsequently, the transcriptome of tumor-derived endothelial cells has been experimentally investigated using serial analysis of gene expression (SAGE) (St Croix et al. 2000) or microarray platforms (Zhang et al. 1999; Ho et al. 2003; Ghilardi et al. 2008) using procedures for the enrichment of endothelial cells or laser capture microdissection of vessels from tissue sections (Roy et al. 2007).

A number of genes have been found to be specifically upregulated in the tumor endothelium, leading to the identification of several novel tumor endothelial markers (TEMs). Since target accessibility from the bloodstream is of fundamental importance for vascular targeting approaches, further work has focused on those genes that encode proteins with predicted transmembrane domains. In a recent analysis, a SAGE approach revealed differences in gene expression patterns in endothelial cells derived from physiological and pathological angiogenic events (Seaman et al. 2007). Interestingly, 13 transcripts were identified in tumor-derived endothelial cells that were undetectable in the angiogenic endothelium of normal, regenerating tissue.

Transcriptomic analyses are able to provide precise information on the quality and quantity of messenger RNAs that are expressed in the cell types and tissues of interest. However, the subsequent validation of the findings is of particular importance, since endothelium-associated targets identified in transcriptomic analyses are not necessarily equally expressed at the protein level and surface-accessible for targeting agents.

As more transcriptomes of solid tumors and associated endothelial cells have become available, investigators have started to compare these databases using bioinformatic procedures for the discovery for novel tumor-associated endothelial markers. One such approach applied a subtractive algorithm to the sequence tag expression data that is available in the public databases to identify novel endothelial-specific genes

(Huminiecki and Bicknell 2000). These were then screened for expression by in situ hybridization, which identified magic roundabout (ROBO4) and an endothelial-specific protein disulphide isomerase (EndoPDI) as tumor endothelial markers (Huminiecki et al. 2002; Sullivan et al. 2003). Another target that came out of this study was the so-called endothelial cells specific molecule 2 (ECSM2), although recently renamed by HUGO as endothelial cell specific chemotaxis regulator (ECSCR). ECSCR is a small (150 kDa) cell surface protein that couples to the actin cytoskeleton through filamin A (Armstrong et al. 2008). There has recently been much interest in ECSCR (Armstrong et al. 2008; Ma et al. 2009) as it is the first identified completely endothelial specific factor to mediate endothelial migration. As endothelial migration is an essential component of angiogenesis and ECSCR is on the cell surface this raises the possibility of therapeutic antibodies. In another study, the crossing of expression databases of in vitro cell culture models of angiogenesis with expression data from diagnostic samples, followed by further prioritization resulted in the identification of Stanniocalcin (STC1) as a putative tumor vascular target (Gerritsen et al. 2002).

A more recent search for novel TEM's has employed knowledge of the human genome sequence (Herbert et al. 2008). In this study each expressed sequence tag from an endothelial or no-endothelial library was uniquely assigned to its best fit in the genome. All genes having only tags from endothelial libraries were then collected and there expression analysed across six normal and tumour tissues. The analysis pulled out known TEM's such as Robo4 but also identified new ones including ECSCR.

In principle, the most direct way to identify novel vascular antigens would involve the in vivo labeling of vascular structures, followed by the isolation and comparative proteomic analysis of proteins. In a search for more systematic discovery methodologies which could provide an Atlas of vascular antigens in normal tissues and at sites of disease, the group of Jan Schnitzer perfused tumor-bearing rodents with silica beads, in order to achieve a physical stripping of membrane proteins from the surface of endothelial cells. The subsequent proteomic analysis of the enriched proteins revealed certain antigens over-expressed in tumor endothelial cells (Oh et al. 2004). Importantly, marker validation included not only immunohistochemical analysis but also in vivo biodistribution studies and/or scintigraphic imaging with radiolabeled antibody preparations. One of the most promising tumor-associated antigens (Annexin A1) was targeted with an ^{125}I-labeled monoclonal antibody, leading to tumor eradication in rodents (Oh et al. 2004). The relevance of these findings is unclear, as the Auger electron emitting radionuclide ^{125}I would not be expected to promote a therapeutic activity at the dose used in the study. Additional preclinical therapeutic data have not been reported, and the product has not progressed to clinical trials.

More recently, a technology for the in vivo chemical labeling of vascular proteins based on the terminal perfusion of tumor-bearing animals with reactive derivatives of biotin has been described (Rybak et al. 2005). This approach allows the biotinylation of proteins on the surface of endothelial cells or in the vessel-associated subendothelial matrix, which are readily accessible from the bloodstream. The purification of biotinylated proteins on a streptavidin column followed by comparative proteomic analysis based on LC-MS/MS methodologies subsequently permits the identification of hundreds of accessible vascular proteins and is able to reveal both quantitative and qualitative differences in the recovery of biotinylated antigens between the tumor and normal organs. This approach has been extended to the ex vivo perfusion of surgically resected human organs with cancer (e.g., kidney and colon; Castronovo et al. 2006; Conrotto et al. 2008), to the discovery of vascular markers of metastasis (Rybak et al. 2007; Villa et al. 2008; Borgia et al. 2010) and to the study of lymphangiogenesis (Rösli et al. 2008).

3 Ligand-Based Pharmacodelivery Applications

Monoclonal antibodies probably represent the only class of binding molecules which can be raised rapidly and with exquisite specificity against virtually any protein target of pharmaceutical interest. The isolation of human monoclonal antibodies has been greatly facilitated by the introduction of antibody phage display technology (Winter et al. 1994). For in vivo antibody-based pharmacodelivery applications only antigens located on the cell surface or in the extracellular space can be considered, since proteins do not generally cross the cell membrane. Antibody internalization into target cells may nonetheless take place for certain antigens located on the cell membrane protein which rapidly recycle.

While monoclonal antibodies in intact IgG format represent the most frequently used antibody type for therapeutic applications (Walsh 2006; Carter 2006), antibody derivatives are increasingly being considered for pharmacodelivery applications (Schrama et al. 2006; Neri and Bicknell 2005; Schliemann and Neri 2007).

Conventional IgG's typically display a therapeutic activity either by modulating the biological function of their target antigens (e.g., by blocking a functional epitope on the target molecule) or by exhibiting biocidal activities mediated by the Fc portion of the antibody molecule (Murphy et al. 2008). In addition to complement activation, the engagement of immune cells such as NK cell via Fcγ receptors (e.g., CD16) appears to be the main avenue for achieving a selective cell killing in vivo (Ferrara et al. 2006; Nimmerjahn and Ravetch 2005).

A large number of antibody derivatives can be considered for pharmacodelivery applications, including antibody-drug conjugates with cleavable linkers (Carter and Senter 2008), radiolabeled antibodies (Sharkey and Goldenberg 2008), antibodies coupled with photosensitizers (Birchler et al. 1999), as well as fusions to enzymes for pro-drug activation (Sharma et al. 2005), mild pro-coagulant factors (Huang et al. 1997) and cytokines. Not only intact IgG molecules can be considered for pharmacodelivery applications, but also scFv fragments and mini-antibodies in the "Small Immune Protein" (SIP) format (Borsi et al. 2002) (Fig. 1). For some antibody derivatives (e.g., radiolabeled antibodies), the therapeutic action is displayed immediately after intravenous administration and the anticancer selectivity directly results from the pharmacokinetic comparison of the areas under the curve for the neoplastic lesions and for normal organs. By contrast, certain therapeutic strategies

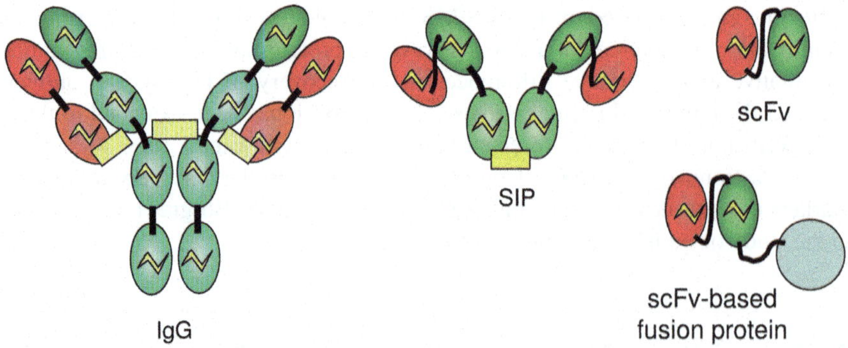

Fig. 1 Schematic representation of antibody formats, including IgG, scFv, scFv fusions and the small immune protein (SIP)

(e.g., Antibody-Directed Enzyme-Prodrug Therapy; ADEPT; Sharma et al. 2005) present a delayed mode of action, at time points when the antibody derivative is still on the tumor but has cleared from circulation and from normal organs. These therapeutic strategies appear to be most promising for the selective killing of tumor cells, while sparing normal tissues.

4 Validated Vascular Tumor Targets

In the following section, we will consider markers of angiogenesis whose suitability for in vivo ligand-based targeting applications has been confirmed by imaging studies, quantitative biodistribution analysis or at least by an ex vivo immunofluorescence analysis following intravenous administration of specific ligands.

4.1 EDA and EDB Domains of Fibronectin

Fibronectin is a large glycoprotein, abundant in blood and in most tissues. Certain alternatively spliced domains of fibronectin (such as the extra-domain A (EDA), the extra-domain B (EDB) and the IIICS region) are usually absent in normal adult tissues (exception made for the endometrium in the proliferative phase and some vessels in the ovaries), but are abundantly expressed with a prominent vascular pattern of staining in conditions of tissue remodeling, such as during tumor formation, wound healing and in placenta (Neri and Bicknell 2005).

The ability of monoclonal antibodies specific to the EDB domain of fibronectin to stain tumor neo-vascular structures (Carnemolla et al. 1989, 1996; Castellani et al. 1994, 2002; Neri et al. 1997; Birchler et al. 2003; Driemel et al. 2007;

Schliemann et al. 2009; Sauer et al. 2009) and to target them in vivo (Tarli et al. 1999; Viti et al. 1999; Borsi et al. 2002; Berndorff et al. 2005; Tijink et al. 2006) has been extensively investigated. The initial characterization of EDA as a tumor-associated antigen for certain cancer pathologies (Borsi et al. 1998) has recently been complemented by the discovery that EDA is an excellent vascular marker of metastasis (Rybak et al. 2007).

The human monoclonal antibodies L19 (specific to EDB; Pini et al. 1998) and F8 (specific to EDA; Villa et al. 2008) have been modified with several different bioactive moieties, including pro-coagulant factors (Nilsson et al. 2001), cytokines (Carnemolla et al. 2002; Halin et al. 2002; Borsi et al. 2003; Ebbinghaus et al. 2005), therapeutic radionuclides (Berndorff et al. 2005; Tijink et al. 2006), enzymes (Heinis et al. 2004) and photosensitizers (Birchler et al. 1999; Fabbrini et al. 2006).

4.2 Extra Domains of Within Tenascin-C

Tenascin-C is a large adhesive glycoprotein, which is abundant in certain tissues. Tenascin-C may contain extra-domains, generated by alternative splicing of the primary transcript, thus leading to the formation of tenascin-C "large" isoforms, which were found to be generally absent in normal adult tissues but abundantly expressed in certain tumor types (e.g., breast cancer; Borsi et al. 1995). More recently, it has been observed that the extra-domain C of tenascin-C displays an even more restricted pattern of expression, while being found in certain tumor types (e.g., high-grade astrocytomas and lung cancer; Carnemolla et al. 1999; Silacci et al. 2006). The human monoclonal antibody F16, specific to the A1 domain of tenascin-C (Brack et al. 2006), and the chimeric antibody 81C6specific to domain D (Zalutsky et al. 2008), have extensively been investigated in biodistribution studies and their derivatives are now in clinical trials (see Chap. 5).

A recent comparative investigation of the immunohistochemical performance of F16 and of the clinical-stage anti-fibronectin antibodies L19 and F8 have revealed that F16 displays the strongest potential for the targeting of human lymphomas (Schliemann et al. 2009) and of thoracic cancer (Pedretti et al. 2009).

4.3 Endoglin

Endoglin (CD105) is a homodimeric transmembrane glycoprotein which acts as co-receptor for TGF-beta and which is overexpressed in neovascular endothelial cells of various solid tumors (Burrows et al. 1995; Wang et al. 1993). Although immunohistochemical studies have revealed that endoglin is also significantly detectable in normal organs (Balza et al. 2001) monoclonal anti-endoglin antibodies have used in biodistribution studies and for imaging and for therapy in rodent and dog models of cancer (Bredow et al. 2000; Fonsatti et al. 2000; Korpanty et al. 2007).

4.4 *Prostate-Specific Membrane Antigen*

PSMA, a membrane glycoprotein with proteolytic activity, was originally found to be over-expressed in prostate cancer. However, several studies have later documented PSMA expression in the neovasculature of several solid tumors (Liu et al. 1997; Silver et al. 1997; Chang et al. 1999), whereas its expression in healthy tissues appears to be restricted to prostatic, duodenal and breast epithelium and renal tubules. Of particular importance for vascular targeting strategies, PSMA appears to be virtually absent in normal blood vessels. The monoclonal antibody J591, labeled with different radionuclides, has demonstrated promising targeting efficacy in patients not only with prostate cancer but also with solid tumors (Bander et al. 2005; Milowsky et al. 2007; Morris et al. 2007).

4.5 *Annexin A1*

Annexins are cytosolic proteins that can associate with plasma membranes in a calcium-dependent manner. Some annexins translocate the lipid bilayer to the outer cell surface. Schnitzer and co-workers have proposed annexin A1 as a target for vascular targeting applications (Oh et al. 2004). A monoclonal antibody to this antigen has been successfully used for the radioimmunoscintigraphic detection of solid tumors in rat model. Furthermore, relatively low doses of the antibody labeled with ^{125}I (50 μCi as a single injection) showed therapeutic efficacy in the same animal model.

4.6 *Phosphatidylserine Phospholipids*

Phosphatidylserine (PS), an anionic phospholipid, is an essential component of the cell membrane, which is preferentially found in the inner leaflet of the lipid bilayer under normal conditions. Under conditions such as cellular stress, apoptosis, and proliferation, PS becomes exposed on the outer surface of the plasma membrane of angiogenic endothelial cells, rendering it accessible for targeting agents (Ran et al. 2005). Targeting experiments using monoclonal antibodies specific to PS have confirmed the accessibility of the target on the external surface of vascular endothelial cells in tumors (Ran et al. 2002, 2005). The PS-antibody 3G4 has been shown to exhibit potent single-agent anti-cancer activity as a naked antibody and to enhance the efficacy of chemotherapy in rodent tumor models (Ran et al. 2005; Huang et al. 2005). Recently, the plasma protein β-2-glycoprotein 1, a member of the complement control protein family, has been identified as a critical co-factor mediating the interaction between 3G4 and surface-exposed PS (Luster et al. 2006).

4.7 VEGF-A and VEGF Receptors

Owing to their well-established functional relevance in angiogenetic processes, VEGF-A and its cognate receptors have been considered as possible targets for antibody-based vascular targeting applications. Most biodistribution studies in rodent models of cancer published so far have exhibited relatively poor tumor:organ ratios over time (e.g., Cooke et al. 2001). However, the Boerman group has recently shown that, in the case of anti-VEGF-A antibodies, targeting results may be strongly dose-dependent and that excellent tumor:organ ratios may be observed when administering low doses of high-specific activity antibodies (Stollman et al. 2008).

4.8 Integrins

Integrins are cell surface proteins each comprised of an alpha and a beta chain. Integrins bind the cell to the extracellular matrix and several of them play a crucial role in angiogenesis. The most studied in angiogenesis are $\alpha 5\beta 1$, $\alpha v\beta 3$ and $\alpha v\beta 5$. $\alpha v\beta 3$ is expressed in newly formed vessels but absent in mature ones (Brooks et al. 1994). For example, anti $\alpha v\beta 3$ antibody showed that it is expressed on the majority of vessels in tumors of the breast, colon, pancreas and lung (Brooks et al. 1995; Max et al. 1997). An anti $\alpha v\beta 3$ antibody (vitaxin) has entered clinical trial but not yet progressed beyond phase II.

The group of Varner have shown that $\alpha 5\beta 1$ integrin is expressed on angiogenic vessels in tumors but absent from quiescent vessels in normal tissue (Kim et al. 2000a). Antagonists of $\alpha 5\beta 1$ integrin have been shown to inhibit angiogenesis leading to tumor regression. It has been shown that these antagonists do not affect cell attachment to vitronectin but instead suppress migration and survival of endothelial cells in this matrix (Kim et al. 2000b).

4.9 Robo4

Robo4 was originally identified through the bioinformatics data-mining of Huminiecki and Bicknell (2000) when they were seeking novel endothelial specific genes. Subsequent studies validated Robo4 as an endothelial gene but also showed that it is expressed only at sites of active angiogenesis, most notably in tumours (Huminiecki et al. 2002). Tumour endothelial expression of Robo4 was independently confirmed by others (Seth et al. 2005). Although there is now much evidence that Robo4, as for the neuronal roundabouts, is involved in filopodia formation (reviewed in Legg et al. 2008; Sheldon et al. 2009) there is little data to date on its use for tumour targeting. Such studies have been delayed by the lack of high affinity antibodies to Robo4.

4.10 Other TEM's Endosialin/TEM1 and TEM7

Of the TEM's identified in the differential SAGE analysis of St. Croix, several have received further validation. Endosialin was first identified by screening antibodies on normal and tumor tissue and was thought to be expressed on tumor endothelium (Rettig et al. 1992). It was independently identified as a tumor marker (TEM1) in the differential SAGE study of St. Croix. However, recent studies have shown that it is more probably expressed on mural cells such a fibroblasts than the tumor endothelium itself (MacFayden et al. 2005). Despite this it remains a validated tumor target.

St Croix et al. (2000) examined TEM7 mRNA expression and found it in the endothelium of tumors of the colon, lung, pancreas, breast, brain and a sarcoma. In contrast, the same group were unable to detect expression in mouse tumors whether homo or xenografts (Carson-Walter et al. 2001). More validation is awaited.

A fusion protein targeting TEM8 has recently been shown to markedly reduce tumor growth in mouse models (Fernando and Fletcher 2009).

5 Products in Clinical Development and Concluding Remarks

The tumor targeting potential of the L19 antibody has been investigated by immunoscintigraphic techniques in patients with cancer, first using the scFv format (Santimaria et al. 2003) and later with the pharmacokinetically superior SIP format (Sauer et al. 2009). SIP(L19), labeled with iodine-131, is currently being investigated for the radioimmunotherapy of solid tumors, with encouraging results in patients with hematological malignancies (Fig. 2; Sauer et al. 2009). The L19 antibody is also being studied in Phase I and Phase II clinical trials as fusion protein with human IL2 or human TNF. L19-IL2 is currently investigated in Phase II clinical studies as monotherapy in patients with renal cell carcinoma and in combination with dacarbazine in patients with metastatic melanoma. Furthermore, L19-IL2 is being used in combination with gemcitabine in Phase Ib studies for the treatment of patients with pancreas cancer. L19-TNF is being investigated as monotherapy in a Phase I trial in patients with different types of malignancies, and in a Phase II trial

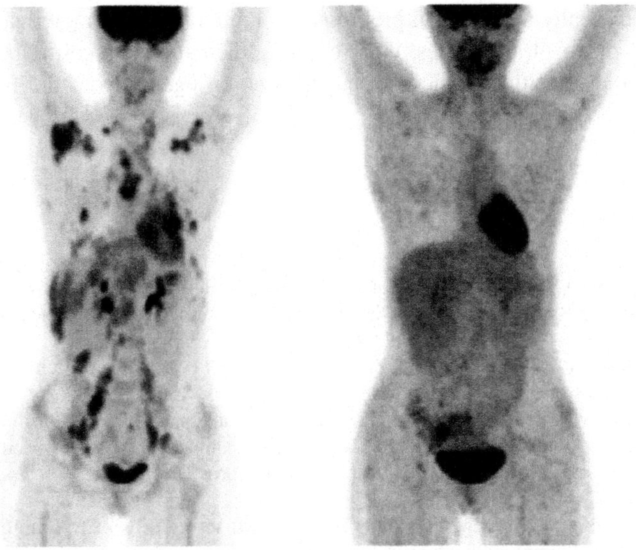

Fig. 2 FDG-PDT analysis of a patient before and 8 months after treatment with SIP(L19) labeled with iodine-131. The patient, affected by Hodgkin lymphoma, had failed six previous lines of chemotherapy, external beam radiation and bone marrow transplantation. Other than physiological glucose uptake in the brain, kidneys, heart and bladder, black spots in the figure indicate the presence of metabolically active neoplastic lesions. A more detailed analysis of the patient's response to treatment can be found in Sauer et al. (2009)

in combination with melphalan in isolated limb perfusion procedures for the treatment of patients with in transit melanoma metastases.

In full analogy to the situation encountered with the L19 antibody, the anti-tenascin F16 antibody is being investigated in Phase Ib studies as fusion protein with IL2, in combination either with doxorubicin (ovarian and breast cancer) or with paclitaxel (lung and breast cancer) or as radioiodinated derivatives for the radioimmunotherapy of patients with both solid and liquid malignancies. Similarly, the murine antitenascin monoclonal antibody 81C6, labeled with ^{131}I or with ^{211}At, has been investigated in several radioimmunotherapy clinical trials for delivery to a surgically-created resection cavity in patients with glioma (Reardon et al. 2006; Zalutsky et al. 2008).

A chimeric version of the anti-phosphatidylserine antibody 3G4, Bavituximab, is currently being investigated in Phase I and Phase II clinical studies either alone or in combination with docetaxel, paclitaxel and/or carboplatin. The same antibody is being studied as anti-viral agent for the therapy of patients with HCV infection (www.peregrinepharmaceuticals.com; Peregrine Pharmaceuticals, Inc.).

The consolidated results of the on-going clinical trials (i.e., at least after Phase II) will shed light on the real therapeutic potential of vascular targeting antibodies and their derivatives. In light of the promising therapeutic results outlined above, it is to be expected that research both on IgG therapeutics and on vascular targeting antibody derivatives will continue, both in pharmaceutical companies and in academic laboratories. The recent guidelines for Phase 0 clinical trials (Kummar et al. 2007) appear to be ideally suited for a preliminary immuno-PET characterization (Tijink et al. 2009) of novel antibodies, thus revealing their tumor targeting potential and facilitating the transition of new vascular targeting agents from the bench to the clinic.

References

Armstrong LJ, Heath VL, Sanderson S, Kaur S, Beesley JFJ, Herbert JMJ, Legg JA, Poulsom R and Bicknell R (2008) ECSM2, an endothelial specific filamin A binding protein that mediates chemotaxis. *Arterio Thromb Vasc Biol*, *28*, 1640–1646.

Balza E, Castellani P, Zijlstra A, Neri D, Zardi L, Siri A (2001) Lack of specificity of endoglin for tumor blood vessels. *Int J Cancer*, *94*, 579–585.

Bander NH, Milowsky MI, Nanus DM, Kostakoglu L, Vallabhajosula S, Goldsmith SJ (2005) Phase I trial of 177lutetium-labeled J591, a monoclonal antibody to prostate-specific membrane antigen, in patients with androgen-independent prostate cancer. *J Clin Oncol*, *23*, 4591–4601.

Berndorff D, Borkowski S, Sieger S, Rother A, Friebe M, Viti F, Hilger CS, Cyr JE, Dinkelborg LM (2005) Radioimmunotherapy of solid tumors by targeting extra domain B fibronectin: identification of the best-suited radioimmunoconjugate. *Clin Cancer Res*, *11*, 7053s–7063s.

Bieker R, Kessler T, Schwoppe C, Padro T, Persigehl T, Bremer C, Dreischauck J, Kolkmeyer A, Heindel W, Mesters RM, Berdel WE (2009) Infarction of tumor vessels by NGR-peptide-directed targeting of tissue factor: experimental results and first-in-man experience. *Blood*, *113*, 5019–5027.

Birchler M, Viti F, Zardi L, Spiess B, Neri D (1999) Selective targeting and photocoagulation of ocular angiogenesis mediated by a phage-derived recombinant antibody. *Nat Biotechnol*, *17*, 984–988.

Birchler MT, Milisavlijevic, Pfaltz DM, Neri D, Odermatt B, Schmid S, Stoeckli SJ (2003) Expression of the extra domain B of fibronectin, a marker of angiogenesis, in head and neck tumors. *Laryngoscope*, *113*, 1231–1237.

Borgia B, Rösli C, Fugmann T, Neri D, Giavazzi R (2010) Accessible markers of liver metastasis revealed by mass spectrometric analysis of vascular structures biotinylated by perfusion of tumor-bearing mice. *Cancer Res*, *70*, 309–318.

Borsi L, Balza E, Gaggero B, Allemanni G and Zardi L (1995) The alternative splicing pattern of the tenascin-C pre-mRNA is controlled by the extracellular pH. *J Biol Chem*, *270*, 6243–6245.

Borsi L, Castellani P, Allemanni G, Neri D, Zardi L (1998) Preparation of phage antibodies to the ED-A domain of human fibronectin, mediator of hepatic fibrogenesis. *Exp Cell Res*, *240*, 244–251.

Borsi L, Balza E, Bestagno M, Castellani P, Carnemolla B, Biro A, Leprini A, Sepulveda J, Burrone O, Neri D, Zardi L (2002) Selective targeting of tumoral vasculature: comparison of different formats of an antibody (L19) to the ED-B domain of fibronectin. *Int J Cancer*, *102*, 75–85.

Borsi L, Balza E, Carnemolla B, Sassi F, Castellani P, Berndt A, Kosmehl H, Biro A, Siri A, Orecchia P, Grassi J, Neri D, Zardi L (2003) Selective targeted delivery of TNF{alpha} to tumor blood vessels. *Blood*, *102*, 4384–4392.

Brack SS, Silacci M, Birchler M, Neri D (2006) Tumor-targeting properties of novel antibodies specific to the large isoform of tenascin-C. *Clin Cancer Res*, *12*, 3200–3208.

Bredow S, Lewin M, Hofmann B, Marecos E, Weissleder R (2000) Imaging of tumour neovasculature by targeting the TGF-beta binding receptor endoglin. *Eur J Cancer*, *36*, 675–681.

Brooks PC, Clark RA and Cheresh DA (1994) Requirement of vascular integrin alpha v beta 3 for angiogenesis. *Science*, *264*, 569–571.

Brooks PC, Stromblad S, Klemke R, Visscher D, Sarkar FH and Cheresh DA (1995) Antiintegrin alpha v beta 3 blocks human breast cancer growth and angiogenesis in human skin. *J Clin Invest*, *96*, 1815–1822.

Burrows FJ, Thorpe PE (1993) Eradication of large solid tumors in mice with an immunotoxin directed against tumor vasculature. *Proc Natl Acad Sci USA*, *90*, 8996–9000.

Burrows FJ, Derbyshire EJ, Tazzari PL, Amlot P, Gazdar AF, King, SW, Letarte M, Vitetta ES, Thorpe PE (1995) Up-regulation of endoglin on vascular endothelial cells in human solid tumors: implications for diagnosis and therapy. *Clin Cancer Res*, *1*, 1623–1634.

Carnemolla B, Balza E, Siri A, Zardi L, Nicotra MR, Bigotti A, Natali PG (1989) A tumor-associated fibronectin isoform generated by alternative splicing of messenger RNA precursors. *J Cell Biol*, *108*, 1139–1148.

Carnemolla B, Neri D, Castellani P, Leprini A, Neri G, Pini A, Winter G, Zardi L (1996) Phage antibodies with pan-species recognition of the oncofoetal angiogenesis marker fibronectin ED-B domain. *Int J Cancer*, *68*, 397–405.

Carnemolla B, Castellani P, Ponassi M, Borsi L, Urbini S, Nicolo' G, Dorcaratto A, Viale G, Winter G, Neri D, Zardi L (1999) Identification of a glioblastoma associated TN-C isoform by a high affinity recombinant antibody. *Am J Pathol*, *154*, 1345–1352.

Carnemolla B, Borsi L, Balza E, Castellani P, Meazza R, Berndt A, Ferrini S, Kosmehl H, Neri D and Zardi L (2002) Enhancement of the antitumor properties of interleukin-2 by its targeted delivery to the tumor blood vessel extracellular matrix. *Blood*, *99*, 1659–1665.

Carson-Walter EB, Watkins DN, Nanda A, Vogelstein B, Kinzler K, St Croix B (2001) Cell surface tumour endothelial markers are conserved in mice and humans. *Cancer Res*, *63*, 5866–73.

Carter PJ (2006) Potent antibody therapeutics by design. *Nat Rev Immunol*, *6*, 343–357.

Carter PJ, Senter P (2008) Antibody-drug conjugates for cancer therapy. *Cancer J*, *14*, 154–169.

Castellani P, Viale G, Dorcaratto A, Nicolo G, Kaczmarek J, Querze G, Zardi L (1994) The fibronectin isoform containing the ED-B oncofetal domain: a marker of angiogenesis. *Int J Cancer*, *59*, 612–618.

Castellani P, Borsi L, Carnemolla B, Biro A, Dorcaratto A, Viale GL, Neri D, Zardi L (2002) Differentiation between high and low grade astrocytoma using a human recombinant antibody to the ED-B domain of fibronectin. *Am J Pathol*, *161*, 1695–1700.

Castronovo V, Waltregny D, Kishel P, Elia G, Rösli C, Rybak J, Neri D (2006) A chemical proteomic approach for the identification of accessible antigens expressed in human kidney cancer. *Mol Cell Proteomics*, *5*, 2083–2091.

Chang SS, O'Keefe DS, Bacich DJ, Reuter VE, Heston WD, Gaudin PB (1999) Prostate-specific membrane antigen is produced in tumor-associated neovasculature. *Clin Cancer Res*, *5*, 2674–2681.

Chaplin DJ, Horsman MR, Siemann DW (2006) Current development status of small-molecule vascular disrupting agents. *Curr Opin Investig Drugs*, *7*, 522–528.

Conrotto P, Rösli C, Rybak JN, Kishel P, Waltregny D, Neri D, Castronovo V (2008) Identification of novel tumor-associated and accessible antigens in human colon cancer by ex vivo protein biotinylation and comparative mass spectrometry analysis. *Int J Cancer*, *123*, 2856–2864.

Cooke SP, Boxer GM, Lawrence L, Pedley RB, Spencer DI, Begent RH, Chester KA. (2001) A strategy for antitumor vascular therapy by targeting the vascular endothelial growth factor: receptor complex. *Cancer Res*, *61*, 3653–3659.

Corti A, Curnis F, Arap W, Pasqualini R (2008) The neovasculature homing motif NGR: more than meets the eye. *Blood*, *112*, 2628–2635.

Dallas NA Samuel S, Xia L, Fan F, Gray MJ, Lim SJ and Ellis LM (2008) Endoglin (CD105): a marker of tumor vasculature and potential target for therapy. *Clin Cancer Res*, *14(7)*, 1931–1937.

Denekamp J (1990) Vascular attack as a therapeutic strategy for cancer. *Cancer Metastasis Rev*, *9*, 267–282.

Driemel O, Kosmehl H, Rosenhahn J, Berndt A, Reichert TE, Zardi L, Dahse R (2007) Expression analysis of extracellular matrix components in brush biopsies of oral lesions. *Anticancer Res*, *27*, 1565–1570.

Ebbinghaus C, Ronca R, Kaspar M, Grabulovski D, Berndt A, Kosmehl H, Zardi L, Neri D (2005) An engineered vascular-targeting antibody-interferon gamma fusion protein for cancer therapy. *Int J Cancer*, *116*, 304–313.

Essler M and Ruoslahti E (2002) Molecular specialization of breast vasculature: a breast-homing phage-displayed peptide binds to aminopeptidase P in breast vasculature. *Proc Natl Acad Sci U S A*, *99*, 2252–2257.

Fabbrini M, Trachsel E, Soldani P, Bindi S, Alessi P, Bracci L, Kosmehl H, Zardi L, Neri D, Neri P (2006) Selective occlusion of tumor blood vessels by targeted delivery of an antibody-photosensitizer conjugate. *Int J Cancer*, *118*, 1805–1813.

Fernando S, Fletcher BS (2009) Targeting tumor endothelial marker 8 in the tumor vasculature of colorectal carcinomas in mice. *Cancer Res*, *69*, 5126–5132.

Ferrara N (2004) Vascular endothelial growth factor as a target for anticancer therapy. Oncologist *9 (Suppl 1)*, 2–10.

Ferrara C, Stuart F, Sondermann P, Brünker P, Umana P (2006) The carbohydrate at FcgammaRIIIa Asn 162. An element required for high affinity binding to non-fucosylated IgG glycoforms. *J Biol Chem*, *281*, 5032–5036.

Folkman J (1990) What is the evidence that tumours are angiogenesis dependant? *J Natl Cancer Inst*, *82*, 4–6.

Fonsatti E, Jekunen AP, Kairemo KJ, Coral S, Snellman M, Nicotra MR, Natali PG, Altomonte M, Maio M (2000) Endoglin is a suitable target for efficient imaging of solid tumors: in vivo evidence in a canine mammary carcinoma model. *Clin Cancer Res*, *6*, 2037–2043.

Gerritsen ME, Soriano R, Yang S, Ingle G, Zlot C, Toy K, Winer J, Draksharapu A, Peale F, Wu FTD, Williams PM (2002) In silico data filtering to identify new angiogenesis targets from a large in vitro gene profiling data set. *Physiol Genomics*, *10*, 13–20.

Ghilardi C, Chiorino G, Dossi R, Nagy Z, Giavazzi R, Bani M (2008) Identification of novel vascular markers through gene expression profiling of tumor-derived endothelium. *BMC Genomics*, *9*, 201.

Halin C, Rondini S, Nilsson F, Berndt A, Kosmehl H, Zardi L, Neri D (2002) Enhancement of the antitumor activity of interleukin-12 by targeted delivery to neovasculature. *Nat Biotechnol*, *20*, 264–269.

Heinis C, Alessi P, Neri D (2004) Engineering a thermostable human prolyl endopeptidase for antibody directed enzyme prodrug therapy (ADEPT). *Biochemistry*, *43*, 6293–6303.

Herbert JM, Stekel D, Sanderson S, Heath VL, Bicknell R (2008) A novel method of differential gene expression analysis using multiple cDNA libraries applied to the identification of tumour endothelial genes. *BMC Genomics*, *9*, 153–174.

Ho M, Yang E, Matcuk G, Deng D, Sampas N, Tsalenko A, Tabibiazar R, Zhang Y, Chen M, Talbi S, Ho YD, Wang J, Tsao PS, Ben-Dor A, Yakhini Z, Bruhn L and Quatermous T (2003) Identification of endothelial cell genes by combined database mining and microarray analysis. *Physiol Genomics*, *13*, 249–62.

Huang X, Molema G, King S, Watkins L, Edgington TS, Thorpe PE (1997) Tumor infarction in mice by antibody-directed targeting of tissue factor to tumor vasculature. *Science*, *275*, 547–550.

Huang X, Bennett M, Thorpe PE (2005) A monoclonal antibody that binds anionic phospholipids on tumor blood vessels enhances the antitumor effect of docetaxel on human breast tumors in mice. *Cancer Res*, *65*, 4408–4416.

Huminiecki L, Bicknell R (2000) In silico cloning of novel endothelial-specific genes. *Genome Res*, *10*, 1796–1806.

Huminiecki L, Gorn M, Suchting S, Poulsom R, Bicknell R (2002) Magic roundabout is a new member of the roundabout receptor family that is endothelial specific and expressed at sites of active angiogenesis. *Genomics*, *79*, 547–552.

Jennewein M, Lewis MA, Zhao D, Tsyganov E, Slavine N, He J, Watkins L, Kodibagkar VD, O'Kelly S, Kulkarni P, Antich PP, Hermanne A, Rösch F, Mason RP, Thorpe PE (2008) Vascular imaging of solid tumors in rats with a radioactive arsenic-labeled antibody that binds exposed phosphatidylserine. *Clin Cancer Res*, *14*, 1377–1385.

Kim S, Bell K, Mousa SA, Varner JA (2000a) Regulation of angiogenesis in vivo by ligation of integrin alpha5 beta 1 with the central cell-binding domain of fibronectin. *Am J Pathol*, *156*, 1345–1362.

Kim S, Harris M and Varner JA (2000b) Regulation of integrin alpha v beta 3 mediated endothelial cell migration and angiogenesis by integrin alpha 5 beta 1 and protein kinase A. *J Biol Chem*, *275*, 33920–33928.

Korpanty G, Carbon JG, Grayburn PA, Fleming JB, Brekken RA (2007) Monitoring response to anticancer therapy by targeting microbubbles to tumor vasculature. *Clin Cancer Res*, *13*, 323–330.

Kummar S, Kinders R, Rubinstein L, Parchment RE, Murgo AJ, Collins J, Pickeral O, Low J, Steinberg SM, Gutierrez M, Yang S, Helman L, Wiltrout R, Tomaszewski JE, Doroshow JH (2007) Compressing drug development timelines using Phase "0" clinical trials. *Nat Rev Drug Disc*, *7*, 131–139.

Legg JA, Herbert JMJ, Clissold P, Bicknell R (2008) Slits and roundabouts in cancer, tumour angiogenesis and endothelial cell migration. *Angiogenesis 11*, 13–21.

Liu H, Moy P, Kim S, Xia Y, Rajasekaran A, Navarro V, Knudsen B, Bander NH (1997) Monoclonal antibodies to the extracellular domain of prostate-specific membrane antigen also react with tumor vascular endothelium. *Cancer Res*, *57*, 3629–3634.

Luster TA, He J, Huang X, Maiti SN, Schroit AJ, de Groot PG, Thorpe PE (2006) Plasma protein beta-2-glycoprotein 1 mediates interaction between the anti-tumor monoclonal antibody 3G4 and anionic phospholipids on endothelial cells. *J Biol Chem*, *281*, 29863–29871.

Ma F, Zhang D, Yang H, Sun H, Wu W, Gan Y, Balducci J, Wei Y, Zhao X, Huang Y (2009) Endothelial cell-specific molecule 2 (ECSM2) modulates actin remodeling and epidermal growth factor receptor signaling. *Genes to Cell*, *14*, 281–293.

MacFayden JR, Haworth O, Roberston D, Hardie D, Webster M-T, Morris HR, Panico M, Sutton-Smith M, Dell A, van der Greer P, Wienke D, Buckley Cd, Isacke CM (2005) Endosialin (TEM1, CD248) is a marker of stromal fibroblasts and is not selectively expressed on tumour endothelium. *FEBS Lett*, *579*, 2569–2575.

Mårlind J, Kaspar M, Trachsel E, Sommavilla R, Hindle S, Bacci C, Giovannoni L, Neri D (2008) The antibody-mediated delivery of interleukin-2 to the stroma of breast cancer strongly enhances the potency of chemotherapy. *Clin Cancer Res*, *14*, 6515–6524.

Max R, Gerritsen RR Nooijen PT, Goodman SL, Sutter A, Keilholz U, Ruiter DJ, De Waal RM (1997) Immunohistochemical analysis of integrin alpha v beta 3 expression on tumor-associated vessels of human carcinomas. *Int J Cancer*, *71*, 320–324.

Milowsky MI, Nanus DM, Kostakoglu L, Sheehan CE, Vallabhajosula S, Goldsmith SJ, Ross JS, Bander NH (2007) Vascular targeted therapy with anti-prostate-specific membrane antigen monoclonal antibody J591 in advanced solid tumors. *J Clin Oncol*, *25*, 540–547.

Morris MJ, Pandit-Taskar N, Divgi CR, Bender S, O'Donoghue JA, Nacca A, Smith-Jones P, Schwartz L, Slovin S, Finn R, Larson S, Scher HI (2007) Phase I evaluation of J591 as a vascular targeting agent in progressive solid tumors. *Clin Cancer Res*, *13*, 2707–2713.

Murphy K, Travers P, Walport M (2008) Janeway's Immunobiology, 7th Ed., Garland Science, New York and London.

Mutuberria R, Satijn S, Huijbers A, Van Der Linden E, Lichtenbeld H, Chames P, Arends JW, Hoogenboom HR (2004) Isolation of human antibodies to tumor-associated endothelial markers by in vitro human endothelial cell selection with phage display libraries. *J Immunol Methods*, *287*, 31–47.

Nanus DM, Milowsky MI, Kostakoglu L, Smith-Jones PM, Vallabahajosula S, Goldsmith SJ, Bander NH (2003) Clinical use of monoclonal antibody HuJ591 therapy: targeting prostate specific membrane antigen. *J Urol*, 170 (Pt 2) S84–S89.

Neri D, Bicknell R (2005) Vascular tumour targeting. *Nat Rev Cancer*, *5*, 436–446.

Neri D, Carnemolla B, Nissim A, Leprini A, Querze G, Balza E, Pini A, Tarli L, Halin C, Neri P, Zardi L, Winter G (1997) Targeting by affinity-matured recombinant antibody fragments of an angiogenesis associated fibronectin isoform. *Nat Biotechnol*, *15*, 1271–1275.

Nilsson F, Kosmehl H, Zardi L, Neri D (2001) Targeted delivery of tissue factor to the ED-B domain of fibronectin, a marker of angiogenesis, mediates the infarction of solid tumours in mice, *Cancer Res*, *61*, 711–716.

Nimmerjahn F, Ravetch JV (2005) Divergent immunoglobulin g subclass activity through selective Fc receptor binding. *Science*, *310*, 1510–1512.

Oh P, Li Y, Yu J, Durr E, Krasinska KM, Carver LA, Testa JE, Schnitzer JE (2004) Subtractive proteomic mapping of the endothelial surface in lung and solid tumours for tissue-specific therapy. *Nature*, *429*, 629–635.

Pedretti M, Soltermann A, Arni S, Weder W, Neri D, Hillinger S (2009) Comparative immunohistochemistry of L19 and F16 in non-small cell lung cancer and mesothelioma: two human antibodies investigated in clinical trials in patients with cancer. *Lung Cancer*, *64*, 28–33

Pini A, Viti F, Santucci A, Carnemolla B, Zardi L, Neri P, Neri D (1998) Design and use of a phage-display library: human antibodies with subnanomolar affinity against a marker of angiogenesis eluted from a two-dimensional gel. *J Biol Chem*, *273*, 21769–21776.

Ran S, Downes A, Thorpe PE (2002) Increased exposure of anionic phospholipids on the surface of tumor blood vessels. *Cancer Res*, *62*, 6132–6140.

Ran S, He J, Huang X, Soares M, Scothorn D, Thorpe PE (2005) Antitumor effects of a monoclonal antibody that binds anionic phospholipids on the surface of tumor blood vessels in mice. *Clin Cancer Res*, *11*, 1551–1562.

Reardon DA, Akabani G, Coleman RE, Friedman AH, Friedman HS, Herndon JE, 2nd, McLendon RE, Pegram CN, Provenzale JM, Quinn JA, Rich JN, Vredenburgh JJ, Desjardins A, Gururangan S, Badruddoja M, Dowell JM, Wong TZ, Zhao XG, Zalutsky MR, Bigner DD (2006) Salvage radioimmunotherapy with murine iodine-131-labeled antitenascin monoclonal antibody 81C6 for patients with recurrent primary and metastatic malignant brain tumors: phase II study results. *J Clin Oncol*, *24*, 115–122.

Rettig WJ, Garin-Chesa P, Healey JH, Su SL, Jaffe EA, Old LJ (1992) Identification of endosialin, a cell surface glycoprotein of vascular endothelial cells in human cancer. *Proc Natl Acad Sci U S A*, *89*, 10832–10836.

Rösli C, Mumprecht VD, Neri D, Detmar M (2008) Identification of the surface-accessible, lineage-specific vascular proteome by two-dimensional peptide mapping. *FASEB J*, *22*, 1933–1944.

Roy S, Patel D, Khanna S, Gordillo GM, Biswas S, Friedman A, Sen CK (2007) Transcriptome-wide analysis of blood vessels laser captured from human skin and chronic wound edge tissue. *Proc Natl Acad Sci U S A*, *104*, 14472–14477.

Ruan W, Sassoon A, An F, Simko JP, Liu B (2006) Identification of clinically significant tumour antigens by selecting phage antibody library on tumor cells in situ using laser capture microdissection. *Mol Cell Proteomics*, *5(12)*, 2364–2373.

Rybak JN, Ettorre A, Kaissling B, Giavazzi R, Neri D, Elia G (2005) In vivo protein biotinylation for identification of organ-specific antigens accessible from the vasculature. *Nat Methods*, *2*, 291–298.

Rybak JN, Roesli C, Kaspar M, Villa A, Neri D (2007) The extra-domain A of fibronectin is a vascular marker of solid tumors and metastases. *Cancer Res*, *67*, 10948–10957.

Santimaria M, Moscatelli G, Viale GL, Giovannoni L, Neri G, Viti F, Leprini A, Borsi L, Castellani P, Zardi L, Neri D, Riva P (2003) Immunoscintigraphic detection of the ED-B domain of fibronectin, a marker of angiogenesis, in patients with cancer. *Clin Cancer Res*, *9*, 571–579.

Sauer A, Erba PA, Petrini M, Menrad A, Giovannoni L, Grana C, Hirsch B, Zardi L, Paganelli G, Mariani G, Neri D, Dürkop H, Menssen HD (2009) Expression of the oncofetal ED-B containing fibronectin isoform in hematologic tumors enables ED-B targeted 131I-L19SIP radioimmunotherapy in Hodgkin lymphoma patients. *Blood*, *113*, 2265–2274.

Schliemann C, Neri D (2007) Antibody-based targeting of the tumor vasculature. *Biochim Biophys Acta*, *1776*, 175–192.

Schliemann C, Palumbo A, Zuberbuhler K, Villa A, Kaspar M, Trachsel E, Klapper W, Menssen HD, Neri D (2009) Complete eradication of human B-cell lymphoma xenografts using rituximab in combination with the immunocytokine L19-IL2. *Blood*, *113*, 2275–2283.

Schliemann C, Wiedmer A, Pedretti M, Szczepanowski M, Klapper W, Neri D (2009) Three clinical-stage tumor targeting antibodies reveal differential expression of oncofetal fibronectin and tenascin-C isoforms in human lymphoma. *Leukemia Res*, *33*, 1718–1722.

Schrama D, Reisfeld RA, Becker JC (2006) Antibody targeted drugs as cancer therapeutics. *Nat Rev Drug Discov*, *5*, 147–159.

Seaman S, Stevens J, Yang MY, Logsdon D, Graff-Cherry C, St Croix B (2007) Genes that distinguish physiological and pathological angiogenesis. *Cancer Cell*, *11*, 539–554.

Seth P, Lin Y, Hanai J, Shivalingappa V, Duyao MP, Sukhatme VP (2005) Magic roundabout, a tumour endothelial marker: expression and signaling. *Biochem Biophys Res Commun*, *332*, 533–541.

Sharkey RM, Goldenberg DM (2008) Novel radiopharmaceuticals for cancer imaging and therapy. *Curr Opin Investig Drugs*, *9*, 1302–1316.

Sharma SK, Pedley RB, Bhatia J, Boxer GM, El-Emir E, Qureshi U, Tolner B, Lowe H, Michael NP, Minton N, Begent RH, Chester KA (2005) Sustained tumor regression of human colorectal cancer xenografts using a multifunctional mannosylated fusion protein in antibody-directed enzyme prodrug therapy. *Clin Cancer Res*, *11*, 814–825.

Sheldon H, Andre M, Legg JA, Heal P, Herbert JM, Sainson R, Sharma AS, Kitajewski JK, Heath VL, Bicknell R (2009) Active involvement of Robo1 and Robo4 in filopodia formation and endothelial cell motility mediated via WASP and other actin nucleation promoting factors. *FASEB J*, *23*, 513–522.

Silacci M, Brack SS, Spaeth N, Buck A, Hillinger S, Arni S, Weder W, Zardi L, Neri D (2006) Human monoclonal antibodies to domain C of tenascin-C selectively target solid tumors in vivo. *Protein Eng Des Sel*, *19*, 471–478.

Silver DA, Pellicer I, Fair WR, Heston WD, Cordon-Cardo C (1997) Prostate-specific membrane antigen expression in normal and malignant human tissues. *Clin Cancer Res*, *3*, 81–85.

Soares MM, King SW, Thorpe PE (2008) Targeting inside-out phosphatidylserine as a therapeutic strategy for viral diseases. *Nat Med*, *14*, 1357–1362.

St Croix B, Rago C, Velculescu V, Traverso G, Romans KE, Montgomery E, Lal A, Riggins GJ, Lengauer C, Vogelstein B, Kinzler KW (2000) Genes expressed in human tumor endothelium. *Science*, *289*, 1197–1202.

Stollman TH, Scheer MGW, Leenders WPJ, Verrijp CN, Soede AC, Oyen WJG, Ruers TJM, Boerman OC (2008) Specific imaging of VEFG-A expression with radiolabeled anti-VEGF monoclonal antibody. *Int J Cancer*, *122*, 2310–2314.

Sullivan DC, Huminiecki L, Moore JW, Boyle JJ, Poulsom R, Creamer D, Barker J, Bicknell R (2003) EndoPDI, a novel protein-disulfide isomerase-like protein that is preferentially expressed in endothelial cells acts as a stress survival factor. *J Biol Chem*, *278*, 47079–47088.

Tarli L, Balza E, Viti F, Borsi L, Castellani P, Berndorff D, Dinkelborg L, Neri D, Zardi L (1999) A high-affinity human antibody that targets tumoral blood vessels. *Blood*, *94*, 192–198.

Tijink BM, Neri D, Leemans CR, Budde M, Dinkelborg LM, Stigter-van Walsum M, Zardi L, van Dongen GA (2006) Radioimmunotherapy of head and neck cancer xenografts using ^{131}I-labeled antibody L19-SIP for selective targeting of tumor vasculature. *J Nucl Med*, *47*, 1127–1135.

Tijink BM, Perk LR, Budde M, van Walsum MS, Visser GWM, Klet RW, Dinkelborg LM, Leemans CR, Neri D, van Dongen GAMS (2009) ^{124}I-L19-SIP for immuno-PET imaging of tumour vasculature and guidance of ^{131}I-L19-SIP radioimmunotherapy. *Eur J Nucl Med Mol Imaging*, *36*, 1235–1244.

Villa A, Trachsel E, Kaspar M, Schliemann C, Sommavilla R, Rybak J, Rösli C, Borsi L, Zardi L and Neri D (2008) A high-affinity human monoclonal antibody specific to the alternatively-spliced EDA domain of fibronectin efficiently targets tumor neo-vasculature in vivo. *Int J Cancer*, *122*, 2405–2413.

Viti F, Tarli L, Giovannoni L, Zardi L, Neri D (1999) Binding affinity and valence determine the tumour targeting performance of anti-angiogenesis antibodies. *Cancer Res*, *59*, 347–352.

Walsh G (2006) Biopharmaceuticals benchmark. *Nat Biotechnol*, *24*, 769–776.

Wang JM, Kumar S, Pye D, van Agthoven AJ, Krupinski J, Hunter RD (1993) A monoclonal antibody detects heterogeneity in vascular endothelium of tumours and normal tissues. *Int J Cancer*, *54*, 363–370.

Winter G, Griffiths AD, Hawkins RE, Hoogenboom HR (1994) Making antibodies by phage display technology. *Annu Rev Immunol*, *12*, 433–455.

Wyder L, Vitaliti A, Schneider H, Hebbard LW, Moritz DR, Wittmer M, Ajmo M, Klemenz R (2000) Increased expression of H/T-cadherin in tumor-penetrating blood vessels. *Cancer Res*, *60*, 4682–4688.

Zalutsky MR, Reardon DA, Akabani G, Coleman RE, Friedman AH, Freidman HS, McLendon RE, Wong TZ and Bigner DD (2008) Clinical experience with alpha particle emitting 211At: treatment of recurrent brain tumor patients with 211At-labeled chimeric antitenascin monoclonal antibody 81C6. *J Nucl Med*, *49*, 30–38.

Zardi L, Carnemolla B, Siri A, Petersen TE, Paolella G, Sebastio G, Baralle FE (1987) Transformed human cells produce a new fibronectin isoform by preferential alternative splicing of a previously unobserved exon. *EMBO J*, *6*, 2337–2342.

Zhang HT, Gorn M, Smith K, Graham AP, Lau KK and Bicknell R (1999) Transcriptional profiling of human microvascular endothelial cells in the proliferative and quiescent state using cDNA arrays. *Angiogenesis*, *3*, 211–219.

The Use of Animal Models in the Assessment of Tumour Vascular Disrupting Agents (VDAs)

R. Barbara Pedley and Gillian M. Tozer

Abstract Tumour vascular disrupting agents (VDAs) are designed to target established tumour blood vessels, with the aim of permanently shutting down tumour blood flow, thereby inducing secondary tumour cell death. The microtubule-disrupting tubulin-binding agents are the largest sub-group of low molecular weight VDAs, a number of which are in advanced clinical development. In addition, a number of putative molecular targets for VDA development are being investigated. In this chapter, we review the role of animal experiments in the pre-clinical assessment of VDAs. We start with considerations of the different rodent tumour models available for study, with an additional section on the potential of the zebrafish. We then review assays of vascular function and morphology, including the use of modern imaging techniques. Throughout, we provide examples of where the techniques have been used and summarise the results obtained. All the models and assay methods have advantages and disadvantages – here, we aim to provide some guidance on their future applications.

1 Introduction

Tumour vascular disrupting agents or VDAs are designed to target *established tumour blood vessels*, with the aim of permanently shutting down tumour blood flow, thereby inducing secondary tumour cell death. This approach is conceptually distinct from anti-angiogenic therapy, where the aim is to prevent the *development of new blood vessels* in tumours, although a single agent may have both vascular disrupting and anti-angiogenic properties. A VDA is characterized by the ability to cause a very rapid (initiated within minutes) shut-down of blood flow that is

R.B. Pedley
UCL Cancer Institute, Paul O'Gorman Building,
University College London, 72 Huntley St, London, WC1E 6BT

T. Meyer (ed.), *Vascular Disruptive Agents for the Treatment of Cancer*,
DOI 10.1007/978-1-4419-6609-4_3,

selective for the tumour and sufficient to cause significant tumour necrosis (within 24 h). Several classes of low molecular weight drugs have innate tumour vascular disrupting properties, of which the largest group is microtubule-disrupting tubulin-binding agents, such as the combretastatins e.g. CA4P/Zybrestat™, CA-1-P (OXi4503), AVE8062, TZT-1027. Others include the cytokine-inducing agent, ASA404, and arsenic trioxide.

In addition, distinct molecular signatures associated with the tumour vasculature are being developed as therapeutic targets for tumour vascular disruption (Neri and Bicknell 2005; Schliemann and Neri 2007) and the search for further molecular targets is on-going. Individual VDAs are at different stages of development, with the lead combretastatin, CA4P and ASA404 already in Phase II/III clinical trial (Rehman and Rustin 2008; Siemann et al. 2009). Animal models play a key role in the assessment of VDAs for a number of reasons:

1. *In vitro* models are inadequate for screening putative VDAs because tumour blood flow cannot be modeled.
2. Mechanistic studies of established VDAs are required for developing better agents and this requires models with an intact vascular system, in addition to *in vitro* models.
3. Animal models are required for biomarker development for use in early clinical trials of new drugs to assess pharmacodynamic end-points, in order to determine whether VDAs are performing as expected.

In this review, we will outline animal models and the specialized techniques that are used for assessing VDAs. We will define the vascular parameters that can be measured by each technique and their most useful applications, with some guidance on advantages and disadvantages.

2 Animal Models

2.1 General Considerations

Numerous rodent models (predominantly mouse) of human cancer have proved valuable research tools, and are the most frequently employed models for assessing the therapeutic efficacy of VDAs. There is evidence that many of these studies are predictive for the clinical situation; Galbraith et al. (2003) demonstrated that data from experimental models, in which rapid reductions in blood flow have been recorded for a variety of tumour types, is consistent with clinical findings. They also showed that the time course of changes following CA4P treatment in rats bearing the P22 rat sarcoma and man was similar, demonstrating the utility of this animal model for preclinical studies of tumour vascular targeting agents. Furthermore, the finding that the effect of CA4P on tumour perfusion was reversible in human tumours (Anderson et al. 2003) again mirrors published results for experimental tumour models.

It is beyond the scope of this review to cover all the animal models employed in the study of VDAs, and therefore typical or novel examples have been selected in order to demonstrate their usefulness.

2.2 *Subcutaneous and Other Ectopic Models*

Sub-cutaneous transplantation of tumour cells from *in vitro* cell cultures or mouse-to-mouse is the conventional means of propagating experimental tumours for therapeutic studies (Twentyman et al. 1980). The advantages of subcutaneous tumour models is that they are rapid to set up, easily accessible, reproducible and synchronised, so that treatment can begin when all the tumours are of an optimal size, and data can easily be quantified. They have been employed since the early development of VDAs, and still remain the most frequently employed model, generally initiated by injection of cells or tumour fragments into the flank or dorsum (Zwi et al. 1989; Laws et al. 1995; Chaplin et al. 1996; Pedley et al. 1996; Dark et al. 1997; Nihei et al. 1999). Other ectopic sites of transplantation, for a range of tumour types, include the mouse foot pad and large muscle groups in the leg, which have been used primarily to facilitate tumour irradiation or hyperthermia for combination therapy studies, most recently for CA4P and OXi4503 (Salmon and Siemann 2006; Hokland and Horsman 2007; Salmon and Siemann 2007). Mouse tumour cells transplanted into immuno-competent syngeneic hosts are now less commonly used than xenotransplanted human tumour cells into immuno-deprived mice (SCID or nude). However, syngeneic systems play an important role for modelling immune interactions and are extremely useful for ensuring a full complement of paracrine interactions between tumour and stromal cells, which may be compromised when these cell types derive from different species. In all cases, tumour cell lines are generally maintained as early passages away from the original primary tumour, in order to minimise genetic drift and clonal selection, although this cannot be altogether avoided.

Use of sub-cutaneous tumours established the vascular disrupting effects of a number of novel agents, which were subsequently found to be active in orthotopically transplanted tumours, spontaneous tumours and metastases in mice. The continued utility of sub-cutaneous models for evaluating VDAs is demonstrated by the close parallels between vascular effects of CA4P in a sub-cutaneous rat tumour model and in man (Galbraith et al. 2003). Sub-cutaneous models also established that, in general, VDAs must be combined with conventional or novel therapies in order to achieve relevant therapeutic efficacy (Pedley et al. 2001, 2002; Horsman and Siemann 2006). Mechanistic studies using sub-cutaneously transplanted tumours helped to demonstrate the importance of endothelial junction instability for the susceptibility of tumour blood vessels to CA4P (Vincent et al. 2005) and the potential importance of bone marrow derived progenitor cells in tumour re-vascularisation after CA4P treatment (Shaked et al. 2006). Sub-cutaneously transplanted tumour models have also been the mainstay for ASA404 studies, recently demonstrating the enhancement of its activity by non-steroidal anti-inflammatory drugs (NSAIDs) (Wang et al. 2008) and its effect on tumour vascular permeability (Zhao et al. 2005).

2.3 Orthotopic and Metastatic Models

While subcutaneous models are easy to establish, and allow the accurate measurement of tumour response to therapy, orthotopically transplanted and metastatic tumour models are considered more clinically relevant for studying the efficacy of cancer therapies, and are increasingly being employed for VDA assessment. In orthotopic animal models the tumour is implanted in its native site (local growth), such as into the colon or caecum for colon cancer, to resemble the natural development of the human disease. Metastatic models may either develop by natural spread from an orthotopic tumour, or from intravenous injection of tumour cells, which home to their clinical site and provide a reproducible system. Both models allow the tumour to interact with the relevant organ environment, and should therefore be better predictors of therapeutic response when treating patients. The disadvantage of these two model systems compared with the subcutaneous site is the inability to monitor tumour growth accurately, but successful spread and subsequent growth can be followed by intravital luminescence imaging of luciferase-expressing tumour cells (see section 5.2 below).

An example is the use of colorectal liver metastases, which can be induced by injecting tumour cells into the spleen or hepatic portal vein, from where they migrate to form discreet deposits in the liver closely resembling the clinical disease. Holwell et al. (2002) reported that OXi4503 displayed greater anti-tumor effects than the A-4 analogue in hepatic deposits of human colon tumors in nude mice. Later studies of multi-dose OXi4503 using the colorectal metastatic model system have shown decrease in tumour perfusion by laser Doppler flowmetry, extensive central necrosis with a thin surviving viable rim (frequently only one cell thick), and significantly improved survival (Pedley et al. 2005; Malcontenti-Wilson et al. 2008). In addition, by optimising the timing of multi-dose delivery, OXi4503 as a single agent can eliminate liver metastases in nude mice bearing the SW1222 colorectal tumour (Pedley et al. 2008), but combination therapy may still be required for complete eradication.

Salmon et al. (2006) established an orthotopic model of renal cell carcinoma by injecting Caki-1 cells into the kidney of nude mice, and employed this to evaluate the effects of CA4P and OXi4503. They found that the VDAs produced extensive central necrosis and left only a small viable rim, resembling that seen in subcutaneous models, which suggested that they may have utility in the treatment of renal cancer; an encouraging result given that current conventional therapies are largely unsuccessful in managing this disease.

2.4 Autochthonous Tumour Models

Spontaneous development of tumours occurs in certain mouse and rat strains. CA4P was active in the T138 spontaneous mouse mammary model (Hill et al. 2002) and its effects were enhanced by administration of the nitric oxide synthase inhibitor, N(omega)-nitro-L-arginine (L-NNA) (Tozer et al. 2009a). Similarly,

CA4P was found to be active in a variety of radiation-induced tumours (Horsman et al. 1998) and TZT-1027 was active in a chemically-induced rat mammary tumour model (Natsume et al. 2007).

Genetically engineered mouse models (GEMMs) for cancer employ transgenic technology to insert or remove genetic material to enhance spontaneous tumour development. For instance, expression of the simian virus 40T antigen oncogene in the retina of transgenic mice produces heritable retinoblastomas (Windle et al. 1990). CA4P was shown to be active in this model (Jockovich et al. 2007). Moreover, the same authors showed that alpha smooth muscle actin positive tumour blood vessels were resistant to treatment with this VDA, confirming previous results in transplanted mouse models of cancer.

2.5 *Isolated Limb Perfusion in Rats*

In early work on VDAs, the P22 rat sarcoma was grown as a 'tissue-isolated' preparation in the right inguinal fat pad of rats, with a blood supply solely from the epigastric vascular pedicle, to investigate the direct effects of CA4 and its prodrug, delivered in a saline-based perfusate (Dark et al. 1997; Tozer et al. 1999). For *ex vivo* perfusion of the VDA, all branching vessels except those feeding the tumour were ligated or cauterised, and effects on vascular resistance measured. Both drugs were found to increase resistance by a factor of at least 3 within 20 min of infusion. However, there was no effect on the vascular resistance of normal hind limb, demonstrating drug selectivity for tumour vasculature. In addition, these studies showed that selectivity for the tumour could be achieved in the absence of systemic effects of the drug and any pro-coagulant activity.

2.6 *Transgenic Knockout Mice*

A knockout mouse is a genetically engineered mouse in which one or more genes have been turned off, allowing researchers to infer its probable function by observing any differences from normal behaviour. They offer a biological and scientific context in which drugs and other therapies can be developed and tested, and have been employed to investigate VDA mode of activity.

The most frequently studied system is ASA404 (formerly DMXAA) in the TNF-receptor 1 knockout mouse. This VDA is known to induce, among other things, tumour necrosis factor (TNF), nitric oxide, serotonin and interferons, causing protracted inhibition of tumour blood flow, followed by extensive haemorrhagic necrosis. These effects are similar to those of TNF, and it was suggested that TNFR1-expressing endothelial cells of the tumour vasculature were the targets for TNF-induced necrosis. The role of TNF in the host response to ASA404 was therefore examined by growing colon 38 carcinomas (TNF positive) in $TNFR1^{-/-}$ and wild type mice (Zhao et al. 2002). They discovered that the antitumour effects following administration of the same dose of ASA404 were substantially reduced in TNFR1$^{-/-}$ mice, but this was accompanied by reduced toxicity. Later work by the same group (Ching et al. 2004) also found, in agreement with the earlier findings, that apoptosis induction and tumour blood flow inhibition following treatment with ASA404 were pronounced in tumours implanted in wild-type mice, but small in tumours implanted in TNF$^{-/-}$ and TNFR1$^{-/-}$ knockout mice. However, the lower toxicity of ASA404 in these knockout mice allowed the use of higher drug doses, which restored both apoptosis induction and tumour blood flow inhibition responses, and also the curative effect of the drug. The results are consistent with the hypothesis that ASA404 can exert an antivascular response both directly and indirectly by induction of TNF, and perhaps of other cytokines, and that multiple mediators of antivascular effects may be involved in providing a selective antitumour effect.

2.7 *Zebrafish*

The zebrafish embryo is becoming an important vertebrate model for assessing drug effects. It has several unique characteristics, including ease of maintenance and drug administration, low cost, and transparency, which permits visual assessment of effects. The subintestinal venous network in the zebrafish is commonly accepted to be formed by angiogenesis (Zheng et al. 2007), making it an excellent model for studying angiogenesis and the effects of antivascular therapy. Parng et al. (2002) treated embryos with SU5416, a potent inhibitor of the VEGF receptors Flt1 (VEGFR-1) and Flk1/KDR (VEGFR-2), which inhibits tumour vascularisation in mammals. Using endogenous alkaline phosphatase staining and a whole animal enzyme assay, they demonstrated that the drug inhibited normal blood vessel growth, reflecting results found in mammals. While this agent is not a true VDA, these results demonstrate that the zebrafish model can be grown in 96-well microtitre plates and thus affords a rapid, high-throughput quantitative assay for vascular-targeted approaches. For tumour vascular studies, tumour cells can be transplanted into zebrafish embryos (Nicoli and Presta 2007) or tumours can be chemically-induced (Spitsbergen et al. 2000). Furthermore, specific gene knockdown in zebrafish is readily achievable by antisense morpholino oligonucleotides (Currie and Ingham 1996). *In vivo* imaging of zebrafish vasculature has been facilitated by the development of transgenics in which endothelial cells express fluorescent proteins under the control of specific vascular promoters e.g. Fli-eGFP (Lawson and Weinstein 2002) and VEGFR2:G-RCFP (Nicoli et al. 2007). VE-cadherin gene inactivation by antisense morpholino oligonucleotide injection into VEGFR2:G-RCFP zebrafish embryos inhibited neovascularisation of transplanted tumours (Nicoli et al. 2007). The Fli-eGFP zebrafish has now been crossed with transgenic zebrafish in which erythrocytes express dsRED (GATA1-dsRED), so that both vascular morphology and function can be imaged on-line, in the same animal (Gray et al. 2007). Further studies are required to fully validate the zebrafish as a model for mammalian tumour angiogenesis and response to vascular-targeted treatments but currently this model has great potential for both mechanistic investigations and development of high throughput assays.

3 Assays for Vascular Function

3.1 General Considerations

Techniques for measuring vascular function are appealing when investigating the effects of VDAs, because they provide quantitative data on the direct target, the tumour blood supply. Blood flow rate is the most obviously relevant vascular parameter for assessing the efficacy of VDAs. It is defined as the rate of delivery of arterial blood to the capillary beds within a particular mass of tissue and so determines the delivery of oxygen and nutrients to tissues, which in turn are key determinants of tumour growth. It is typically measured in units of milliliters of blood per gram of tissue per minute ($ml\,g^{-1}\,min^{-1}$), or, alternatively, per unit volume of tissue ($ml\,ml^{-1}\,min^{-1}$). However, quantitative estimates of blood flow rate are relatively difficult to obtain in small animals (see section 3.2 below) and other parameters such as blood volume ($ml\,g^{-1}$ or $ml\,ml^{-1}$ or simply relative changes from baseline) and red cell velocity ($\mu m\,s^{-1}$ in individual/groups of blood vessels or relative changes) are often-used alternatives (see sections 3.4 to 3.6 below). These estimates are useful and offer a practical approach for assessing response to VDAs but care should be taken in interpreting results, as no direct inferences regarding blood flow rate can be made from them. This is illustrated by considering that tissue blood flow rate (*F in* $ml\,g^{-1}\,min^{-1}$) is related to fractional blood volume of the tissue (*V in* $ml\,g^{-1}$) by the average time taken for blood to pass through a particular capillary bed (capillary mean transit time, τ). This classical relationship is known as the *central volume principle* (Stewart 1894):

$$\tau = V / F$$

A reduction in V following administration of a VDA suggests a reduction in F but this would not be the case or the effect would be diminished if τ decreased as well (e.g. by an increase in the tissue perfusion pressure).

3.2 Blood Flow Rate

In order to estimate blood flow rate, F, the most accurate approach is to measure the rate of delivery of an agent carried to the tissue by the blood. A contrast agent is injected into the blood-stream, and its concentration time-course in arterial blood (input function) together with the kinetics of its uptake into tissue (tissue response function) are measured. *F* is then estimated from a mathematical model relating the tissue response function to the input function (Tozer et al. 2009b). The contrast agent can be radio-active, whereby tissue concentrations can be measured by gamma or scintillation counting or by an external imaging system (e.g. a positron emitter for positron emission tomography, see section 5.4). Alternatively, a contrast agent that is suitable for external magnetic resonance imaging, computed tomography or ultrasound imaging can be used (see section 5.3 below). Radio-active agents have the advantage that they can be administered at true tracer concentrations, therefore not interfering with physiological processes, and they do not necessarily need sophisticated imaging technology.

Small, lipid-soluble, metabolically inert molecules, which rapidly cross the vascular wall and diffuse through the extra-vascular space, are useful as blood flow markers. In this case, the fraction of marker crossing the capillary vascular wall from the blood in a single pass through the tissue (extraction fraction) is close to 1.0 and, for fully perfused tissue, the accessible volume fraction of the tissue is also close to 1.0. The small, lipid soluble, inert molecule, iodo-antipyrine (labeled with ^{14}C or ^{125}I) dissolved in saline has been used as a blood flow tracer for investigating the effect of CA4P on tumour and normal tissue blood flow rate, using a mathematical model based on that devised by Kety (Kety 1960; Tozer et al. 1994). In the case of this type of tracer, net uptake rate into tissue over a short time (seconds) after intra-venous injection is determined primarily by blood flow rate, making the mathematics relatively straightforward (Tozer et al. 2009a). Using this approach, studies on CA4P identified its selective effect on the P22 rat sarcoma compared with a wide range of normal rat tissues (Prise et al. 2002) (Fig. 1a). In addition, combining this technique with an autoradiographic approach identified spatial inhomogeneity of tumour blood flow response, which confirmed that survival of tumour cells in the tumour periphery related to resistance of peripheral blood vessels to shut-down (Fig. 1b). Other fully quantitative methods for estimating blood flow rate in animal models, for instance using labelled microspheres that are trapped in the microcirculation, have not been applied to studies of VDAs. However, fluorescent microspheres have been used in a semi-quantitative mode (Sheng et al. 2004). Quantitative estimation of tumour blood flow rate is invaluable for accurately determining response to VDAs and also useful for validating other methods. However, experiments are relatively complex and longitudinal estimates in the same animal are only possible if sophisticated imaging technology is available, making other less quantitative methods complementary (see below).

3.3 High Frequency Micro-ultrasound

Doppler ultrasound is being evaluated for determining vascular function, as it provides the facility for serial measurements non-invasively. The effect of VDAs on perfusion in superficial tumours has been monitored in experimental mouse

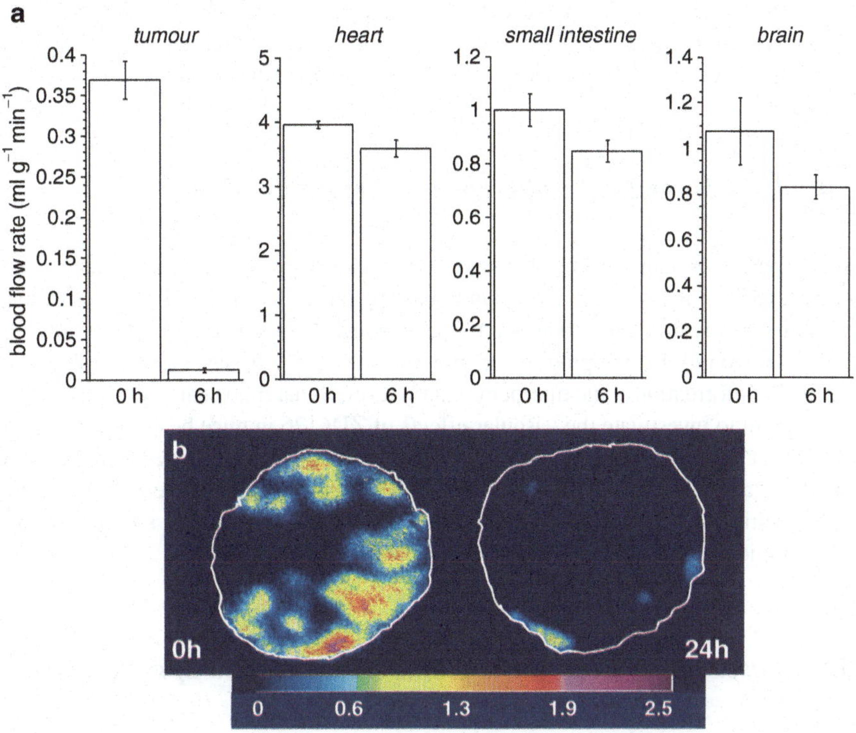

Fig. 1 (**a**) Effect of CA4P (30 mg kg^{-1}) on blood flow rate (*F*) in the P22 tumour and a range of normal rat tissues estimated using the uptake of ^{125}I-iodoantipyrine, either with no treatment (0 h) or 6 h following treatment. (**b**) Blood flow rate (*F*) in ml g^{-1} min^{-1} in the P22 tumour estimated using the uptake of ^{14}C-iodoantipyrine combined with autoradiography to access spatial distribution of radioactivity C_{tiss} either with no treatment (0 h) or 24 h following a single intraperitoneal 100 mg kg^{-1} dose of CA-4-P

tumours using high-frequency (>20 MHz) three-dimensional Doppler ultrasound (HFD) techniques (Goertz et al. 2002). MeWo human melanoma cells were injected orthotopically into the skin of nude mice, tumour growth monitored, and subsequently treated with the VDA ZD6126. Ultrasound studies (serial sections of the same tumour at baseline, 4 and 24 h post treatment) were then performed and compared with controls. These provided information on the relative spatial distribution of blood velocities and moving blood volume, and results were compared with measurements of tumour perfusion histologically (Hoechst 33342, Sect. Multifluorescence Microscopy). Volumetric imaging showed a significant reduction in perfusion at 4 h post ZD2616 and recovery at 24 h, correlating with Hoechst 33342 staining. This demonstrated the feasibility of HFD for following, longitudinally, the effect of VDAs on blood perfusion. High-frequency ultrasound imaging has also been used to follow the vascular effects of OXi4503 in MeWo melanoma xenografts in mice (Shaked et al. 2006). The initial decrease in perfusion seen at 4 h was subsequently followed by a surge in perfusion in peripheral functional vessels by 3 days, although whether this was a result of re-perfusion of existing vessels or development of new vessels is difficult to assess.

3.4 Doppler Optical Coherence Tomography (DOCT)

Blood perfusion can also be assessed non-invasively in anaesthetised mice using DOCT. OCT is analogous to ultrasound imaging, but uses near-IR light waves instead of sound waves to form subsurface tissue images. Its Doppler extension, known as DOCT, is a dual-imaging platform giving microstructural tissue details overlaid with perfusion information at the microcirculation level. Skliarenko et al. (2006) employed this system to investigate the vascular effects of ZD6126 in mice bearing intradermal tumours. Continuous imaging for 30 min following treatment showed a rapid fall in perfusion at 7 min, followed by cessation, and was consistent with the early reduction in interstitial fluid pressure (IFP) also observed. These data showed strong evidence of the rapid vascular damage following ZD1626 treatment.

3.5 Laser Doppler Flowmetry and Near Infrared Spectroscopy

Laser Doppler flowmetry (LDF) provides a means of estimating relative changes in red cell velocity e.g. following treatment, via surface or tissue-inserted probes. This measures a frequency shift in light reflected from moving red cells, which is a measure of average red cell velocity (Stern 1975). LDF and near infrared spectroscopy (NIRS) have been used to detect and evaluate acute effects of different VDAs on perfusion and blood volume in tumors (Kragh et al. 2002). Mouse mammary carcinomas were treated with FAA, CA4P and ASA404, and tumour perfusion before and after treatment was evaluated by non-invasive LDF using a 41°C heated probe, while tumour blood volume was estimated by NIRS using light guide coupled reflectance measurements at 800+10 nm. The VDAs significantly decreased tumour perfusion by 50%, 73% and 47% respectively. In addition, FAA and ASA404 reduced the blood volume within the tumour, indicating that they shunted blood from tumour to adjacent tissue. This was not found for CA4P, suggesting that the mechanism of action in this case was vascular shut-down with the blood pool trapped within the tumour.

3.6 Multifluorescence Microscopy

The fluorescent DNA-binding dye, Hoechst 33342, certain carbo-cyanine dyes and fluorescent lectins are examples of rapidly binding agents that have been used to determine a 'perfused vascular volume' (as a fraction of the total tissue volume) in tumours. In this case, tissues are excised after several circulation times, following intra-venous injection of the dye, and functional vessels appear in tissue sections as fluorescent halos. Conventional Chalkley point counting (Chalkley 1943; Vermeulen et al. 2002) or image analysis provides the fractional tissue volume occupied by fluorescence. This is a useful measure of vascular function in many circumstances bearing in mind that these methods are relatively insensitive because they cannot discriminate between perfused vessels with different flow rates.

The heterogeneous pathophysiology of solid tumours has a major influence on VDA therapy. Multiparameter quantitative microscopy of the tumor microenvironment before and after treatment can be employed to follow the complex therapeutic-tumor interactions, determine which tumor regions are being successfully treated, and to optimize combined cancer therapies. To accomplish this, a range of biomarkers have been used to demonstrate effects of VDA therapy on blood vessel number and perfusion, hypoxia, and tumour damage, concomitantly, over whole tumour sections. An example of this is given in El Emir et al. (El-Emir et al. 2005), where mice bearing subcutaneous colorectal tumours were treated with CA4P and results compared with untreated controls. Following treatment, and prior to killing the mice, markers for hypoxia (pimonidazole) and perfusion (Hoechst 33342) were injected. The relationship between fluorescence parameters was investigated on the same frozen tumor section by switching to the appropriate filter for each of the biomarkers and then co-registering the images for quantification to show the inter-relationship of tumor biomarkers before and after treatment (Fig. 2). Sections were subsequently stained with H&E to compare fluorescence images with their corresponding morphology. This work demonstrated the rapid drop in perfusion and increase in hypoxia after CA4P, followed by reduction in total blood vessel numbers. By 24 h the majority of the tumour was necrotic but the remaining peripheral rim was actively perfused, demonstrating how this region remains viable and able to continue growth.

The distribution and efficacy of antivascular antibodies can be incorporated into the pathophysiology images, by fluorescently labeling the antibody. El-Emir et al. (2007) employed Cy3-NHS labeled L19-SIP, an antibody to the EDB domain of fibronectin, to demonstrate the highly selective perivascular localization of the antibody in colorectal tumours.

An ingenious use of fluorescence microscopy was described in Shaked et al. (2006), who studied the recruitment of circulating endothelial progenitor cells (CEPs) into Lewis Lung carcinomas in mice which had been lethally irradiated, and transplanted with green fluorescent protein-positive (GFP^+) bone marrow cells. These cells exist in low numbers in tumours of untreated animals, but treatment with OXi-4503 led to acute mobilisation of GFP^+ bone marrow cells, which homed to the remaining viable rim and were incorporated into the tumour vasculature. Prior treatment with the antiangiogenic antibody DC101 to VEGFR-2 reduced the number of CEPs incorporated into the tumour, and reduced the size of the surviving rim and blood flow, providing a mechanistic rationale for the enhanced efficiency of VDAs when combined with antiangiogenic drugs.

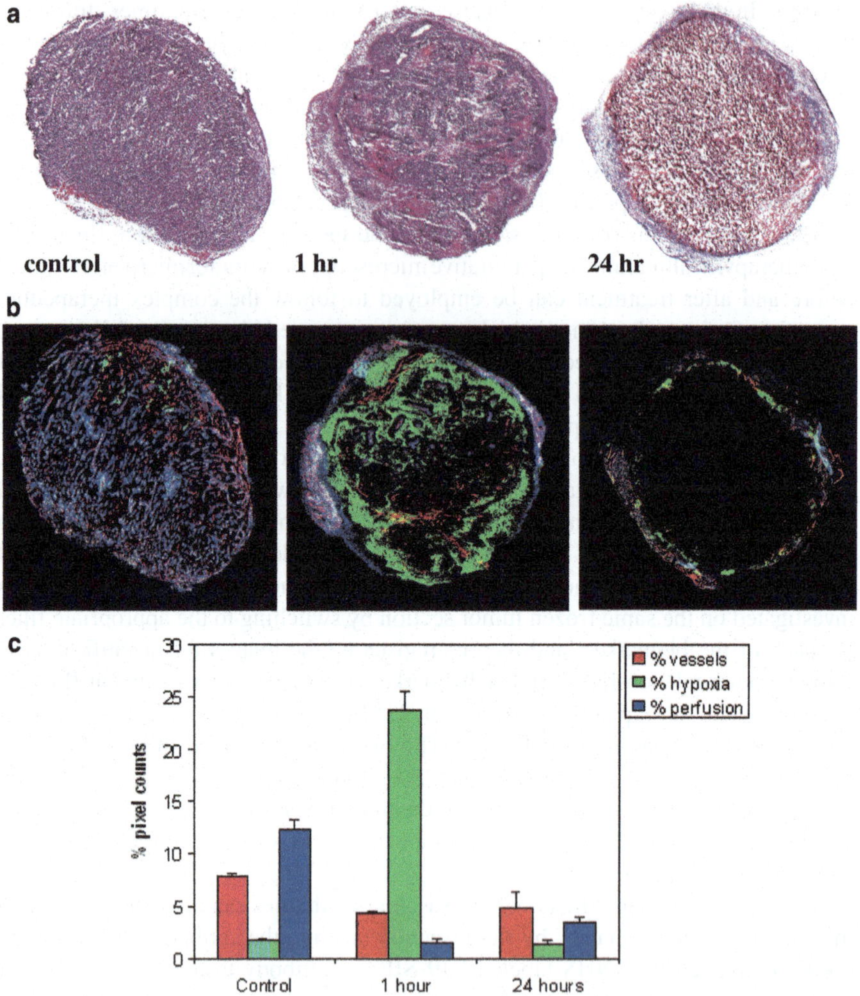

Fig. 2 Effect of CA4P over time in the human colorectal adenocarcinoma xenograft SW1222 grown in nude mice. (**a**) H&E montaged images of control tumour, and CA4P-treated tumours at 1 and 24 h. (**b**) Corresponding co-registered montaged fluorescence images of the same tumour sections: blood vessels (*red*), hypoxia (*green*), perfusion (*blue*). All images at ×200 magnification. (**c**) Histogram showing quantitative analysis of blood vessel distribution, perfusion and hypoxia over time for the same treatments. Means ± SD for 4 mice/group

3.7 *Matrigel Plug Assay*

Recently, the Matrigel plug assay has been used for testing effects of VDAs on angiogenic blood vessels. In this assay, test angiogenesis-inducing compounds or tumor cells are introduced into cold liquid Matrigel, which is a laminin-rich reconstituted matrix. After subcutaneous injection, the Matrigel solidifies, permitting penetration by host cells and the formation of new blood vessels. Assessment of drug effects on vessels in the Matrigel plug can then be performed.

An example of this is the evaluation of the VDA ZD6126 using a Matrigel pellet containing FGF (Micheletti et al. 2003; Giavazzi et al. 2007). The matrigel was injected s.c. in mice and after 7 days a strong angiogenic response could be seen in the pellet, with numerous functional, perfused vessels, particularly abundant at the periphery. Treatment with ZD6126 caused an almost complete shut-down in the vessels by 1 h, demonstrated by confocal microscopy following injection of FITC-isolectin B4. This effect was reversible, and by 22 h after treatment vessels in the Matrigel were re-perfused, primarily in the periphery. This is also a useful model for investigating relative delivery of combined therapies (VDAs or antiangiogenic agents) for optimal efficacy (Giavazzi et al. 2007).

3.8 Intravital Video Microscopy

Intravital video microscopy (IVM) of tumours growing in dorsal skin-fold 'window chambers' provides a means for real-time observation, monitoring, recording and quantitative analysis of specific variables and events in the same tumour, over periods of minutes to weeks (Vajkoczy et al. 2000; Dewhirst et al. 2002; Fukumura and Jain 2008). These chronic observation chambers were first developed for the rabbit ear, in the first part of the twentieth century (Sandison 1924) and subsequently adapted for the mouse (Algire 1943). Removal of overlying tissue from the tumour, as part of the window chamber surgery, greatly reduces signal attenuation and scatter, allowing imaging of individual capillaries. Modern advances in molecular biology, whereby both tumour and stromal cells, including the host vasculature, can be genetically modified to constitutively or conditionally express fluorescent proteins, combined with availability of novel fluorescent probes and advanced techniques for fluorescence microscopy, has led to sustained interest in window chamber preparations (Koehl et al. 2009 for a recent review). Valuable quantitative information can be extracted from IVM images by use of video post-processing and image analysis techniques. This information includes morphological parameters such as vascular diameter, length, density and branching patterns, as well as functional parameters such as red blood cell velocity and oxygenation status (Sorg et al. 2005; Iga et al. 2006; Makale 2008; Reyes-Aldasoro et al. 2008a). IVM has been used to directly establish the extent and time-course of vascular shut-down after treatment with CA4P (Tozer et al. 2001), AVE8062 (Hori et al. 2002) and ASA404 (Seshadri et al. 2007), as well as establishing an apoptotic mode of tumour cell death for arsenic trioxide by imaging the tumour uptake of a fluorescently labeled caspase inhibitor (Griffin et al. 2007). Imaging the kinetics of extravasation of a fluorescently labeled dextran, in a rat window chamber model using multi-photon fluorescence microscopy, established that CA4P further disrupts the already compromised barrier function of tumour blood vessels (Reyes-Aldasoro et al. 2008b). In a mouse window chamber model, expression of different isoforms of VEGF-A in genetically modified tumours was found to influence tumour vascular maturity and thus susceptibility to CA4P, in terms of tumour vascular response (Tozer et al. 2008). Technological advances in IVM make it a very powerful technique for mechanistic studies of VDAs, which remain to be fully exploited.

4 Assays for Vascular Morphology

4.1 Microvascular Corrosion Casting of Tumour Architecture

Quantitative microvascular corrosion casting has been employed to examine the effect of VDAs on the 3D vascular architecture of tumours. Briefly, mice are anaesthetised and infused with the casting agent, and after polymerisation of the resin the surrounding tissue is removed and the microvascular casts viewed by scanning electron microscopy (for details of the procedure see Konerding et al. 1999; El Emir et al. 2007). The model allows quantification of vessel parameters such as size and diameter, intervessel and interbranch distances, and branching angles. This has also helped to validate the use of animal models by demonstrating the vascular similarities between pre-clinical and clinical tumours (Folarin et al. 2010).

Using their orthotopic renal cell carcinoma model, Salmon et al. (2006) have employed corrosion casting to quantify the effects of both CA4P and OXi4503 on tumour vasculature. They demonstrated that the vascular density within the remaining viable rim, which survived after treatment with both VDAs, was significantly greater than that found in the tumours of untreated mice. A detailed investigation into the effect of OXi4503 on the vascular architecture of colorectal liver metastases has also been carried out by Malcontenti-Wilson et al. (2008). Untreated tumour deposits showed a dense microvascular network of tortuous vessels with direct sinusoidal supply. SEMs of microvascular casts following treatment with OXi4503 showed large filling defects, indicating patterns of vascular shut-down, and extravasation of resin from some preserved vessels indicative of vascular leakage. There was a pronounced dose-dependent effect, with destruction of vessels in the centre, and flattening and dilation of vessels at the periphery. Higher doses led to almost complete destruction of vessels both centrally and at the host–tumour interface.

4.2 Transmission Electron Microscopy (TEM)

Because TEM is capable of imaging at a significantly higher resolution than light microscopy, it has been employed to gain insight into the mechanisms of action of VDAs.

An example of this is the VDA ZD6126, where TEM was used to investigate damage to tumour blood vessels at high resolution in the Hras5 tumour model in nude mice (Blakey et al. 2002). The drug was shown to cause rapid effects on the

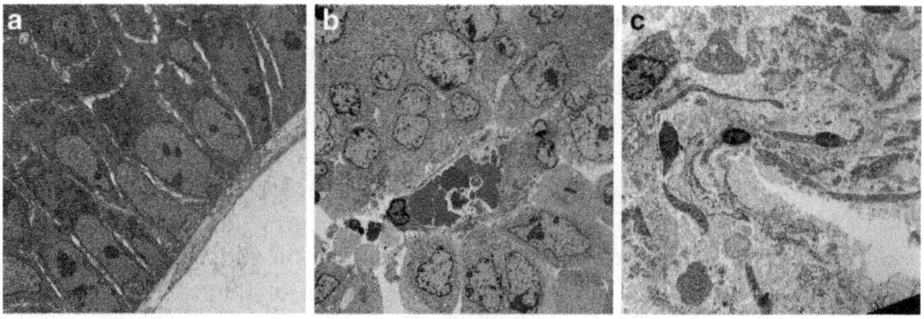

Fig. 3 Transmission electron micrographs showing the effect of OXi4503 (40 mg kg^{-1}) on SW1222 colorectal xenograft tumour vasculature over time. (**a**) Untreated tumour. (**b**) 6 h post treatment. (**c**) 24 h post treatment. Magnification, ×4,400

tumour endothelium, leading to exposure of the basement membrane and accumulation of platelets, with deposition of fibrin. Subsequently there was extensive loss of endothelial cells and thrombosis. This is consistent with the rapid morphological effects reported in vitro. A similar study was performed on the effect of OXi4503 over time in the SW1222 colorectal model (Pedley, unpublished data). The untreated tumours were well organised into acini of columnar/palisade shaped cells, with large intercellular gaps (Fig. 3a). The capillaries were relatively normal, possessing an intact endothelium and overlying pericytes. By 3 h post OXi4503 there was loss of endothelial coverage around the whole vascular wall and accumulation of platelets within the vessels, while inter-tumour cell gaps were widening and basal blebbing was occurring. By 6 h there was overall thinning of the endothelial lining and loss of integrity, with frequent appearance of swollen erythrocytes and platelets, and extensive evidence of dead and dying tumour cells (Fig. 3b). By 24 h some surviving tumour cells and vessels were observed in the tumour periphery, but there was massive central necrosis with no intact vessels, although endothelial cell remnants could be observed throughout the necrotic regions (Fig. 3c).

4.3 *Confocal Laser Scanning Microscopy (CLSM) and Multi-Photon Fluorescence Microscopy (MPFM)*

CLSM can be employed for 3D image analysis of tumour microvessels, and is described by Natsume et al. (2007) for investigating the effects of TZT-1027 in nude mice bearing MX-1 breast tumour xenografts. A FITC-labeled gelatine probe was injected into the mice at selected times after VDA, which were subsequently dipped into iced saline solution to solidify the gelatine. Tumours and normal tissues were resected and examined by CLSM in order to visualise the vasculature in 3D. This showed disruption of tumour microvessels at 1 h and destruction of the tumour microvessel network at 3 h after TZT-1027 administration. They were also able to demonstrate that the VDA effects were tumour-specific.

In MPFM, intense near-infrared (NIR) light is used to induce non-linear absorption in a probe fluorophore such that excitation of the fluorophore is only achieved at the focal plane of the imaging lens. This inherent sectioning capability allows the collection of 3-D data without the use of a confocal aperture. The long wavelength excitation laser light used in MPFM makes it particularly useful for in vivo imaging, where good tissue penetration is an advantage. Use of MPFM for *in vivo* imaging of rodent tumours growing in dorsal skin flap window chambers has been used for longitudinal investigations of tumour vascular morphology, via intravenous administration of fluorescent macromolecular contrast agents (Tozer et al. 2005). Furthermore, leakage kinetics of the markers from blood to tissue was measured via MPFM to estimate tumour vascular permeability and its increase in response to CA4P, in a rat tumour model (Reyes-Aldasoro et al. 2008a, b).

5 Non-invasive Imaging

5.1 General Considerations

Anatomical, physiological and molecular noninvasive *in vivo* imaging techniques are now commonly employed in animal models for the assessment of cancer therapies, including VDAs, and are providing a useful platform for the translation of knowledge from preclinical studies to clinical trials. A major advantage is the ability to follow the outcome of therapy in individual animals rather than averaging the results from groups. Results are frequently confirmed by subsequent immunohistochemistry.

5.2 Bioluminescence/Fluorescence Imaging

Bioluminescence imaging is a useful tool for the long-term, non-invasive visualisation of cell populations in live animals, and uses internal biological sources of light as reporters of tumour growth, sites of metastatic disease and the response to treatment over time. Tumour cells are constitutively transfected to express luciferase (e.g. firefly luciferase) and injected into the mouse at the relevant site. At selected time points a luciferin substrate is injected, which is oxidised by the enzyme to produce light, and visualised by highly sensitive CCD cameras using a light-proof cabinet. Luciferase and its substrate luciferin are non-toxic to mammalian cells and negligible functional differences have been reported between expressing and non-expressing cells. A novel use of BLI is the evaluation of antivascular effects of CA4P in the luciferase-expressing breast cancer xenograft MDA-MB-231 (Zhao et al. 2008), based on the fact that light-emitting dynamics would be related to vascular delivery of the substrate. In untreated mice, following injection of luciferin substrate there was a rapid increase in light emission, peaking at 6 min and decreasing over the following 20 min. After administration of CA4P, the detected light emission was delayed and reduced between 50% and 90%, with some recovery seen by 24 h following further administration of luciferin. This acute pharmacodynamic study followed the pattern of vascular shut-down created by the VDA, and combines the potential for long-term chronic assessment of tumour control following therapy. Results were confirmed by dynamic contrast-enhanced MRI and by histology.

In an alternative system, (Valentini et al. 2008) used the fluorescent contrast agent indocyanine green (ICG) to evaluate *in vivo* the vascular disruption caused by ZD6126. The blood perfusion of the MDA-MB-435 tumor model transplanted in nude mice was estimated from the ICG signal measured via a fibre-based single photon counting system immediately after its systemic injection into mice. Subsequent optical measurements were performed at 3 h after VDA treatment, using a fluorescence imaging setup. After 24 h the mice were killed, tumors excised, and the extent of necrosis was evaluated using standard histological analysis. Fluorescence emission from treated tumours was significantly lower than that from controls, and histology confirmed significantly higher necrosis in treated tumours. These supportive findings indicate that this is a useful system for monitoring the anti-vascular effects induced by VDAs.

5.3 Nuclear Magnetic Resonance Spectroscopy (MRS) and Imaging (MRI)

Some nuclei e.g. 1H, 31P, 19F and 13C, when placed in a magnetic field, can absorb radiofrequency energy of a specific strength depending on the nuclear type. This resonant state provides a means for detection in living tissues. The resonance signal varies in energy depending on the chemical environment, providing the opportunity to measure the relative abundance of specific nuclei, most commonly 31P and 1H, in different chemical states (MRS). In MRI, image contrast is achieved through application of magnetic field gradients across the body. 1H MRI is an established diagnostic technique in the clinic for many conditions but a variety of radiofrequency and gradient pulse sequences, as well as the dependence of the resonance signal on the relaxation times T1, T2 and T2* make MRI a very versatile technique, with continuing technological advances and increasing applicability to tumour vascular studies. MRS and MRI are particularly important because new techniques can be developed and validated in pre-clinical models for direct translation into man (Fig. 4).

1H-MRI and 31P-MRS were first applied to studies of experimental tumours in the early 1970s (Damadian 1971; Zaner and Damadian 1975). In the late 1990s, both techniques were used to investigate and monitor longitudinal changes in ectopically transplanted tumours in mice following treatment with CA4P (Beauregard et al. 1998; Maxwell et al. 1998). 31P-MRS clearly showed a decrease in concentration of high energy phosphate metabolites following treatment, consistent with

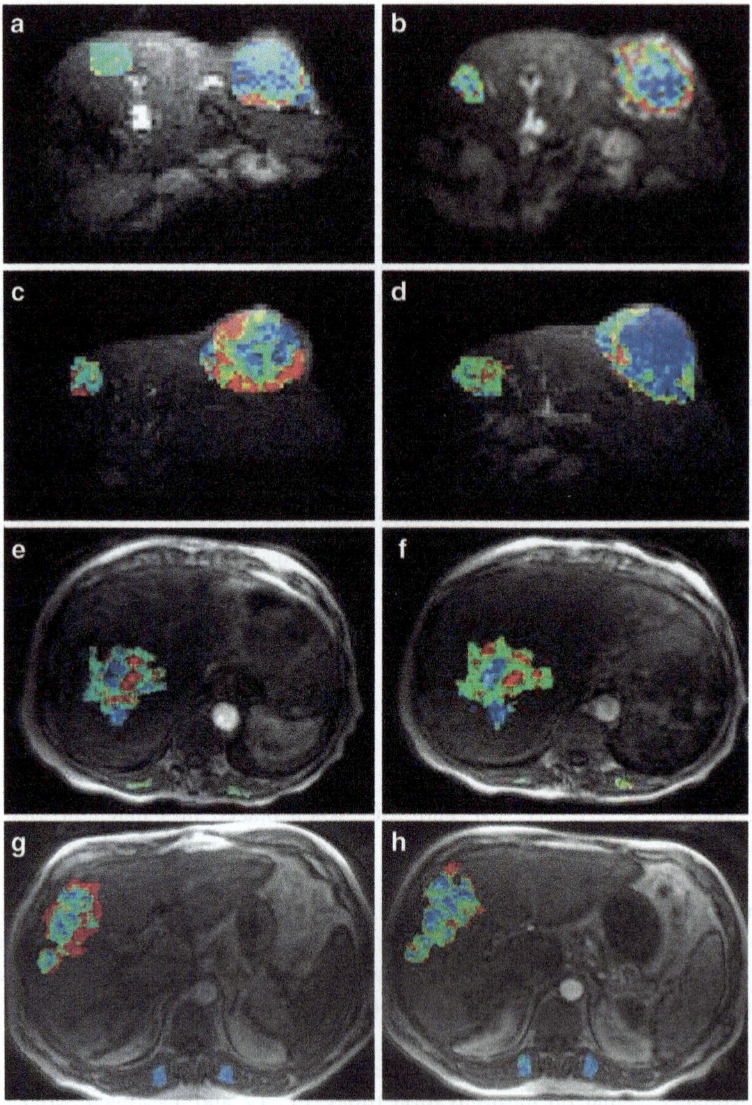

Fig. 4 Representative MR images from single slices through the following: a transplanted C38 colon tumor in a C57/BL6 mouse, pre- and posttreatment with 0 $mg\,kg^{-1}$ ZD6126 (**a** and **b**); as above, pre- and posttreatment with 200 $mg\,kg^{-1}$ ZD6126 (**c** and **d**), a human liver metastasis scanned twice 2 days apart with no intervening treatment (**e** and **f**); and a human liver metastasis pre- and posttreatment with 56 $mg\,m^{-2}$ ZD6126 (**g** and **h**). The IAUC color scale increases from *green* to *yellow* to *red* (Reproduced from Evelhoch et al. 2004. With permission)

vascular disruption. In addition, a chelated gadolinium (Gd-DTPA), which is paramagnetic and enhances the signal from T1-weighted 1H-MRI images, was used as an exogenous contrast agent to monitor tumour vascular changes (dynamic contrast-enhanced MRI or DCE-MRI) (Beauregard et al. 1998). Tumour uptake kinetics of Gd-DTPA following its intravenous administration can be monitored and vascular parameters extracted by applying suitable mathematical models (Tofts et al. 1999). This technique has been used extensively for VDA studies in animal models (Beauregard et al. 2002; Maxwell et al. 2002; Robinson et al. 2003; McPhail et al. 2005, Breidahl 2006 #2815; Salmon and Siemann 2006) and is the most commonly used technique for testing for vascular effects of VDAs in early clinical trials, firstly used for ASA404 and CA4P (Dowlati et al. 2002; Galbraith et al. 2002, 2003; Stevenson et al. 2003), then shortly after for ZD6126 (Evelhoch et al. 2004). However, uptake of Gd-DTPA into tissue is rather complex to model because the vascular wall can form a significant barrier. Therefore, the uptake constant (usually termed k_{trans}) reflects a combination of parameters, including blood flow rate and vascular permeability. In a pre-clinical study of CA4P comparing the uptake kinetics of Gd-DTPA with those of a well-established radio-tracer for blood flow, Gd-DTPA MRI was found to provide an accurate estimate of the time-course of vascular disruption but underestimated the extent of blood flow reduction (Maxwell et al. 2002). High molecular weight gadolinium-based contrast agents, such as albumin-GdDTPA and ultrasmall superparamagnetic iron oxides have also been used to study tumour response and susceptibility to VDAs in pre-clinical studies (Beauregard et al. 2001; Robinson et al. 2007; Vogel-Claussen et al. 2007; Howe et al. 2008; Seshadri et al. 2008). In this case, the vascular wall provides a greater barrier for tumour uptake than it does for Gd-DTPA and K_{trans} is less influenced by blood flow rate, such that estimates of tumour blood volume and even vascular permeability to the particular contrast agent can be obtained.

Other MRI techniques exploit endogenous tissue characteristics for providing image contrast. Diffusion-weighted 1H-MRI relies on the reduction of signal in a field gradient due to water diffusion, which is affected by blood flow, cellular density, of cell membranes etc. This method is potentially important for clinical drug development (Padhani et al. 2009) and may be particularly useful for detecting necrosis after VDA treatment (Thoeny et al. 2005). R2* (= 1/T2*) is sensitive to levels of deoxyhaemoglobin in the blood and significant changes were found in a rat tumour model following treatment with ZD6126 (Robinson et al. 2005), ASA404 and CA4P (McPhail et al. 2007). Whereas R2* tended to increase at early times after treatment, consistent with a reduction in blood flow and increase in deoxyhaemoglobin levels, it subsequently decreased at 24 h after treatment, when perfusion measured by Hoechst 33342 was still severely compromised and necrosis was apparent. This may relate to absence of blood in necrotic regions and illustrates the complexity of interpreting some MRI signals.

MRS and MRSI are set to continue to be important for bio-marker studies, associated with clinical trials of VDAs and other vascular-targeted strategies. The intrinsically poor sensitivity of these methods may be overcome by novel nuclear hyper-polarisation techniques, which are now being evaluated in animal tumour models (Day et al. 2007).

5.4 Positron Emission Tomography (PET)

PET imaging using fluorine-18 fluorodeoxyglucose (^{18}F-FDG) has been widely used to evaluate tumour glucose metabolism before and after conventional therapies. Zhao, Moore, Waller et al. 1999 studied the effects of CA4P over time in a liver metastatic model of a murine mammary carcinoma in B6D2F$_1$ mice, investigating whether it was a useful predictor of therapeutic outcome by radiotracer uptake into remaining viable tumour cells. They found that small-animal PET image analysis was concordant with histological measurements, a single dose of CA4P resulting in an average 30% volume destruction of metastatic mass by 24 hours after administration. A similar study has been performed by Kim, Ravoori, Landen et al. 2007, who employed ^{18}F-FDG uptake to assess the effect of the VDA AVE8062 on the metabolic activity of the HeyA8 ovarian tumour in nude mice. 18F-FDG uptake was assessed pre-treatment, and 2 and 24 hours post treatment, by non-invasive PET imaging. Treated mice demonstrated a rapid decrease in metabolic activity compared with controls, with ^{18}F-FDG uptake decreasing by 83% (2 hours) and 82% (24 hours) compared to pre-treatment images, thus providing an early indicator of therapeutic response. Effects were again confirmed by immunohistochemistry, which showed decreased microvessel density and proliferation, induction of apoptosis in tumour-vessel endothelial cells, and rapid development of central necrosis, followed by a significant reduction in tumour size as measured by MRI (see section 5.3). These studies indicate that ^{18}F-FDG-PET imaging is a useful functional predictor of tumour response to VDAs.

An alternative use of PET imaging with micro-CT has recently been reported for a novel 18F-RGD peptide (^{18}F-AH111585), which can monitor tumour vascularity non-invasively (Morrison et al. 2009). This has been employed to assess the effects of the VEGFR-2 inhibitor ZD4190 (not a true VDA, but worth reporting for its relevance to this field), on microvessel density in mice bearing Calu-6 non-small cell lung cancer xenografts. The therapy resulted in a significant (31.8%) decrease in tracer uptake compared with an increase of 26.9% in controls, indicating that this offers a new approach to noninvasively image the response of antivascular therapies.

15O-labeled water and 15O-labeled carbon monoxide were used in the early clinical trials of CA4P to unequivocally demonstrate compromised blood flow and blood volume respectively, in human tumours (Anderson et al. 2003). Other PET tracers that may prove useful for tumour vascular targeting include 18F-labelled fluoro-L-thymidine (FLT) for cell proliferation, 18F-labelled misonidazole for hypoxia, and various angiogenesis and apoptosis markers that are in development (Pantaleo et al. 2008).

5.5 Scintigraphic Imaging of Tumour Hypoxia

One of the major features of VDA treatment is the induction of hypoxia within the tumour, as blood flow is reduced (Fig. 2). This is potentially a useful alternative, or additional, tumour response marker to blood flow for monitoring VDA efficacy.

Siim et al. (2000) investigated whether a marker for tissue hypoxia, in this case ^{99m}Technetium-labeled 2,2'-(1,4-Diaminobutane)bis(2-methyl-3-butanone) Dioxime (^{99m}Tc-labeled HL-91; Prognox), could be employed for scintigraphic monitoring of tumour response to ASA404. Mice bearing RIF-1 fibrosarcomas in the gastrocnemius muscle (see section 2.2 Subcutaneous and Other Ectopic Models) were administered the VDA and ^{99m}Tc-labeled HL-91 concomitantly, scanned by gamma camera at 3 h, and radioactivity in each tumour determined by comparing tumour-bearing and contralateral leg. This showed a dose-dependent increase in uptake of the hypoxia marker in tumours following treatment with ASA404, correlating with survival, and although this biomarker is no longer available, it does indicate the potential of hypoxic markers for non-invasive imaging of blood flow inhibition.

6 Other Assays

6.1 Hollow Fibre Assay

Suggitt et al. (2004) described the use of the hollow fibre assay as a rapid means of investigating the effects of OXi4503. This assay involves the short-term growth of tumour cells within biocompatible hollow fibres implanted in the s.c and/or i.p. sites in mice, so that the pharmacological capacity of a drug to reach different physiological compartments can be assessed while also demonstrating the therapeutic effects at these sites. One mouse can support up to six cell lines, so reducing the cost of xenograft studies. A549 lung carcinoma cells were grown in the hollow fibres, which were then implanted in the mice, and the mice treated with VDA after 4 days. Tumour cells were retrieved from the fibres at 24 h, for both flow cytometry and immunostaining of drug damage. A greater proportion of cells were held in mitosis after treatment, and exhibited microtubule disruption. The normal nuclear structure was also disrupted, with fragmented nuclei and blebbing, characteristic of apoptosis. It was suggested that this model could provide a cost effective *in vivo* model for the development of 'personalised' cancer treatments.

6.2 Wick-in-Needle Method for the Measurement of Interstitial Fluid Pressure (IFP)

IFP is elevated in tumours due to abnormal vasculature and lymphatic drainage, and has been linked to poor drug delivery and response to treatment. This can be measured by the wick-in-needle technique, which consists of a hypodermic needle connected to a pressure transducer via a tube filled with saline. The needle is then placed in the tumor where the pressure is to be measured, the needle hole being filled with sutures to improve the fluid communication between probe and tumor. The pressure transducer converts the pressure to a voltage which is logged by a computer. The method was employed by Skliarenko et al. (2006) to investigate the effect of ZD6126 on tumour IFP, and the response of tumours with different IFPs to VDA treatment. Tumours were grown intramuscularly in the hind limbs of mice, and measurements were taken before, and at set times after, treatment. They also measured oxygen partial pressure (pO_2), using a fibre optic probe, which was inserted near the centre of the tumour. They showed that tumour IFP was reduced by ZD6126, and found a link between high IFP and reduced response to VDA treatment. They were also able to demonstrate a concomitant drop in pO_2 to 0 mmHg at 30 min, the time of drug-induced complete blood flow shut-down.

References

Algire GH (1943) An adaptation of the transparent-chamber technique to the mouse. J Nat Cancer Inst 4: 1–11.

Anderson HL, Yap JT, Miller MP et al. (2003) Assessment of pharmacodynamic vascular response in a phase I trial of combretastatin A4 phosphate. J Clin Oncol 21: 2823–30.

Beauregard DA, Thelwall PE, Chaplin DJ et al. (1998) Magnetic resonance imaging and spectroscopy of combretastain A_4 prodrug-induced disruption of tumour perfusion and energetic status. Br J Cancer 77: 1761–67.

Beauregard DA, Hill SA, Chaplin DJ et al. (2001) The susceptibility of tumors to the antivascular drug combretastatin A4 phosphate correlates with vascular permeability. Cancer Res 61: 6811–5.

Beauregard DA, Pedley RB, Hill SA et al. (2002) Differential sensitivity of two adenocarcinoma xenografts to the anti-vascular drugs combretastatin A4 phosphate and 5,6-dimethylxanthenone-4-acetic acid, assessed using MRI and MRS. NMR Biomed 15: 99–105.

Blakey DC, Westwood FR, Walker M et al. (2002) Antitumor activity of the novel vascular targeting agent ZD6126 in a panel of tumor models. Clin Cancer Res 8: 1974–83.

Breidahl T, Nielsen FU, Stødkilde-Jørgensen H, Maxwell RJ, Horsman MR (2006) The effects of the vascular disrupting agents combretastatin A-4 disodium phosphate, 5,6-dimethylxanthenone-4-acetic acid and ZD6126 in a murine tumour: a comparative assessment using MRI and MRS. Acta Oncol 45: 306–16.

Chalkley HW (1943) Method for quantitative morphologic analysis of tissues. J Natl Cancer Inst 4: 47–53.

Chaplin DJ, Pettit GR, Parkins CS et al. (1996) Antivascular approaches to solid tumour therapy: evaluation of tubulin binding agents. Br J Cancer 74 (Suppl. XXVII): S86–8.

Ching LM, Zwain S and Baguley BC (2004) Relationship between tumour endothelial cell apoptosis and tumour blood flow shutdown following treatment with the antivascular agent DMXAA in mice. Br J Cancer 90: 906–10.

Currie PD and Ingham PW (1996) Induction of a specific muscle cell type by a hedgehog-like protein in zebrafish. Nature 382: 452–5.

Damadian R (1971) Tumor detection by nuclear magnetic resonance. Science 171: 1151–3.

Dark GD, Hill SA, Prise VE et al. (1997) Combretastatin A-4, an agent that displays potent and selective toxicity toward tumor vasculature. Cancer Res 57: 1829–34.

Day SE, Kettunen MI, Gallagher FA et al. (2007) Detecting tumor response to treatment using hyperpolarized 13C magnetic resonance imaging and spectroscopy. Nat Med 13: 1382–7.

Dewhirst MW, Shan S, Cao Y et al. (2002) Intravital fluorescence facilitates measurement of multiple physiologic functions and gene expression in tumors of live animals. Dis Markers 18: 293–311.

Dowlati A, Robertson K, Cooney M et al. (2002) A phase I pharmacokinetic and translational study of the novel vascular targeting agent combretastatin a-4 phosphate on a single-dose intravenous schedule in patients with advanced cancer. Cancer Res 62: 3408–16.

El Emir E, Qureshi U, Dearling JL et al. (2007) Predicting response to radioimmunotherapy from the tumor microenvironment of colorectal carcinomas. Cancer Res 67: 11896–905.

El-Emir E, Boxer GM, Petrie IA et al. (2005) Tumour parameters affected by combretastatin A-4 phosphate therapy in a human colorectal xenograft model in nude mice. Eur J Cancer 41: 799–806.

El-Emir E, Dearling JL, Huhalov A et al. (2007) Characterisation and radioimmunotherapy of L19-SIP, an anti-angiogenic antibody against the extra domain B of fibronectin, in colorectal tumour models. Br J Cancer 96: 1862–70.

Evelhoch JL, LoRusso PM, He Z et al. (2004) Magnetic resonance imaging measurements of the response of murine and human tumors to the vascular-targeting agent ZD6126. Clin Cancer Res 10: 3650–7.

Folarin AA, Konerding MA, Timonen J et al. (2010) Three-dimensional analysis of tumour vascular corrosion casts using stereoimaging and micro-computed tomography. Microvascular Research 80:89–98.

Fukumura D and Jain RK (2008) Imaging angiogenesis and the microenvironment. APMIS 116: 695–715.

Galbraith SM, Rustin GJ, Lodge MA et al. (2002) Effects of 5,6-dimethylxanthenone-4-acetic acid on human tumor microcirculation assessed by dynamic contrast-enhanced magnetic resonance imaging. J Clin Oncol 20: 3826–40.

Galbraith SM, Maxwell RJ, Lodge MA et al. (2003) Combretastatin A4 phosphate has tumor antivascular activity in rat and man as demonstrated by dynamic magnetic resonance imaging. J Clin Oncol 21: 2831–42.

Giavazzi R, Bani MR and Taraboletti G (2007) Tumor-host interaction in the optimization of paclitaxel-based combination therapies with vascular targeting compounds. Cancer Metastasis Rev 26: 481–8.

Goertz DE, Yu JL, Kerbel RS et al. (2002) High-frequency Doppler ultrasound monitors the effects of antivascular therapy on tumor blood flow. Cancer Res 62: 6371–5.

Gray C, Packham IM, Wurmser F et al. (2007) Ischemia is not required for arteriogenesis in zebrafish embryos. Arterioscler Thromb Vasc Biol 27: 2135–41.

Griffin RJ, Williams BW, Bischof JC et al. (2007) Use of a fluorescently labeled poly-caspase inhibitor for in vivo detection of apoptosis related to vascular-targeting agent arsenic trioxide for cancer therapy. Technol Cancer Res Treat 6: 651–4.

Hill SA, Chaplin DJ, Lewis G et al. (2002) Schedule dependence of combretastatin A4 phosphate in transplanted and spontaneous tumour models. Int J Cancer 102: 70–4.

Hokland SL and Horsman MR (2007) The new vascular disrupting agent combretastatin-A1-disodium-phosphate (OXi4503) enhances tumour response to mild hyperthermia and thermoradiosensitization. Int J Hyperthermia 23: 599–606.

Holwell SE, Cooper PA, Thompson MJ et al. (2002) Anti-tumor and anti-vascular effects of the novel tubulin-binding agent combretastatin A-1 phosphate. Anticancer Res 22: 3933–40.

Hori K, Saito S and Kubota K (2002) A novel combretastatin A-4 derivative, AC7700, strongly stanches tumour blood flow and inhibits growth of tumours developing in various tissues and organs. Br J Cancer 86: 1604–14.

Horsman MR and Siemann DW (2006) Pathophysiologic effects of vascular-targeting agents and the implications for combination with conventional therapies. Cancer Res 66: 11520–39.

Horsman M, Ehrnrooth E, Ladekarl M et al. (1998) The effect of combretastatin A-4 disodium phosphate in a C3H mouse mammary carcinoma and a variety of murine spontaneous tumors. Int J Radiat Oncol Biol Phys 42: 895–98.

Howe FA, McPhail LD, Griffiths JR et al. (2008) Vessel size index magnetic resonance imaging to monitor the effect of antivascular treatment in a rodent tumor model. Int J Radiat Oncol Biol Phys 71: 1470–6.

Iga AM, Sarkar S, Sales KM et al. (2006) Quantitating therapeutic disruption of tumor blood flow with intravital video microscopy. Cancer Res 66: 11517–9.

Jockovich ME, Bajenaru ML, Pina Y et al. (2007) Retinoblastoma tumor vessel maturation impacts efficacy of vessel targeting in the LH(BETA)T(AG) mouse model. Invest Ophthalmol Vis Sci 48: 2476–82.

Kety SS (1960) Theory of blood tissue exchange and its application to measurements of blood flow. Methods Med Res 8: 223–27.

Kim TJ, Ravoori M, Landen CN et al. (2007) Antitumor and antivascular effects of AVE8062 in ovarian carcinoma. Cancer Res 67: 9337–45.

Koehl GE, Gaumann A and Geissler EK (2009) Intravital microscopy of tumor angiogenesis and regression in the dorsal skin fold chamber: mechanistic insights and preclinical testing of therapeutic strategies. Clin Exp Metastasis 26: 329–44.

Konerding MA, Malkusch W, Klapthor B et al. (1999) Evidence for characteristic vascular patterns in solid tumours: quantitative studies using corrosion casts. Br J Cancer 80: 724–32.

Kragh M, Quistorff B, Horsman MR et al. (2002) Acute effects of vascular modifying agents in solid tumors assessed by noninvasive laser Doppler flowmetry and near infrared spectroscopy. Neoplasia 4: 263–7.

Laws AL, Matthew AM, Double JA et al. (1995) Preclinical in vitro and in vivo activity of 5,6-dimethylxanthenone-4-acetic acid. Br J Cancer 71: 1204–9.

Lawson ND and Weinstein BM (2002) Arteries and veins: making a difference with zebrafish. Nat Rev Genet 3: 674–82.

Makale M (2008) Chapter 8. Noninvasive imaging of blood vessels. Methods Enzymol 444: 175–99.

Malcontenti-Wilson C, Chan L, Nikfarjam M et al. (2008) Vascular targeting agent Oxi4503 inhibits tumor growth in a colorectal liver metastases model. J Gastroenterol Hepatol 23: e96-e104.

Maxwell RJ, Nielsen FU, Breidahl T et al. (1998) Effects of combretastatin on murine tumours monitored by 31P MRS, 1H MRS and 1H MRI. Int J Radiat Oncol Biol Phys 42: 891–94.

Maxwell RJ, Wilson J, Prise VE et al. (2002) Evaluation of the anti-vascular effects of combretastatin in rodent tumours by dynamic contrast enhanced MRI. NMR Biomed 15: 89–98.

McPhail LD, Chung YL, Madhu B et al. (2005) Tumor dose response to the vascular disrupting agent, 5,6-dimethylxanthenone-4-acetic acid, using in vivo magnetic resonance spectroscopy. Clin Cancer Res 11: 3705–13.

McPhail LD, Griffiths JR and Robinson SP (2007) Assessment of tumor response to the vascular disrupting agents 5,6-dimethylxanthenone-4-acetic acid or combretastatin-A4-phosphate by intrinsic susceptibility magnetic resonance imaging. Int J Radiat Oncol Biol Phys 69: 1238–45.

Micheletti G, Poli M, Borsotti P et al. (2003) Vascular-targeting activity of ZD6126, a novel tubulin-binding agent. Cancer Res 63: 1534–7.

Morrison MS, Ricketts SA, Barnett J et al. (2009) Use of a novel Arg-Gly-Asp radioligand, 18F-AH111585, to determine changes in tumor vascularity after antitumor therapy. J Nucl Med 50: 116–22.

Natsume T, Watanabe J, Ogawa K et al. (2007) Tumor-specific antivascular effect of TZT-1027 (Soblidotin) elucidated by magnetic resonance imaging and confocal laser scanning microscopy. Cancer Sci 98: 598–604.

Neri D and Bicknell R (2005) Tumour vascular targeting. Nat Rev Cancer 5: 436–46.

Nicoli S and Presta M (2007) The zebrafish/tumor xenograft angiogenesis assay. Nat Protoc 2: 2918–23.

Nicoli S, Ribatti D, Cotelli F et al. (2007) Mammalian tumor xenografts induce neovascularization in zebrafish embryos. Cancer Res 67: 2927–31.

Nihei Y, Suzuki M, Okano A et al. (1999) Evaluation of antivascular and antimitotic effects of tubulin binding agents in solid tumor therapy. Jpn J Cancer Res 90: 1387–96.

Padhani AR, Liu G, Koh DM et al. (2009) Diffusion-weighted magnetic resonance imaging as a cancer biomarker: consensus and recommendations. Neoplasia 11: 102–25.

Pantaleo MA, Nannini M, Maleddu A et al. (2008) Conventional and novel PET tracers for imaging in oncology in the era of molecular therapy. Cancer Treat Rev 34: 103–21.

Parng C, Seng WL, Semino C et al. (2002) Zebrafish: a preclinical model for drug screening. Assay Drug Dev Technol 1: 41–8.

Pedley RB, Boden JA, Boden R et al. (1996) Ablation of colorectal xenografts with combined radioimmunotherapy and tumor blood flow-modifying agents. Cancer Res 56: 3293–300.

Pedley RB, Hill SA, Boxer GM et al. (2001) Eradication of colorectal xenografts by combined radioimmunotherapy and combretastatin a-4 3-O-phosphate. Cancer Res 61: 4716–22.

Pedley RB, El-Emir E, Flynn AA et al. (2002) Synergy between vascular targeting agents and antibody-directed therapy. Int J Radiat Oncol Biol Phys 54: 1524–31.

Pedley RB, El Emir E, Sharma SK et al. (2005) Therapeutic effects of the antivascular agent combretastatin A-1 phosphate on orthotopic and subcutaneous colorectal tumours in nude mice. Proc AACR 46:943.

Pedley RB, Qureshi U, El-Emir E et al. (2008) OXi4503 shows efficacy as a single agent in colorectal liver metastases in nude mice, and potential for enhancing antibody-targeted therapies. NCRI Cancer Conference.

Prise VE, Honess DJ, Stratford MRL et al. (2002) The vascular response of tumor and normal tissues in the rat to the vascular targeting agent, combretastatin A-4-phosphate, at clinically relevant doses. Int J Oncol 21: 717–726.

Rehman F and Rustin G (2008) ASA404: update on drug development. Expert Opin Investig Drugs 17: 1547–51.

Reyes-Aldasoro CC, Akerman S and Tozer GM (2008a) Measuring the velocity of fluorescently labelled red blood cells with a keyhole tracking algorithm. J Microsc 229: 162–73.

Reyes-Aldasoro CC, Wilson I, Prise VE et al. (2008b) Estimation of apparent tumor vascular permeability from multiphoton fluorescence microscopic images of P22 rat sarcomas in vivo. Microcirculation 15: 65–79.

Robinson SP, McIntyre DJ, Checkley D et al. (2003) Tumour dose response to the antivascular agent ZD6126 assessed by magnetic resonance imaging. Br J Cancer 88: 1592–7.

Robinson SP, Kalber TL, Howe FA et al. (2005) Acute tumor response to ZD6126 assessed by intrinsic susceptibility magnetic resonance imaging. Neoplasia 7: 466–74.

Robinson SP, Howe FA, Griffiths JR et al. (2007) Susceptibility contrast magnetic resonance imaging determination of fractional tumor blood volume: a noninvasive imaging biomarker of response to the vascular disrupting agent ZD6126. Int J Radiat Oncol Biol Phys 69: 872–9.

Salmon HW and Siemann DW (2006) Effect of the second-generation vascular disrupting agent OXi4503 on tumor vascularity. Clin Cancer Res 12: 4090–4.

Salmon BA and Siemann DW (2007) Characterizing the tumor response to treatment with combretastatin A4 phosphate. Int J Radiat Oncol Biol Phys 68: 211–7.

Salmon HW, Mladinich C and Siemann DW (2006) Evaluations of vascular disrupting agents CA4P and OXi4503 in renal cell carcinoma (Caki-1) using a silicon based microvascular casting technique. Eur J Cancer 42: 3073–8.

Sandison JC (1924) A new method for the microscopic study of living growing tissues by the introduction of a transparent chamber in the rabbit's ear. Anat Rec 28: 281–87.

Schliemann C and Neri D (2007) Antibody-based targeting of the tumor vasculature. Biochim Biophys Acta 1776: 175–92.

Seshadri M, Spernyak JA, Maiery PG et al. (2007) Visualizing the acute effects of vascular-targeted therapy in vivo using intravital microscopy and magnetic resonance imaging: correlation with endothelial apoptosis, cytokine induction, and treatment outcome. Neoplasia 9: 128–35.

Seshadri M, Bellnier DA and Cheney RT (2008) Assessment of the early effects of 5,6-dimethylxanthenone-4-acetic acid using macromolecular contrast media-enhanced magnetic resonance imaging: ectopic versus orthotopic tumors. Int J Radiat Oncol Biol Phys 72: 1198–207.

Shaked Y, Ciarrocchi A, Franco M et al. (2006) Therapy-induced acute recruitment of circulating endothelial progenitor cells to tumors. Science 313: 1785–7.

Sheng Y, Hua J, Pinney KG et al. (2004) Combretastatin family member OXI4503 induces tumor vascular collapse through the induction of endothelial apoptosis. Int J Cancer 111: 604–10.

Siemann DW, Chaplin DJ and Walicke PA (2009) A review and update of the current status of the vasculature-disabling agent combretastatin-A4 phosphate (CA4P). Expert Opin Investig Drugs 18: 189–97.

Siim BG, Laux WT, Rutland MD, Palmer BN, Wilson WR (2000) Scintigraphic imaging of the hypoxia marker (99m) technetium-labeled 2,2′-(1,4-diaminobutane)bis(2-methyl-3-butanone) dioxime (99mTc-labeled HL-91; prognox): noninvasive detection of tumor response to the antivascular agent 5,6-dimethylxanthenone-4-acetic acid. Cancer Res 60: 4582–8.

Skliarenko JV, Lunt SJ, Gordon ML et al. (2006) Effects of the vascular disrupting agent ZD6126 on interstitial fluid pressure and cell survival in tumors. Cancer Res 66: 2074–80.

Sorg BS, Moeller BJ, Donovan O et al. (2005) Hyperspectral imaging of hemoglobin saturation in tumor microvasculature and tumor hypoxia development. J Biomed Opt 10: 44004.

Spitsbergen JM, Tsai HW, Reddy A et al. (2000) Neoplasia in zebrafish (Danio rerio) treated with 7,12-dimethylbenz[a]anthracene by two exposure routes at different developmental stages. Toxicol Pathol 28: 705–15.

Stern MD (1975) In vivo evaluation of microcirculation by coherent light scattering. Nature 254: 56–58.

Stevenson JP, Rosen M, Sun W et al. (2003) Phase I trial of the antivascular agent combretastatin A4 phosphate on a 5-day schedule to patients with cancer: magnetic resonance imaging evidence for altered tumor blood flow. J Clin Oncol 21: 4428-38.

Stewart GN (1894) Researches on the circulation time in organs and on the infulenced which affect it. J Physiol (London) 15: Parts I–III.

Suggitt M, Swaine DJ, Pettit GR et al. (2004) Characterization of the hollow fiber assay for the determination of microtubule disruption in vivo. Clin Cancer Res 10: 6677–85.

Thoeny HC, De Keyzer F, Chen F et al. (2005) Diffusion-weighted MR imaging in monitoring the effect of a vascular targeting agent on rhabdomyosarcoma in rats. Radiology 234: 756–64.

Tofts PS, Brix G, Buckley DL et al. (1999) Estimating kinetic parameters from dynamic contrast-enhanced T(1)-weighted MRI of a diffusable tracer: standardized quantities and symbols. J Magn Reson Imaging 10: 223–32.

Tozer GM, Shaffi KM, Prise VE et al. (1994) Characterisation of tumour blood flow using a 'tissue-isolated' preparation. Br J Cancer 70: 1040–46.

Tozer GM, Prise VE, Wilson J et al. (1999) Combretastatin A-4 phosphate as a tumor vascular-targeting agent: early effects in tumors and normal tissues. Cancer Res 59: 1626–34.

Tozer GM, Prise VE, Wilson J et al. (2001) Mechanisms associated with tumor vascular shutdown induced by combretastatin A-4 phosphate: intravital microscopy and measurement of vascular permeability. Cancer Res 61: 6413–22.

Tozer GM, Ameer-Beg SM, Baker J et al. (2005) Intravital imaging of tumour vascular networks using multi-photon fluorescence microscopy. Adv Drug Deliv Rev 57: 135–52.

Tozer GM, Akerman S, Cross NA et al. (2008) Blood vessel maturation and response to vascular-disrupting therapy in single vascular endothelial growth factor-A isoform-producing tumors. Cancer Res 68: 2301–11.

Tozer GM, Prise VE and Cunningham VJ (2009) Quantitative estimation of tissue blood flow rate. Methods Mol Biol 467: 271–86.

Tozer GM, Prise VE, Lewis G et al. (2009) Nitric oxide synthase inhibition enhances the tumor vascular-damaging effects of combretastatin a-4 3-o-phosphate at clinically relevant doses. Clin Cancer Res 15: 3781–90.

Twentyman PR, Brown JM, Gray JW et al. (1980) A new mouse tumor model system (RIF-1) for comparison of end-point studies. J Natl Cancer Inst 64: 595–604.

Vajkoczy P, Ullrich A and Menger MD (2000) Intravital fluorescence videomicroscopy to study tumor angiogenesis and microcirculation. Neoplasia 2: 53–61.

Valentini G, D'Andrea C, Ferrari R et al. (2008) In vivo measurement of vascular modulation in experimental tumors using a fluorescent contrast agent. Photochem Photobiol 84: 1249–56.

Vermeulen PB, Gasparini G, Fox SB et al. (2002) Second international consensus on the methodology and criteria of evaluation of angiogenesis quantification in solid human tumours. Eur J Cancer 38: 1564–79.

Vincent L, Kermani P, Young LM et al. (2005) Combretastatin A4 phosphate induces rapid regression of tumor neovessels and growth through interference with vascular endothelial-cadherin signaling. J Clin Invest 115: 2992–3006.

Vogel-Claussen J, Gimi B, Artemov D et al. (2007) Diffusion-weighted and macromolecular contrast enhanced MRI of tumor response to antivascular therapy with ZD6126. Cancer Biol Ther 6: 1469–75.

Wang LC, Ching LM, Paxton JW et al. (2009) Enhancement of the action of the antivascular drug 5,6-dimethylxanthenone-4-acetic acid (DMXAA; ASA404) by non-steroidal anti-inflammatory drugs. Invest New Drugs 27: 280–4.

Windle JJ, Albert DM, O'Brien JM et al. (1990) Retinoblastoma in transgenic mice. Nature 343: 665–9.

Zaner KS and Damadian R (1975) Phosphorus-31 as a nuclear probe for malignant tumors. Science 189: 729–31.

Zhao S, Moore JV, Waller ML et al. (1999) Positron emission tomography of murine liver metastases and the effects of treatment by combretastatin A-4. Eur J Nucl Med 26: 231–8.

Zhao L, Ching LM, Kestell P et al. (2002) The antitumour activity of 5,6-dimethylxanthenone-4-acetic acid (DMXAA) in TNF receptor-1 knockout mice. Br J Cancer 87: 465–70.

Zhao L, Ching LM, Kestell P et al. (2005) Mechanisms of tumor vascular shutdown induced by 5,6-dimethylxanthenone-4-acetic acid (DMXAA): Increased tumor vascular permeability. Int J Cancer 116: 322–6.

Zhao D, Richer E, Antich PP et al. (2008) Antivascular effects of combretastatin A4 phosphate in breast cancer xenograft assessed using dynamic bioluminescence imaging and confirmed by MRI. FASEB J 22: 2445–51.

Zheng L, Ling P, Wang Z et al. (2007) A novel polypeptide from shark cartilage with potent anti-angiogenic activity. Cancer Biol Ther 6: 775–80.

Zwi LJ, Baguley BC, Gavin JB et al. (1989) Blood flow failure as a major determinant in the antitumor action of flavone acetic acid. J Natl Cancer Inst 81: 1005–13.

Combination Therapy with Chemotherapy and VDAs

Giulia Taraboletti, Katiuscia Bonezzi, and Raffaella Giavazzi

Abstract A growing body of preclinical and clinical evidence substantiates the feasibility of combining vascular disrupting agents (VDAs) and conventional anticancer therapies. The enhanced disease response to this combination is attributable to the respective activity of VDAs on the tumor vasculature and of the cytotoxic drug on proliferating tumor cells. However, the nature of the mode of action of VDAs is likely to cause pathophysiological modifications in the tumor microenvironment that can influence the delivery and the activity of the drug with which is combined. A full understanding of the action of VDAs, together with the pharmacological interactions with cytotoxic drugs, will expedite approaches aiming to maximize the antitumor effects of combination therapy. This review focuses on the rationales underpinning the combination of small molecule VDAs with chemotherapy, discussing the pathophysiological changes associated with VDA activity and implication of these for combination modalities.

1 Introduction

Preclinical and clinical experiences have clearly evinced the potential of vascular disrupting agents (VDAs) in combination with other therapeutic approaches. The first indication supporting the need for combination therapy was the limited activity shown by these agents when used alone in preclinical models. Despite the massive tumor necrosis induced by a single administration of VDAs, the actual effect on tumor growth was negligible; only with repeated treatments or in combination regimens (radio- or chemotherapy) was a relevant antineoplastic effect

R. Giavazzi (✉)
Mario Negri Institute for Pharmacological Research,
via Giuseppe La Masa 19, 20156, Milano, Italy
e-mail: raffaella.giavazzi@marionegri.it

T. Meyer (ed.), *Vascular Disruptive Agents for the Treatment of Cancer*,
DOI 10.1007/978-1-4419-6609-4_4,

observed. This result was further upheld by clinical investigations, which, using imaging techniques, confirmed that VDAs affected the tumor vasculature. However, these same studies also showed that in most cases the alterations in vascular parameters were transient, with values reverting to baseline by 24 h after treatment. These findings clearly pointed to the need for an optimized employment of VDAs through either a change in the administration schedule or their use in combination therapies and, indeed, clinical trials with VDAs in combination with conventional chemotherapeutic agents are currently being conducted.

Vascular disrupting agents include two types of compounds: low molecular weight compounds and ligand-directed VDAs (antibodies, peptides or small molecules directed against selected vascular targets) (Chaplin et al. 2006; Hinnen and Eskens 2007; Lippert 2007; Neri and Bicknell 2005; Tozer et al. 2005). This review will focus mainly on small molecule VDAs, which comprise flavone acetic acid derivatives (namely, DMXAA/ASA404) and tubulin binding agents. The latter compounds include combretastatin A-4P (CA4P, Zybrestat, Fosbretabulin), combretastatin A-1P (OXi4503, CA1P), TZT-1027 (Soblidotin), ZD6126, AVE8062 (AC-7700), ABT-751, and NPI-2358. The antitumor activity and mechanism/s of action of these molecules are reviewed elsewhere in this book. Here we will discuss the state of the art for their use in combination with chemotherapy in preclinical studies (Table 1). A number of agents considered cytotoxic in nature have also shown vascular disrupting activity, but these are beyond of the scope of this review.

2 Combining VDAs and Chemotherapy

The rationale for combining VDAs and chemotherapeutic agents is grounded on:

1. The complementary targeting of different regions of the tumor or different cell types
2. Synergistic activity on the same tumor compartment
3. The increased sensitivity to the combined drug as a result of microenvironmental changes induced by VDAs
4. The increased activity of VDAs by agents that reduce resistance to them or their toxicity
5. Modifications of drug distribution induced by VDAs

2.1 Complementary Targeting of Different Regions of the Tumor (Spatial Cooperation)

The ability of VDAs to destroy tumor regions usually poorly responsive to radio- and/or chemotherapy is the main rationale for their addition to other therapies. Vascular disrupting agents typically induce necrosis in the central region of the tumor

Table 1 Summary of preclinical studies on combinations of VDA with chemotherapeutic drugs

VDA	Dose VDA	Chemotherapeutic	Dose chemo	Tumor type	Schedule	Notes	References
DMXAA	*80 μmol/kg*	Melphalan	*34 μmol/kg ip*	Mouse breast	Different sequences compared (–4 h → +8 h)	Best activity: VDA before chemo	Pruijn et al. (1997)
				MDAH-Mca-4		Evaluation by tumor growth delay	
						PK analysis	
	17.5 mg/kg	Cisplatin	*2.5–10 mg/kg ip*	Murine KHT sarcoma	Different sequences compared (–2 h → +8 h)	Best activity: VDA given 1 h after chemo	Siemann et al. (2002)
				Human breast SKBR3		No synergy if VDA given 2 h before chemo	
				Human ovarian OW-1		Evaluation by clonogenic assay	
						No additional bone marrow toxicity	
	80 μmol/kg	5-FU, Cisplatin	*Different doses*	Mouse breast	Different sequences compared (–4 h → +4 h)	No synergy if VDA given 4 h before paclitaxel	Siim et al. (2003)
		Doxorubicin	*Up to the MTD*	MDAH-Mca-4			
		Cyclophosphamide					
		Carboplatin, Etoposide			With paclitaxel	Evaluation by tumor growth delay	
		Vincristine			Coadministration with all agent	Different therapeutic gain with different drugs	
		Paclitaxel, Docetaxel				PK analysis	

(continued)

Table 1 (continued)

VDA	Dose VDA	Chemotherapeutic	Dose chemo	Tumor type	Schedule	Notes	References
	100 mg/kg	CA4P Cisplatin Cyclophosphamide	*2.5–10 mg/kg ip* *2.5–15 mg/kg ip*	Human breast SKBR3 Human ovarian OW-1 Murine KHT sarcoma	Different sequences compared (−1 h → +8 h)	Best activity: VDA 1 h after chemo No synergy with VDA given 1 h before chemo Evaluation by clonogenic assay No additional bone marrow toxicity	Siemann et al. (2002)
	125 mg/kg	Cisplatin Vinblastine	*5–20 mg/kg ip* *1–15 mg/kg ip*	Human Kaposi's (KSY-1)	VDA 1 h after chemo VDA 1,3,5 days after single dose cisplatin	Evaluation by clonogenic assay Tumor growth delay	Li et al. (2002)
	227 µmol/kg	Paclitaxel	*23.7 µmol/kg ip*	Mouse breast MDAH-Mca-4	Different sequences compared (−4 h → +4 h)	No potentiating effect of combination	Siim et al. (2003)
	25 mg/kg	Irinotecan	*45 mg/kg ip*	Rat rabdomiosarcoma	Different sequences compared (−1 h → +1 h)	Activity with all schedules PK analysis	Wildiers et al. (2004)
	200 mg/kg	Carboplatin Paclitaxel	*50 mg/kg ip* *15 mg/kg ip*	Human ovarian TOV21G, TOV112D, ES-2	VDA 0.5 – 1 h before chemo Q7x3 (or Q7x4)		Staflin et al. (2006)
	100 mg/kg	Paclitaxel Carboplatin	*15 mg/kg ip* *50 mg/kg ip*	ARO e KAT-4 Anaplastic tyroid	VDA 24 h before chemo (7-day cycles)		Yeung et al. (2007)

OXi4503/CA1P	*100 mg/kg*	Cisplatin	*6 mg/kg ip*	Colon MAC 29	VDA 20 min after chemo	Negligible toxicity	Shnyder et al. (2003)
	25 mg/kg	Carboplatin Paclitaxel	*50 mg/kg ip* *15 mg/kg ip*	Human ovarian TOV21G, TOV112D, ES-2	VDA 0.5 – 1 h before chemo		Staflin et al. (2006)
	25 mg/kg	Doxorubicin	*5 mg/kg ip*	Ewing's sarcoma TC-32	VDA 1 h after chemo, twice weekly	Not well tolerated after repeated treatments	Dalal and Burchill (2009)
ZD6126	*Up to 150 mg/kg*	Cisplatin	*Up to 15 mg/kg ip*	Murine KHT sarcoma	Different sequences compared (–24 h →+24 h)	No additional bone marrow toxicity	Siemann and Rojiani (2002)
				Human renal Caki-1		Evaluation by clonogenic assay	
	100 mg/kg	Cisplatin	*4 mg/kg ip*	Human lung Calu-6	Cisplatin once then ZD6126 Q1x5		Blakey et al. (2002)
	125 mg/kg	Paclitaxel	*15 mg/kg ip*	Human pharynx FaDu	VDA 15 min after chemo		Davis et al. (2002)
	200 mg/kg	Cisplatin	*6 mg/kg iv*	Human lung PC14PE6	VDA 1 h after chemo (apoptosis studies) Cisplatin once, then VDA daily (metastasis studies)	Apoptosis of tumor and endothelial cells Activity on artificial (i.v.) metastasis	Goto et al. (2004)
	75 mg/kg	Gemcitabine	*100 mg/kg ip*	Human pancreas L3.6pl	VDA daily, chemo twice weekly	Analysis of primary tumor and metastasis	Kleespies et al. (2005)
	200 mg/kg	Paclitaxel	*20 mg/kg iv*	Human MDA-MB-435	Different sequences compared	No synergy if VDA 2–24 h after paclitaxel Best activity: VDA before chemo Best activity increasing interval between treatments	Martinelli et al. (2007)

(continued)

Table 1 (continued)

VDA	Dose VDA	Chemotherapeutic	Dose chemo	Tumor type	Schedule	Notes	References
TZT-1027	*1 mg/kg*	Cisplatin Gemcitabine Irinotecan Paclitaxel Docetaxel 5-FU	*4 mg/kg iv* *250 mg/kg iv* *100 mg/kg iv* *82.9 mg/kg iv* *100 mg/kg iv* *67 mg/kg iv*	Murine leukemia P388 Human NSCLC A549	Different sequences compared (−24 h → +24 h)	Different therapeutic gain with different drugs Evaluation by ILS	Natsume et al. (2006)
	2 mg/kg	Docetaxel	*40 mg/kg iv*	Murine colon26	VDA 10 min after chemo	VDA effect on tumor prefusion prevented by chemo	Watanabe et al. (2007)
AVE8062	*20, 80 mg/kg*	Cisplatin	*2.5–5 mg/kg iv*	Murine colon26 Murine sarcoma S180 Murine lung M109 Human lung LX1 Human colon LS180	Concomitant, Q4x3 Different sequences compared (−24 h → +24 h) on Colon26	Some toxicity Best activity: concomitant PK analysis	Morinaga et al. (2003)
	30 mg/kg	Docetaxel	*1.4–2 mg/kg ip*	Human ovarian HeyA8, HeyA8-MDR and SKOV3ip1	VDA twice weekly Docetaxel once weekly	Activity also on non-responsive HeyA8-MDR	Kim et al. (2007)
MN-029	*100 mg/kg*	Cisplatin	*2–10 mg/kg ip*	Murine KHT sarcoma	VDA 1 h after chemo	Evaluation by clonogenic assay	Shi and Siemann (2005)
ABT-751	*75, 100 mg/kg*	Cisplatin 5-FU	*10 mg/kg ip* *30 mg/kg ip*	Human NSCLC Calu-6 Human colon HT-29 and HCT-116	VDA daily from day 10 DDP single dose on day 10 5FU Q1x5 from day 10		Jorgensen et al. (2007)

(Tozer et al. 2005), which is less perfused and hypoxic, and therefore less responsive to the action of radiotherapy or chemotherapy. Conversely, the highly proliferating tumor cells remaining in the viable regions after VDA treatment become an optimal target for cytoxic agents.

In addition to tumor cells, other VDA-recruited host cells in the viable tumor periphery might also be responsible for tumor regrowth/escape, and therefore be a target for the cytotoxic agent (Fig. 1). Bone marrow-derived circulating endothelial progenitors (CEPs) can be transiently mobilized by VDAs and home in on the perivascular space of tumors where they promote neoangiogenesis ("vasculogenic

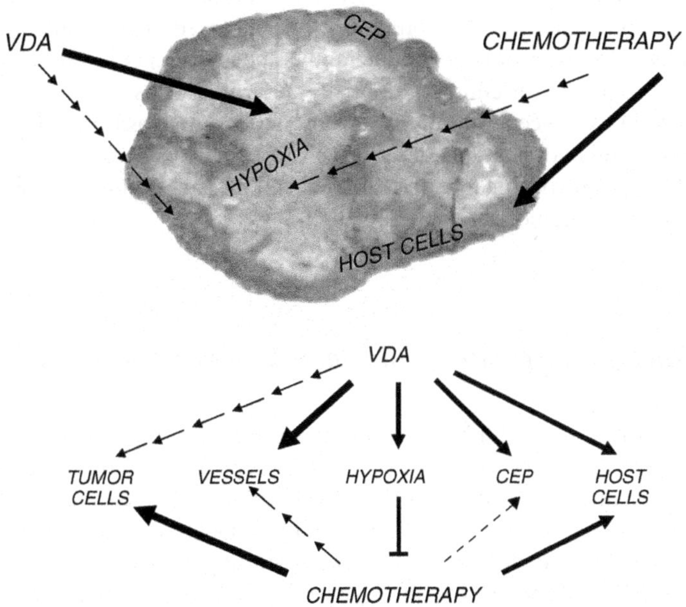

Fig. 1 Proposed targets for the antineoplastic effect of combined therapies with VDAs and chemotherapy. VDAs and chemotherapy target distinct tumor compartments. VDAs mainly target tumor vessels and induce necrosis in the central region of the lesion, leaving a rim of viable cells at the tumor periphery, which is responsible for the rapid repopulation of tumors after VDA administration and the consequent failure to achieve significant response. In contrast, cytotoxic drugs preferentially affect the highly proliferating, well-perfused tumor periphery that remains after VDA treatment. VDAs and cytotoxic agents might also influence the tumor microenviroment and induce the recruitment of host cells. VDAs may also mobilize bone marrow-derived circulating endothelial progenitors (CEPs) in the viable rim of the tumor that contribute to rapid tumor regrowth. Some cytotoxic agents administered at conventional doses/schedules also mobilize CEPs whereas the same drugs given at low, metronomic doses, target CEPs. These changes caused by the VDA in the tumor environment, including hypoxia and recruited host cells, might provide targets and opportunities for combinations therapies

rebounds"), thus favoring tumor re-growth (Shaked et al. 2006; Shaked and Kerbel 2007). CA4P or OXi-4503 induced a rapid mobilization of CEPs. Interestingly, antiangiogenic agents were shown to prevent a CEP spike in response to VDAs, and to markedly suppress tumor growth (Shaked et al. 2006). The increase in CEPs following treatment with VDAs was confirmed in cancer patients treated with AVE8062 (Farace et al. 2007) and ZD6126 (Beerepoot et al. 2006). Some (though not all) chemotherapy administered according to the MTD schedule have been reported to mobilize CEPs, whereas the same agents given frequently at lower doses (metronomic chemotherapy) actually target CEPs (Bertolini et al. 2003; Shaked et al. 2008). These findings highlight the need for carefully designed combination regimens of VDAs with these drugs in order to prevent the possible detrimental synergy in mobilizing CEPs and optimize the antitumor activity of biologicals and chemotherapy. Indeed, based on available results, the metronomic administration of the chemotherapeutic agents seems to represent the optimal schedule for combination therapies with VDAs.

The bulk of evidence at our disposal substantiates the feasibility of a combination of VDAs with radiotherapy (described elsewhere in this book) or chemotherapy that would simultaneously target the different compartments of the tumor, resulting in an enhanced antitumor activity.

2.2 Synergistic Activity on the Same Tumor Compartment

Combination therapies with VDAs could be designed with the aim to achieve an enhanced activity on the same tumor compartment. Potentiated targeting of the vascular compartment is accomplished by combining VDAs with inhibitors of angiogenesis (described elsewhere in this book). Notably, some classes of cytotoxic agents – including tubulin-targeting agents such as taxanes – are able to target endothelial cells (Belotti et al. 1996; Giavazzi et al. 2008; Taraboletti et al. 2002), and, thus making them the best candidates for combination with VDAs, provided the correct administration schedule is used. Indeed, to maximize their vascular targeting effect, ad hoc schedules of administration of chemotherapeutics (metronomic chemotherapy) have been proposed (Klement et al. 2000). The increase in endothelial cell apoptosis induced by the combination of ZD6126 with cisplatin (Goto et al. 2004) or AVE8062 with paclitaxel (Kim et al. 2007) confirms that the vascular compartment is conceivably the target of combinations of VDAs with chemotherapy.

It should likewise be remembered that most VDAs also have a direct cytotoxic activity on tumor cells (Kim et al. 2007; Micheletti et al. 2003; Nicholson et al. 2006). The implications of this observation in the development of combination therapies, particularly with certain classes of chemotherapeutics, remain to be explored.

2.3 Combination with Agents That Exploit the Microenvironmental Changes Induced by VDAs

It has been hypothesized that the profound effects of VDAs on the tumor might generate an environment favorable to the activity of specific agents. A typical example of this action is found in bioreductive drugs, inactive prodrugs that are converted into cytotoxic agents under conditions of low oxygen tension (Horsman and Siemann 2006). Such compounds would inevitably benefit from the hypoxic/anoxic conditions induced by VDAs. Another example is the potentiating effect of DMXAA on melphalan, in part ascribed to hypoxia and lowered pH, which increase the cytotoxic activity of melphalan in vitro (Pruijn et al. 1997).

The ability of VDAs, such as DMXAA, to activate tumor-associated inflammatory cells and cause the release of cytokines and chemokines creates a tumor environment that is likely to influence the response to other therapies (Jassar et al. 2005).

It should be borne in mind, however, that VDAs might also affect the tumor environment by making it less responsive to chemotherapy. CA4P has been reported to increase expression of the glucose-regulated stress protein GRP78 in the tumor, an endoplasmic reticulum chaperone induced by glucose depletion, acidosis and hypoxia. Since GRP78 protects cells against endoplasmic reticulum stress and topoisomerase inhibitors, it might represent a mechanism of possible drug resistance induced by VDAs (Dong et al. 2005).

2.4 Combination with Agents That Potentiate the Activity of VDAs, Reduce Resistance to Them or Limit Their Toxicity

Non-steroidal anti-inflammatory drugs (NSAIDs) potentiate the antitumor activity of DMXAA. An antagonizing activity of NSAIDs on the protective effects of prostaglandins released in response to vascular injury caused by VDAs has been indicated as the mechanisms of this effect (Wang et al. 2009).

Pharmacological inhibition of nitric oxide (NO) potentiates VDA activity. Resistance to VDAs has been associated with overexpression of iNOS (Cullis et al. 2006). Nitric oxide synthase inhibitors of different structural classes has been shown to augment the activity of CA4P in terms of reduction in perfused vascular volume and increased necrosis (Davis et al. 2002). Nitric oxide synthase inhibitor N-nitro-L-arginine methyl ester (L-NAME) is known to potentiate the vascular effect of CA4P (Tozer et al. 1999), and likewise, the NO inhibitor L-NNA to enhance the effect of ZD6126 (Wachsberger et al. 2005). This improvement of VDA activity is likely to impact the overall activity of a combination with conventional chemotherapy.

Still another mechanism is the reduction of VDA toxicity – for example with antihypertensives (see below) (Gould et al. 2007) – that would favor the tolerability of cytotoxic chemotherapy.

2.5 Modification in Blood Flow: Effects on Cytotoxic Drug Pharmacokinetics

The possibility that vascular alterations caused by VDAs would improve rather than hinder the distribution of the combined chemotherapeutic agent has long been debated.

Clinical trials with dynamic contrast enhanced magnetic resonance imaging (DCE-MRI) have confirmed preclinical results indicating that VDAs reduce blood flow in tumors. In KHT tumors, perfusion at the tumor periphery was shown to decrease 4 h after treatment with CA4P, but to return to baseline 20 h later (Salmon and Siemann 2007). Siim et al. reported that vessel shut down induced by DMXAA was not reversed 24 h after injection, whereas CA4P-induced flow shutdown was (Siim et al. 2003). Similarly to CA4P, we found that the occlusion of blood vessels by ZD6126 was reversible, and 22 h after treatment, vessels were again perfused (Micheletti et al. 2003).

In keeping with the mechanism of action of VDAs, vessel density has been shown to decrease in the center of the tumor, not in the periphery, where it actually tends to increase (Salmon and Siemann 2007).

How do these effects of VDAs on tumor blood flow affect chemotherapy? On the one hand, the decrease in perfusion may lead to reduced tissue oxygenation (which could raise concerns over a diminished activity of the cytotoxic agent). On the other, the vascular shutdown induced by VDAs could affect the distribution of other drugs to the tumor, either by reducing their delivery or, conversely, with VDAs given afterwards, by enhancing the concentration of the administered agents via a "trapping" effect.

Several authors have investigated how VDAs influence the pharmacokinetics (PK) and distribution of other therapeutics. Studies with different tumor models have consistently shown that VDAs have no effect on the *plasma* PK of chemotherapeutics: the co-administration of DMXAA was reported to have no influence on the PK of carboplatin or paclitaxel in plasma (Siim et al. 2003), or on the plasma PK of melphalan (Pruijn et al. 1997). Similarly, CA4P left the plasma PK of irinotecan (Wildiers et al. 2004) and 5-FU (Grosios et al. 2000) unaltered, as did AVE8062 with the distribution of cisplatin in plasma and kidney (Morinaga et al. 2003). For our part, we found that ZD6126 had no impact on the PK of paclitaxel in plasma of mice (unpublished observation).

By contrast, PK in *tumors* is often described to be affected by VDAs, although there is no general agreement on whether the agents increase or reduce the distribution of cytotoxic drugs to the tumors. It is reasonable to hypothesize that the administration of a VDA *before* or simultaneously with chemotherapy would, because of vessel shutdown, impair the distribution of the latter to the tumor. This has been described for combinations of DMXAA with paclitaxel (Siim et al. 2003) and Ca4P with irinotecan (Wildiers et al. 2004), but not for DMXAA with melphalan (Pruijn et al. 1997) or AVE8062 with 5-FU (Morinaga et al. 2003).

On the other hand, the administration of a VDA *after* a cytotoxic drug is expected to increase the concentration of the latter in the tumor thanks to a "trapping effect." The finding that Ca4P given together or shortly after irinotecan increased tumor levels of the metabolite SN-38 seems to support this hypothesis (Wildiers et al. 2004). In a combination with therapeutic antibodies, CA4P administered 48 h after iodine-labeled antibodies against carcinoembryonic antigen caused the increased retention of the antibody in experimental colorectal tumors (Pedley et al. 2001), even at doses too low to cause vessel shutdown (Lankester et al. 2007). This trapping effect resulted in greater antitumor activity of the combination compared to VDA administration or radioimmunotherapy alone (Pedley et al. 2001). Whether this favorable effect is due to the nature of a large molecule – the antibody – compared to small molecules – the chemotherapeutic – remains to be investigated. Indeed, Ca4P given 20 min after 5-FU caused a decrease of 5-FU distribution in tumors (Grosios et al. 2000). Therefore, although the hypothesis of a "trapping effect" is indeed intriguing and no doubt reserves promising clinical applications of VDAs, it still needs to be upheld by experimental evidence.

It is important to underline that most studies have reported no correlation between the final antitumor activity of the combination and VDA-induced changes in the PK of the cytotoxic drugs used. Instead, in many cases an enhanced antitumor activity of the combination compared to single agents was observed, despite a decreased tumor accumulation of chemotherapeutics.

In our study on the combination of ZD6126 and paclitaxel, we found that, regardless of the increased antitumor activity, the VDA administered 24–96 h before paclitaxel caused a decreased distribution of the drug in tumors, evident 1–24 h after its administration (Martinelli et al. 2007 and data not published). A detailed analysis, however, showed that pretreatment with the VDA resulted in an increased ratio between paclitaxel levels at the tumor periphery and in the central region, suggesting that, while the VDA does not increase the total amount of chemotherapy within the tumor, it might favor the distribution of the cytotoxic drug in the vital regions of tumors where it is more likely to be active.

It is worth noting that the nature of the PK/antitumor activity relationship of a given chemotherapeutic agent might account for the final outcome of its combination with VDAs.

3 Sequencing and Timing

Because VDAs affect vessel structure and functionality and potentially influence the tumor distribution and activity of cytotototoxic drugs, the critical issue is how to avoid a negative effect on the therapy with which it is combined. Several preclinical studies have addressed this point, and, with few exceptions (Wildiers et al. 2004), these studies have shown that the efficacy of the combination depends on the sequence of administration of the two agents.

As a general rule, studies comparing different sequences of administration have pointed to a greater efficacy when the *VDA was given after the chemotherapeutic agent* (Table 1). DMXAA or CA4P given 1 h after cisplatin had a greater than additive effect on mouse KHT sarcoma, assessed by clonogenic assay, whereas no additive activity was observed when the VDA was given 1–2 h before cisplatin (Siemann et al. 2002). In combinations with DMXAA and paclitaxel on a mouse breast model, a more than additive antineoplastic activtity was observed when the VDA was given shortly before or up to 8 h after paclitaxel, while no additive activity was observed if the VDA was given 4 h before paclitaxel (Siim et al. 2003). In a study comparing TZT-1027 given together, 24 before or 24 h after cisplatin, gemcitabine or irinotecan, the general best sequential treatment was reported to be with the VDA given after the chemotherapeutics (Natsume et al. 2006).

Other studies, although not specifically comparing different sequences of administration, reported a relevant antitumor activity of the combination with VDAs given after cytotoxic agents. Combinations of DMXAA or CA4P given 1 h after cisplatin or cyclophosphamide were more active than single agents on breast and ovarian cancer models (Siemann et al. 2002). CA4P increased the activity of 5-FU on the Mac 29 colon carcinoma when given 20 min after the cytotoxic drug (Grosios et al. 2000), and OXi4503 given 1 h after doxorubicin was more active than single agents on Ewing's sarcoma (Dalal and Burchill 2009). Finally, the activity of cisplatin and vinblastin on Kaposi's sarcoma was potentiated by CA4P administrated 1 h after the chemotherapy (Li et al. 2002).

Preclinical studies have indicated that, in particular cases, administration of a *VDA before a cytotoxic agent* could increase the activity of the combination or might even be necessary to avoid possible negative interactions between the two agents. In time course experiments, the most enhanced activity was observed with DMXAA given before melphalan in a mouse mammary carcinoma (Pruijn et al. 1997). In this case the effect was ascribed to the lower pH induced by pretreatment with the VDA, which increased the cytotoxic activity of melphalan.

A unique case is the combination of tubulin targeting VDAs with taxanes, since this latter class of compounds cause an opposite effect on the same molecular target, i.e., the microtubules. Indeed, we described a potential negative interaction between the two types of compounds: in vitro, endothelial cells exposed to paclitaxel or docetaxel – but not to other, non tubulin-targeting cytotoxic agents cisplatin and doxorubicin – become unresponsive to the vascular disrupting activity of N-acetylcolchinol, the active drug of ZD6126; in vivo, pretreatment of mice with paclitaxel prevented vessel shutdown and tumor necrosis induced by ZD6126 (Taraboletti et al. 2005), suggesting that the administration of the VDA after the taxane would not be beneficial, since pretreatment with the taxane would protect the tumor vasculature against the activity of ZD6126. Another study corroborated these findings, reporting that docetaxel given 10 min before TZT-1027 prevented the activity of the VDA, assessed by measuring the reduction of tumor perfusion in Colon26 tumors and the permeability of endothelial cells in vitro (Watanabe et al. 2007). When testing the antitumor activity of a combination of ZD6126 and paclitaxel administered with different schedules, we found that the VDA given 2 or 24 h after the cytotoxic drug showed no significant benefit, whereas when it was administered 24 and 72 h before chemotherapy the therapeutic activity of paclitaxel was improved (Martinelli et al. 2007). This activity was paralleled by a VDA-induced increase in cell proliferation in the viable tumor tissue, suggesting that the administration of the VDA before paclitaxel not only eludes the protective effect of the latter, but also increases the number of tumor cells potentially responsive to the taxane (Martinelli et al. 2007). As mentioned above (Complementary Targeting of Different Regions of the Tumor (Spatial Cooperation)), in addition to tumor cells, other VDA-recruited host cells present in viable tumor regions, including CEPs (Shaked et al. 2006), might also provide targets for the cytotoxic agent.

Our study also indicated the potential benefit of increasing the interval between the administration of the two compounds (Martinelli et al. 2007). This finding found further support from other studies, which showed the superior activity of ZD6126 given either before or after – but not concomitantly with – cisplatin (Siemann and Rojiani 2002) and the lack of potentiating activity of CA4P given a few hours before or after paclitaxel (Siim et al. 2003).

Other studies have reported activity achieved through the *co-administration of VDAs and cytotoxic drugs* (Siim et al. 2003). For example, co-administration of AVE8062 with 5-FU was reported to be more active than sequential administrations (6 and 24 h before or after) (Morinaga et al. 2003). Differences in the agents used or the experimental models studied might account for the discrepancies in these results. Nonetheless, the correct scheduling of drug administration in combination regimes remains a crucial issue for the clinical development of VDAs, since the therapeutic potential of these agents will most likely take place in combination with conventional treatments.

4 Toxicity

Increases of toxicity or appearances of additional side effects not observed with conventional chemotherapy need to be considered in combination therapy. Preclinical studies have in general shown improved antitumor effects without increases in toxicity caused by either VDAs or cytotoxic drugs. In fact, no additional toxicity has been described with DMXAA or CA4P in combination with cisplatin and ciclophosphamide (Siemann et al. 2002), or with ZD6126 in combination with cisplatin (Siemann and Rojiani 2002) or paclitaxel (Martinelli et al. 2007). In contrast, high dose combinations of AVE8062 with cisplatin (Morinaga et al. 2003) and OXi4503/CA1P with doxorubicin were not well tolerated (Dalal and Burchill 2009).

Clinical experiences thus far reported have nonetheless highlighted that toxicity is an important issue limiting the clinical development of VDAs. Early phase clinical trials have depicted a characteristic toxicity profile, different from that of the cytotoxic agents, and consistent with a vascular activity (Beerepoot et al. 2006; van Heeckeren et al. 2006). Adverse cardiovascular effects include transient hypertension, myocardial infarction, cardiac ischemia, and increased blood levels of markers of cardiac damage (e.g., troponins). Acute hemodynamic changes induced by tubulin-targeting VDAs are responsible, at least in part, for adverse cardiac events (Gould et al. 2007).

This toxicity is indicative of an effect of VDAs on the normal vasculature, pointing to a limited selectivity of these agents for the tumor vasculature and to the need to develop more selective agents. Experimental models have shown that anti-hypertensive therapy prevents the cardiac side effects of tubulin-targeting VDAs without compromising their antitumor efficacy (Gould et al. 2007). Nonetheless, toxicity remains a relevant issue for the clinical application of these compounds and an important question to consider in the design of combination therapies. Toxicity may result from additive toxicity of the two agents or from the alteration of the cytotoxic drug's PK induced by the VDA. For example, a phase I trial of CA4P with carboplatin evinced a dose-limiting thrombocytopenia caused by VDA-induced changes in carboplatin PK (Bilenker et al. 2005).

5 Conclusions

The majority of preclinical studies have documented an increased benefit that stems from the combination of VDAs with conventional chemotherapy (Table 1). For most of the combinations, the enhanced response is most likely attributable to the fact that VDAs and cytotototoxic agents target distinct tumor compartments. By destroying the more central part of the tumor, VDAs affect the area of the tumor that is less vascularized and, consequently, where the delivery of chemotherapeutic drugs is limited. These cytotoxic drugs are more likely to kill tumor cells in the viable rim that remains after VDA treatment, because this region is better vascularized, less hypoxic, and presents a high proliferation index. However, this putative explanation should take into consideration the complex interaction among tumor cells, angiogenic vessels, and host cells, which are ultimately affected by the altered milieu caused by VDAs (Fig. 1). Because of their vascular effects, VDAs are likely to influence positively or negatively the delivery and the activity of the drug with which it is combined; timing and sequencing, as well as the nature of the cytotoxic drug, thus take on major implications in the outcome of such combinations.

The translation of VDA-based combination therapies to the clinic raises the need for the identification of circulating, tissue and imaging biomarkers to be used as pharmacodynamic indicators of activity. As discussed elsewhere in this book, changes in dynamic MRI vascular measures represent one of the major pharmacodynamic biomarkers to be assessed after VDA delivery; likewise, circulating endothelial cells (CECs) are promising markers of VDA-induced tumor vascular damage to be used in the clinic. Preclinical studies aimed at evaluating these aspects will inevitably prove helpful in the design of clinical trials combining VDAs and conventional chemotherapy.

Acknowledgements Part of the work presented here was supported by grants from the Italian Ministry of Health, Contract N.RO Strategici 11/07, the Italian Association for Cancer Research (AIRC), and the European Union, IP-FP6-LSHC-CT-2003-STROMA, 503233 and IP-FP7-HEALTH-2007-ADAMANT, 201342.

We thank Tom Wiley for editing assistance and Valentina Scarlato for technical assistance.

References

Beerepoot LV, Radema SA, Witteveen EO et al (2006) Phase I clinical evaluation of weekly administration of the novel vascular-targeting agent, ZD6126, in patients with solid tumors. J Clin Oncol 24: 1491–1498
Belotti D, Vergani V, Drudis T et al (1996) The microtubule-affecting drug paclitaxel has antiangiogenic activity. Clin Cancer Res 2: 1843–1849
Bertolini F, Paul S, Mancuso P et al (2003) Maximum tolerable dose and low-dose metronomic chemotherapy have opposite effects on the mobilization and viability of circulating endothelial progenitor cells. Cancer Res 63: 4342–4346
Bilenker JH, Flaherty KT, Rosen M et al (2005) Phase I trial of combretastatin a-4 phosphate with carboplatin. Clin Cancer Res 11: 1527–1533
Blakey DC, Westwood FR, Walker M et al (2002) Antitumor activity of the novel vascular targeting agent ZD6126 in a panel of tumor models. Clin Cancer Res 8: 1974–1983
Chaplin DJ, Horsman MR and Siemann DW (2006) Current development status of small-molecule vascular disrupting agents. Curr Opin Investig Drugs 7: 522–528
Cullis ER, Kalber TL, Ashton SE et al (2006) Tumour overexpression of inducible nitric oxide synthase (iNOS) increases angiogenesis and may modulate the anti-tumour effects of the vascular disrupting agent ZD6126. Microvasc Res 71: 76–84
Dalal S and Burchill SA (2009) Preclinical evaluation of vascular-disrupting agents in Ewing's sarcoma family of tumours. Eur J Cancer 45: 713–722
Davis PD, Tozer GM, Naylor MA et al (2002) Enhancement of vascular targeting by inhibitors of nitric oxide synthase. Int J Radiat Oncol Biol Phys 54: 1532–1536
Dong D, Ko B, Baumeister P et al (2005) Vascular targeting and antiangiogenesis agents induce drug resistance effector GRP78 within the tumor microenvironment. Cancer Res 65: 5785–5791
Farace F, Massard C, Borghi E et al (2007) Vascular disrupting therapy-induced mobilization of circulating endothelial progenitor cells. Ann Oncol 18: 1421–1422
Giavazzi R, Bonezzi K and Taraboletti G (2008) Microtubule targeting agents and angiogenesis. In: Fojo T (ed) Microtubules as Targets for Cancer Therapies. Humana Press,Totowa, pp 519–530
Goto H, Yano S, Matsumori Y et al (2004) Sensitization of tumor-associated endothelial cell apoptosis by the novel vascular-targeting agent ZD6126 in combination with cisplatin. Clin Cancer Res 10: 7671–7676
Gould S, Westwood FR, Curwen JO et al (2007) Effect of pretreatment with atenolol and nifedipine on ZD6126-induced cardiac toxicity in rats. J Natl Cancer Inst 99: 1724–1728
Grosios K, Loadman PM, Swaine DJ et al (2000) Combination chemotherapy with combretastatin A-4 phosphate and 5-fluorouracil in an experimental murine colon adenocarcinoma. Anticancer Res 20: 229–233
Hinnen P and Eskens FA (2007) Vascular disrupting agents in clinical development. Br J Cancer 96: 1159–1165
Horsman MR and Siemann DW (2006) Pathophysiologic effects of vascular-targeting agents and the implications for combination with conventional therapies. Cancer Res 66: 11520–11539
Jassar AS, Suzuki E, Kapoor V et al (2005) Activation of tumor-associated macrophages by the vascular disrupting agent 5,6-dimethylxanthenone-4-acetic acid induces an effective CD8+ T-cell-mediated antitumor immune response in murine models of lung cancer and mesothelioma. Cancer Res 65: 11752–11761
Jorgensen TJ, Tian H, Joseph IB et al (2007) Chemosensitization and radiosensitization of human lung and colon cancers by antimitotic agent, ABT-751, in athymic murine xenograft models of subcutaneous tumor growth. Cancer Chemother Pharmacol 59: 725–732
Kim TJ, Ravoori M, Landen CN et al (2007) Antitumor and antivascular effects of AVE8062 in ovarian carcinoma. Cancer Res 67: 9337–9345
Kleespies A, Kohl G, Friedrich M et al (2005) Vascular targeting in pancreatic cancer: the novel tubulin-binding agent ZD6126 reveals antitumor activity in primary and metastatic tumor models. Neoplasia 7: 957–966

Klement G, Baruchel S, Rak J et al (2000) Continuous low-dose therapy with vinblastine and VEGF receptor-2 antibody induces sustained tumor regression without overt toxicity. J Clin Invest 105: R15–R24

Lankester KJ, Maxwell RJ, Pedley RB et al (2007) Combretastatin A-4-phosphate effectively increases tumor retention of the therapeutic antibody, 131I-A5B7, even at doses that are sub-optimal for vascular shut-down. Int J Oncol 30: 453–460

Li L, Rojiani AM and Siemann DW (2002) Preclinical evaluations of therapies combining the vascular targeting agent combretastatin A-4 disodium phosphate and conventional anticancer therapies in the treatment of Kaposi's sarcoma. Acta Oncol 41: 91–97

Lippert JW, 3rd (2007) Vascular disrupting agents. Bioorg Med Chem 15: 605–615

Martinelli M, Bonezzi K, Riccardi E et al (2007) Sequence dependent antitumour efficacy of the vascular disrupting agent ZD6126 in combination with paclitaxel. Br J Cancer 97: 888–894

Micheletti G, Poli M, Borsotti P et al (2003) Vascular-targeting activity of ZD6126, a novel tubulin-binding agent. Cancer Res 63: 1534–1537

Morinaga Y, Suga Y, Ehara S et al (2003) Combination effect of AC-7700, a novel combretastatin A-4 derivative, and cisplatin against murine and human tumors in vivo. Cancer Sci 94: 200–204

Natsume T, Watanabe J, Horiuchi T et al (2006) Combination effect of TZT-1027 (Soblidotin) with other anticancer drugs. Anticancer Res 26: 1145–1151

Neri D and Bicknell R (2005) Tumour vascular targeting. Nat Rev Cancer 5: 436–446

Nicholson B, Lloyd GK, Miller BR et al (2006) NPI-2358 is a tubulin-depolymerizing agent: in-vitro evidence for activity as a tumor vascular-disrupting agent. Anticancer Drugs 17: 25–31

Pedley RB, Hill SA, Boxer GM et al (2001) Eradication of colorectal xenografts by combined radioimmunotherapy and combretastatin a-4 3-O-phosphate. Cancer Res 61: 4716–4722

Pruijn FB, van Daalen M, Holford NH et al (1997) Mechanisms of enhancement of the antitumour activity of melphalan by the tumour-blood-flow inhibitor 5,6-dimethylxanthenone-4-acetic acid. Cancer Chemother Pharmacol 39: 541–546

Salmon BA and Siemann DW (2007) Characterizing the tumor response to treatment with combretastatin A4 phosphate. Int J Radiat Oncol Biol Phys 68: 211–217

Shaked Y and Kerbel RS (2007) Antiangiogenic strategies on defense: on the possibility of blocking rebounds by the tumor vasculature after chemotherapy. Cancer Res 67: 7055–7058

Shaked Y, Ciarrocchi A, Franco M et al (2006) Therapy-induced acute recruitment of circulating endothelial progenitor cells to tumors. Science 313: 1785–1787

Shaked Y, Henke E, Roodhart JM et al (2008) Rapid chemotherapy-induced acute endothelial progenitor cell mobilization: implications for antiangiogenic drugs as chemosensitizing agents. Cancer Cell 14: 263–273

Shi W and Siemann DW (2005) Preclinical studies of the novel vascular disrupting agent MN-029. Anticancer Res 25: 3899–3904

Shnyder SD, Cooper PA, Pettit GR et al (2003) Combretastatin A-1 phosphate potentiates the antitumour activity of cisplatin in a murine adenocarcinoma model. Anticancer Res 23: 1619–1623

Siemann DW and Rojiani AM (2002) Antitumor efficacy of conventional anticancer drugs is enhanced by the vascular targeting agent ZD6126. Int J Radiat Oncol Biol Phys 54: 1512–1517

Siemann DW, Mercer E, Lepler S et al (2002) Vascular targeting agents enhance chemotherapeutic agent activities in solid tumor therapy. Int J Cancer 99: 1–6

Siim BG, Lee AE, Shalal-Zwain S et al (2003) Marked potentiation of the antitumour activity of chemotherapeutic drugs by the antivascular agent 5,6-dimethylxanthenone-4-acetic acid (DMXAA). Cancer Chemother Pharmacol 51: 43–52

Staflin K, Jarnum S, Hua J et al (2006) Combretastatin A-1 phosphate potentiates the antitumor activity of carboplatin and paclitaxel in a severe combined immunodeficiency disease (SCID) mouse model of human ovarian carcinoma. Int J Gynecol Cancer 16: 1557–1564

Taraboletti G, Micheletti G, Rieppi M et al (2002) Antiangiogenic and antitumor activity of IDN 5390, a new taxane derivative. Clin Cancer Res 8: 1182–1188

Taraboletti G, Micheletti G, Dossi R et al (2005) Potential antagonism of tubulin-binding anticancer agents in combination therapies. Clin Cancer Res 11: 2720–2726

Tozer GM, Prise VE, Wilson J et al (1999) Combretastatin A-4 phosphate as a tumor vascular-targeting agent: early effects in tumors and normal tissues. Cancer Res 59: 1626–1634

Tozer GM, Kanthou C and Baguley BC (2005) Disrupting tumour blood vessels. Nat Rev Cancer 5: 423–435

van Heeckeren WJ, Bhakta S, Ortiz J et al (2006) Promise of new vascular-disrupting agents balanced with cardiac toxicity: is it time for oncologists to get to know their cardiologists? J Clin Oncol 24: 1485–1488

Wachsberger PR, Burd R, Marero N et al (2005) Effect of the tumor vascular-damaging agent, ZD6126, on the radioresponse of U87 glioblastoma. Clin Cancer Res 11: 835–842

Wang LC, Ching LM, Paxton JW et al (2009) Enhancement of the action of the antivascular drug 5,6-dimethylxanthenone-4-acetic acid (DMXAA; ASA404) by non-steroidal anti-inflammatory drugs. Invest New Drugs 27: 280–284

Watanabe J, Natsume T and Kobayashi M (2007) The inhibitory effect of docetaxel and p38 MAPK inhibitor on TZT-1027 (Soblidotin)-induced antivascular activity. Anticancer Res 27: 3909–3918

Wildiers H, Ahmed B, Guetens G et al (2004) Combretastatin A-4 phosphate enhances CPT-11 activity independently of the administration sequence. Eur J Cancer 40: 284–290

Yeung SC, She M, Yang H et al (2007) Combination chemotherapy including combretastatin A4 phosphate and paclitaxel is effective against anaplastic thyroid cancer in a nude mouse xenograft model. J Clin Endocrinol Metab 92: 2902–2909

Lessons from Animal Imaging in Preclinical Models

Lesley D. McPhail and Simon P. Robinson

Abstract Biomarkers are now an essential component of the process of drug development. Numerous biomarkers are being generated by a diverse range of disciplines but this chapter focuses specifically on the development of in vivo imaging biomarkers of tumour response to VDA therapy in preclinical models. In vivo imaging techniques are particularly attractive to monitor VDA therapies as they (1) are non-invasive, (2) enable longitudinal studies to be performed, (3) can provide functional measurements of tumour perfusion and (4) can be used in the clinic. So far, magnetic resonance has dominated the in vivo imaging area of VDA research, and dynamic contrast-enhanced magnetic resonance imaging (DCE-MRI) has been the most popular method of choice to evaluate VDAs both preclinically and in the clinic. Nevertheless, alternative MR and non-MR imaging modalities are continually being sought, and existing methodology developed to provide the best possible means to assess efficacy of VDAs in vivo with a view to translating these advances to the clinic, and also gaining further insight into their mechanism of action. This chapter describes the methodology of the different imaging modalities that have been used to assess VDAs in experimental rodent models and discusses the key findings of these studies.

1 Magnetic Resonance Imaging of Tumour Vasculature

Magnetic resonance imaging (MRI) is a technique whereby a powerful magnet is used to generate high resolution images of tissues. It works on the principle that certain nuclei of compounds from which tissue is composed possess an odd number of protons and neutrons. It is the magnetic-dipole moment caused by unequal pairing of these protons and neutrons that makes magnetic resonance possible (Howe et al. 1993). When such nuclei are placed in an external magnetic

---

L.D. McPhail (✉)
Cancer Research Technology, The Beatson Institute for Cancer Research,
Garscube Estate, Switchback Road, Bearsden, Glasgow, G61 1BD, UK
e-mail: lmcphail@cancertechnology.com

T. Meyer (ed.), *Vascular Disruptive Agents for the Treatment of Cancer*,
DOI 10.1007/978-1-4419-6609-4_5,

field, the nuclear dipoles line up parallel and anti-parallel to the direction of the magnetic field, resulting in net magnetisation. A radiofrequency pulse can then be used to alter the alignment of magnetisation causing the nuclei to precess. This precessing magnetisation induces an oscillating current in a receiver coil which can be detected (this is the NMR signal, which can be processed as an image or spectrum). The signal typically observed in MR is from the hydrogen atoms (protons) on water and lipids. This is because hydrogen is the most abundant nucleus in the body and it also has the strongest magnetic dipole moment of any nucleus.

MRI predominantly assesses the behaviour of water in tissue. Tumour tissue is physiologically distinct from normal anatomical structures as it has an irregular and leaky vascular network and areas of hypoxia and necrosis (Vaupel et al. 1989; Carmeliet and Jain 2000; Carmeliet 2003). Therefore, the movement of water molecules in tumour tissue differs to that of normal tissue. Consequently, MRI can be used to obtain a wealth of information regarding tumour vascularisation, metabolism and pathophysiology (Gillies et al. 2000; Evelhoch et al. 2000; Padhani 2003).

Tumour blood vessels are poorly formed, have large endothelial cell gaps, incomplete basement membranes and a lack of pericyte coverage (Carmeliet and Jain 2000; Carmeliet 2003). These abnormalities present a hyperpermeable blood vessel phenotype which can be exploited by MR contrast agents. Contrast agents/medium are paramagnetic substances that can be used to evaluate vascularisation. They leak through the blood vessels and shorten the MR relaxation times of the water in the tissues to which they have access. Thus, perfused tumour tissue should enhance more quickly than normal tissue in an MR image due to the more permeable nature of the vasculature. This has underpinned the large clinical success of contrast enhanced MRI in tumour detection and diagnosis. The uptake of contrast agent into the tumour tissue reflects tumour perfusion and vessel permeability and can be characterised by either semi-quantitative or quantitative analysis (Padhani and Husband 2001; Choyke et al. 2003).

Contrast agents are normally paramagnetic gadolinium chelates and are classified as either low-molecular weight or high-molecular weight agents (also known as macromolecular contrast medium (MMCM), or blood pool agents). Low-molecular weight contrast agents (<1,000 Da) diffuse more rapidly from the intravascular space into the extravascular–extracellular space (EES) (Padhani 2003). MMCM (>30,000 Da) has prolonged intravascular retention due to its larger size (Brasch and Turetschek 2000; Padhani 2003; Barrett et al. 2006). Currently, low-molecular weight agents are routinely used in the clinic and MMCMs have yet to be approved for routine use in humans. However, clinical trials for MMCMs are underway.

2 Why Use MRI for VDA Assessment?

VDA therapy works by altering tumour perfusion and permeability. Thus, MRI is an ideal technique to assess the efficacy of VDAs, as it allows functional measurements of changes in these physiological parameters. Moreover, changes in perfusion and permeability are found to occur at early time-points, before the onset of necrosis or any changes in tumour volume. This means that MRI can be used for early detection of VDA effectiveness. It has been well documented that when used as a monotherapy, VDAs characteristically induce central necrosis but leave a proliferating rim of cells at the tumour periphery (Siemann et al. 2004; Tozer et al. 2005). Consequently, tumour size can remain unaltered. Therefore, it is pertinent that along side the development of VDAs, techniques are also developed that can measure changes in vascular response, other than tumour anatomical size, in response to therapy.

The importance of imaging biomarkers in oncology drug development has now been recognised by the FDA (FDA Critical Path Initiative. http://www.fda.gov/cder/regulatory/medimaging). MRI can be used to generate alternative, functional biomarkers of tumour response, which is especially important with regards to the more novel therapies being developed, such as VDAs. The non-invasive and non-destructive nature of MRI allows for longitudinal studies and multiple biomarker measurements to be made, and perhaps the most attractive aspect of MRI is that it is a clinically transferable technique. The following sections describe specific MRI methods that have been used in the preclinical evaluation of VDAs.

3 Dynamic Contrast-Enhanced MRI

To date, dynamic contrast enhanced MRI (DCE-MRI) has been the most popular imaging method used to monitor VDAs in both rodent and human tumours. DCE-MRI involves the acquisition of magnetic resonance images before, during and after the intravenous administration of a contrast agent. The contrast agent most commonly used is low-molecular weight gadolinium-diethylenetriamine penta-acetic acid (Gd-DTPA). Pharmacokinetic modelling of the serial DCE-MRI data can be used to calculate parameters based on physiological models that assess contrast agent uptake into the tumour tissue (Leach et al. 2005). If the arterial input function is known, DCE-MRI data can be quantitatively analysed to yield the transfer constant K^{trans} (s^{-1}) (Gillies et al. 2002) and the integrated area under the gadolinium-time curve (IAUGC) (mM Gd min). These are the two primary DCE-MRI biomarkers recommended for the evaluation of antiangiogenic and antivascular therapies in the clinic (Leach et al. 2005).

K^{trans} is a modelling parameter that describes the transendothelial transport of low molecular weight contrast agent into the extravascular extracellular space (EES) (Tofts et al. 1999). K^{trans} is related mathematically to the modelling parameters K_{ep} and V_e ($K_{ep} = K^{trans}/V_e$). K_{ep} is a rate constant between EES and blood plasma, and V_e is the volume of EES per unit volume of tissue (Tofts et al. 1999). The physiological interpretation of K^{trans} is dependent on both the permeability of the capillaries and the blood flow of the tissue being imaged. When the capillaries are highly permeable, uptake of contrast agent into the tissue is flow limited and K^{trans} is equal to the blood flow per unit volume of tissue. In low permeability situations, uptake of contrast agent into the tissue is permeability limited and K^{trans} is equal to the permeability surface area of the capillaries between blood plasma and the EES per unit volume of tissue.

Uptake of contrast agent into tissue can be limited by both blood flow and permeability at the same time, which is most likely to be the situation found in heterogeneous tumour tissue. Therefore, it is too difficult to determine if K^{trans} is equal to either tumour blood flow or vessel permeability in the tumour microenvironment, as it is probably a combination of both. Nevertheless, an effective VDA would be expected to reduce some of these physiological parameters, reducing K^{trans}.

IAUGC is calculated from the area under the gadolinium concentration curve up to a specified cut-off time (usually 60 s). IAUGC is a simpler, more robust method than K^{trans} as it does not assume any physiological model, or require any curve-fitting and is therefore not prone to fit-failures. However, the precise relationship between IAUGC and tumour physiology is unclear.

When the arterial input function is not known, semi-quantitative analysis can be used to describe tissue enhancement. Methods of semi-quantitative analysis include the gradient of the signal–intensity–time curve, the maximum increase in signal intensity normalised to baseline signal intensity (enhancement) and the enhancing fraction (Galbraith et al. 2002a; O'Connor et al. 2007).

3.1 Preclinical Assessment of ZD6126 Using DCE-MRI

DCE-MRI was used to establish tumour dose–response to ZD6126 in a rat GH3 prolactinoma model (Robinson et al. 2003a). Both 25 and 50 mg/kg ZD6126 were found to significantly reduce IAUGC and the mean fraction of highly enhancing pixels in the tumour tissue, which was indicative of a reduction in perfusion (Fig. 1). The study also incorporated multigradient recalled echo MRI measurements of R_2* (an MR parameter sensitive to tissue deoxyhaemoglobin) and necrosis was assessed by histology. Importantly, both the MRI biomarkers were associated with the induction of massive central tumour necrosis assessed histologically, which increased in a dose-dependent manner. A strong inverse correlation was found between IAUGC and necrosis 24 h post ZD6126 treatment. These results are consistent with a dose-dependent reduction in tumour perfusion and vascular collapse.

The duration of ZD6126-induced vascular shutdown has also been investigated using the same rat GH3 prolactinoma model (McIntyre et al. 2004). IAUGC and highly enhancing fraction measurements were made prior to and 24, 48, 60, 72 and 96 h post-treatment with a single dose ZD6126, and tumour necrosis was assessed by histology. Somewhat surprisingly, the results showed that even at 96 h post-treatment there was no recovery in tumour perfusion in this tumour model. Evelhoch et al. conducted a parallel preclinical and clinical DCE-MRI study of ZD6126 (Evelhoch et al. 2004). Both mice bearing C38 colon carcinoma xenografts and human tumours showed a reduction in IAUGC 24 h and 6 h respectively after ZD6126 treatment, again confirming a reduction in tumour perfusion and efficacy of the drug, with some evidence of dose response in the Phase 1 trial.

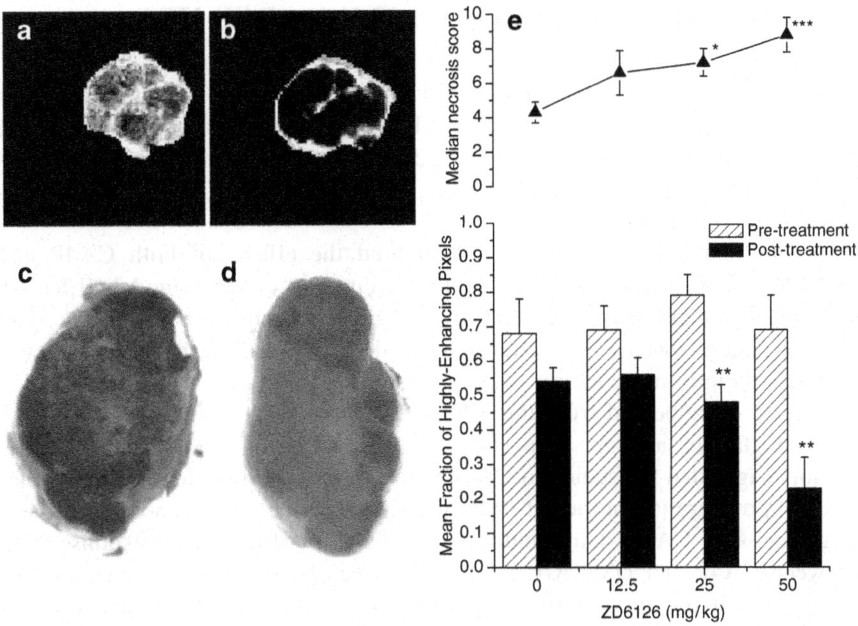

Fig. 1 T_1-weighted DCE-MRI images acquired from a subcutaneous rat GH3 prolactinoma (**a**) prior to and (**b**) 24 h post-treatment with 50 mg/kg ZD6126. Following treatment, the highly-enhancing fraction was clearly limited to the tumour periphery. Haematoxylin and eosin stained histological sections from (**c**) a control and (**d**) ZD6126-treated GH3 prolactinoma are also shown. Treatment with ZD6126 caused massive central tumour necrosis, with the central necrotic core being surrounded by a viable rim of tumour cells. The dose response of GH3 prolactinomas to ZD6126 evaluated by DCE MRI and qualified by necrosis scoring is summarised in (**e**). Treatment with ZD6126 induced a dose-dependent decrease in the mean fraction of highly enhancing pixels in the GH3 prolactinomas (lower graph), and this was associated with a dose-dependent increase in tumour necrosis (upper graph) (Robinson et al. 2003b)

The studies discussed so far use DCE-MRI to measure biomarkers of tumour blood flow and permeability that are altered by VDA treatment. However, these are the acute anti-vascular effects induced by VDAs, and an initial reduction in blood flow and vascular collapse results in tumour necrosis. A preclinical ZD6126 study by Bradley et al. investigated the relationship between tumour necrosis and DCE-MRI measurements with a view to identify any DCE-MRI biomarkers of drug-induced necrosis (Bradley et al. 2007). The Hras5 transformed NIH3T3 mouse fibroblast cell line grown in nude rats was selected as the tumour model due to its reproducibly low level of background necrosis. An extensive range of MRI measurements were made prior to and 24 h after a number of clinically relevant doses of ZD6126, and correlates were sought with necrosis assessed by histology. The results demonstrated that both the enhancing fraction and non-enhancing non-fitted voxels showed a good correlation with ZD6126-induced necrosis, suggesting their use as imaging biomarkers of necrosis.

3.2 *Preclinical Assessment of CA4P Using DCE-MRI*

CA4P was first assessed using DCE-MRI by Beauregard et al. in a mouse tumour model (Beauregard et al. 1998). DCE-MRI revealed that perfusion was reduced 3 h post-treatment with 100 mg/kg CA4P, and a reduction in tumour energetics determined by ^{31}P-MRS of the same tumours aided confirmation that CA4P compromised tumour blood flow.

A subsequent DCE-MRI study compared the effects of both CA4P and DMXAA on perfusion against two colon carcinoma xenograft models (LS174T and HT29) (Beauregard et al. 2002). A significant reduction in IAUGC, and thus perfusion, was seen 3 h after a single dose of CA4P in the LS174T xenografts (although the reduction was less than for DMXAA), but not the HT29 xenografts. It appeared from the MR images shown that the LS174T tumours had a higher basal level of perfusion compared to the HT29 tumours. The authors suggested resistance to CA4P could be due to lower levels of endothelial cell proliferation in the HT29 tumours, as endothelial cells are the primary target cells of CA4P. This could also explain the differential response seen between CA4P and DMXAA, as the two drugs have distinct mechanisms of action, and it remains unproven that endothelial cells are the primary target cells of DMXAA.

Maxwell et al. used radiolabelled iodoantipyrine uptake and DCE-MRI to assess CA4P-induced reductions in tumour blood flow in a rat P22 carcinosarcoma model (Maxwell et al. 2002). A low dose of 10 mg/kg CA4P significantly reduced iodoantipyrine uptake, and hence tumour blood flow, 6 h post-treatment, but by 24 h this had recovered to baseline. A higher dose of 100 mg/kg CA4P induced a significant reduction in tumour blood flow and which showed no recovery by 24 h. DCE-MRI demonstrated a smaller magnitude of changes in K^{trans} compared to iodoantipyrine uptake. Nevertheless, the time-course and dose-dependent patterns were similar between the two measurements. A further DCE-MRI study compared K^{trans} and IAUGC measurements after CA4P treatment in the same rat P22 carcinosarcoma model, and in the tumours of 18 patients in the Phase I clinical trial (Galbraith et al. 2003). There was a 64% reduction of K^{trans} 6 h post-treatment in the rat tumour model. The patient tumours showed an overall K^{trans} reduction of 34% and 29%, at 4 and 24 h post-treatment respectively.

CA4P is a first generation VDA, and second generation analogues are currently under investigation. OXi4503 (CA1P) is one such analogue that has been assessed by DCE-MRI (Salmon and Siemann 2006). In this study, both CA4P and OXi4503 showed a similar reduction in K^{trans} of 80–90% 4 h post-treatment in a mouse KHT sarcoma model. However, recovery of perfusion by 48 h was significantly slower for OXi4503 than CA4P. These findings were corroborated by tumour uptake of the histological perfusion marker Hoechst 33342, as tumours treated with OXi4503 had significantly less perfused vessels than tumours treated with CA4P. Interestingly, no significant differences in necrosis were found between the OXi4503 and CA4P treated tumours.

3.3 *Preclinical Assessment of DMXAA Using DCE-MRI*

The first preclinical DCE-MRI study of DMXAA assessed perfusion of murine HT29 and LS174T xenografts 3 h after a single 27.5 mg/kg dose (Beauregard et al. 2002). The study concluded that DMXAA caused a significant reduction in IAUGC and therefore perfusion in both tumour types. These results were reinforced by ^{31}P-MRS, which demonstrated a reduction in tumour energetics and was used as an indirect measurement of perfusion.

A more extensive DCE-MRI study to evaluate dose response to DMXAA was later performed on a well perfused GH3 prolactinoma tumour model in rats (McPhail et al. 2006). K^{trans} and IAUGC were measured 4 and 24 h after treatment with a range of DMXAA doses. 5-hydroxyindole-acetic acid (5-HIAA, a metabolite of serotonin) levels in blood taken from the same rats were also measured as an index of vascular damage induced by DMXAA (Kestell et al. 2001), and following MRI, the tumours were assessed for drug-induced necrosis by histology. Both 5-HIAA measurements and histology showed that an intermediate dose of 200 mg/kg DMXAA induced significant anti-vascular and anti-tumour effects. However, there were no significant changes in K^{trans} and IAUGC at this dose. It was only the highest dose of DMXAA used (350 mg/kg) that caused a significant reduction in K^{trans} and IAUGC. This result was unexpected as necrosis induced by DMXAA is thought to be attributed to reduced blood flow/perfusion, which should have been detected by DCE-MRI.

Analysis of individual rats in the intermediate cohort showed both decreases and increases in tumour K^{trans} and IAUGC. Although unexpected, the results are actually similar to those of the clinical DCE-MRI studies of DMXAA, which have shown both significant increases in K^{trans}, as well as significant reductions in IAUGC and an overall lack of dose response (Galbraith et al. 2002b; McKeage et al. 2006). Taken together, these results question the sensitivity of K^{trans} and IAUGC for use as suitable imaging biomarkers to assess DMXAA. K^{trans} is a composite measurement of both perfusion and vessel permeability. DMXAA has been shown to both increase vessel permeability and decrease vessel perfusion (Zwi et al. 1994; Lash et al. 1998 and Zhao et al. 2005), so it could be that at intermediate doses these opposing effects counterbalance each other, and hence no apparent change in K^{trans}.

Contrast agent choice is another factor that could compromise the sensitivity of MR measurements. Low molecular weight contrast agents are most commonly used for preclinical DCE-MRI studies as they are approved for use in humans. However, low molecular weight contrast agents pass through the endothelial membranes of the vasculature rapidly and as a result K^{trans} reflects both perfusion and permeability (Perini et al. 2008). MMCM are essentially impermeable to endothelial membranes of vessels in normal tissues, but not the hyperpermeable vessels of tumour tissue (Barrett et al. 2006; Perini et al. 2008). Hence, MMCM provide greater selectivity for tumour tissue (Barrett et al. 2006). With MMCM, permeability is the limiting factor of transfer of contrast agent from the intravascular space to the EES. Therefore, if MMCM is used, DCE-MRI measurements of K^{trans} could be easier to interpret as K^{trans} would more accurately reflect permeability rather than a combination of both permeability and perfusion (Barrett et al. 2006).

In a recent study, MMCM-enhanced MRI was used to assess the effects of DMXAA against fibrosarcomas grown either subcutaneously or orthotopically in the leg muscle of mice (Seshadri et al. 2008). Twenty-four hours after a single high dose of DMXAA, vascular volume and permeability were calculated from changes in the longitudinal MR relaxation rate R_1 after administration of the MMCM albumin-(Gd-DTPA)$_{35}$. The results demonstrated a significant decrease in ΔR_1, and thus permeability and vascular volume, after treatment with 30 mg/kg DMXAA. It appears that conflicting K^{trans} measurements occur at intermediate doses of DMXAA that are more clinically relevant, rather than at high doses of the drug for which reduced perfusion has already been established. Therefore, it would be extremely informative if a DMXAA dose–response study was performed using MMCM-enhanced MRI.

One theory of why DMXAA increases vascular permeability is attributed to its ability to induce TNF-α. TNF-α increases blood vessel permeability and after longer exposure, it ultimately induces vascular collapse (Watanabe et al. 1988; Kallinowski et al. 1989; Ferrero et al. 1996; Lejeune, 2002; Kerkar et al. 2006). Thus, it could be hypothesised that there may be earlier time-points at which DMXAA-induced TNF-α predominantly increases vessel permeability rather than vascular occlusion and collapse. If MMCM-enhanced MRI does truly provide a sensitive measurement of permeability, then the introduction of early time-points would be a good test to measure any increases in vascular permeability caused by DMXAA.

3.4 Preclinical DCE-MRI Summary

It is clear why DCE-MRI has been the imaging method of choice to assess VDAs in the clinic. It has the power to generate non-invasive biomarkers of response that can measure anti-vascular effects, and it is a widely accessible technique. The preclinical studies discussed in this section have successfully demonstrated significant reductions in tumour perfusion after VDA treatment as measured by DCE-MRI. In many of the studies the DCE-MRI data was also validated by combining it with other techniques, such as measuring tumour blood flow using radiolabelled iodoantipyrene, or indirectly measuring perfusion using ^{31}P-MRS to assess tumour energetics. Correlates between histological measurements of tumour necrosis and perfusion have also helped qualify DCE-MRI biomarkers.

The two tubulin-binding agents ZD6126 and CA4P both demonstrated dose-dependent reductions in DCE-MRI biomarkers (Maxwell et al. 2002; Robinson et al. 2003a). However, DCE-MRI failed to establish dose–response for DMXAA (McPhail et al. 2006). The combination of the complex nature of (1) DMXAA, (2) heterogeneous tumour tissue, and (3) the K^{trans} measurement could be responsible for the inconsistent results. The results of the DMXAA DCE-MRI studies highlight the need to investigate alternative imaging methods that allow more sensitive data interpretation.

4 Susceptibility Contrast MRI

Susceptibility contrast MRI involves measuring tumour uptake of intravenously administered ultrasmall superparamagnetic iron oxide (USPIO) nanoparticles (Wu et al. 2004). USPIO particles create large susceptibility effects that increase the regional transverse MRI relaxation rate R_2*, and their long intravascular half-life enables acquisition of steady-state, high-resolution tumour maps of R_2*, compared to K^{trans} or IAUGC maps derived from DCE MRI, in which the images must be acquired far more rapidly at the expense of spatial resolution. A USPIO-induced increase in R_2* provides an imaging biomarker for tumour fractional blood volume (Robinson et al. 2003b). In addition, the ratio of the change in transverse relaxivities, $\Delta R_2^*/\Delta R_2$, can be used to derive maps of capillary diameter (vessel size index), and which has shown good agreement with histologically determined vessel size (Dennie et al. 1998; Tropres et al. 2001).

4.1 Preclinical Assessment of VDAs Using Susceptibility Contrast MRI

Susceptibility contrast MRI revealed a significant reduction in ΔR_2*, and hence fractional blood volume, of murine C3H mammary carcinomas 1 h after treatment with CA4P (Bentzen et al. 2005). A similar approach confirmed that ZD6126 reduced tumour blood volume 24 h post-treatment (Robinson et al. 2007). A significant positive correlation between post-treatment fractional tumour blood volume and Hoechst 33342 uptake was obtained, providing qualification of the MRI-derived imaging biomarker.

More recently, DMXAA was assessed using susceptibility contrast MRI, in which both fractional blood volume and vessel size index were determined 24 h post-treatment in the rat GH3 prolactinoma model (Howe et al. 2008). Histogram analysis of the MRI data helped take into account the heterogeneity of the tumour vasculature and response to treatment, and the results demonstrated that DMXAA caused both a reduction in tumour blood volume and vessel size. The reduction in fractional blood volume correlated with increased tumour necrosis, which suggests that fractional blood volume determined by this method could be potentially used as imaging biomarker of tumour response to DMXAA. These studies highlight the potential of susceptibility contrast MRI to provide a more specific quantitative imaging biomarker of fractional tumour blood volume at high spatial resolution. A number of USPIO contrast agents are currently in development, and once clinically approved, should provide a powerful additional MRI approach for use in clinical trials of VDAs.

5 Intrinsic Susceptibility MRI

In addition to the use of intravenously administered exogenous contrast agents to assess tumour vascularity, endogenous contrast in the form of paramagnetic deoxygenated blood, or deoxyhaemoglobin, can also be used as a method to assess mature and immature vessels and their response to VDA therapy. This method is known as intrinsic susceptibility MRI, or blood oxygenation level dependent MRI (BOLD MRI) (Robinson et al. 2003b; Robinson et al. 2005; Padhani and Choyke 2006; McPhail et al. 2007). Intrinsic susceptibility MRI exploits the paramagnetic properties of deoxyhaemoglobin in the blood to create contrast in an MR image (Padhani and Choyke 2006). The presence of deoxyhaemoglobin creates magnetic susceptibility perturbations around blood vessels, which in turn increases the transverse magnetic resonance relaxation rate R_2* of the surrounding tissue in proportion to the tissue deoxyhaemoglobin concentration. In the absence of changes to R_2 and R_2' (the irreversible and reversible transverse MR relaxation rates in tissue in the absence of deoxyhaemoglobin), R_2* depends on tissue deoxyhaemoglobin concentration and may provide an acute index of changes in tissue oxygenation (Robinson et al. 2005). This means that in a tumour R_2* map, deoxygenated tissue appears brighter as it has a higher concentration of paramagnetic deoxyhaemoglobin. VDAs induce vascular collapse, which should theoretically increase tumour deoxyhaemoglobin concentration and hence R_2*, due to the lack of oxygenated blood flowing to the tumour.

5.1 Preclinical Assessment of VDAs Using Intrinsic Susceptibility MRI

ZD6126 was the first VDA to be preclinically assessed using intrinsic susceptibility MRI (Robinson et al. 2005). Tumour R_2* measurements were made acutely over the first 35 min after administration, and then again 24 h later. As hypothesised, a hyperacute increase in R_2* was observed after ZD6126 treatment, consistent with ischemia caused by vascular collapse. However, by 24 h post-treatment, R_2* had significantly decreased below baseline measurements (Fig. 2). Histological assessment of tumour perfusion using Hoechst 33342 uptake revealed that there was a significant reduction in perfusion at both 35 min and 24 h post-treatment, implying that reduction in R_2* at 24 h could not be due to tumour re-oxygenation. It was hypothesised that the reduction in R_2* seen at this later time point could instead be due to prolonged vascular collapse and blood flow deprivation, which would reduce tumour blood volume.

CA4P and DMXAA were assessed by intrinsic susceptibility MRI using the same GH3 prolactinoma tumour model as for the ZD6126 study, and results for the three VDAs were compared (McPhail et al. 2007). Over the first 35 min of challenge, tumour R_2* response for each drug was different. CA4P caused no significant

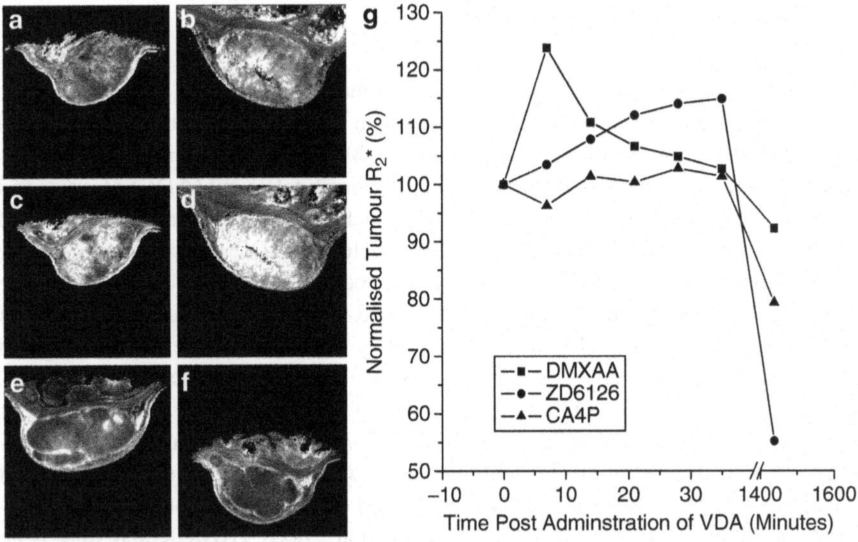

Fig. 2 Rat tumour R_2* maps acquired (**a** and **b**) prior to and (**c** and **d**) 14 min and 35 min post intravenous administration of 350 mg/kg DMXAA and 50 mg/kg ZD6126 respectively. Tumour regions exhibiting relatively fast (intense) R_2* are consistent with the presence of paramagnetic deoxyhaemoglobin. Note the apparent hyperacute increase in R_2* following challenge with these VDAs. Calculated tumour R_2* maps acquired 24 h post-treatment with (**e**) 100 mg/kg CA4P or (**f**) 50 mg/kg ZD6126 are also shown. At this time point, R_2* is reduced, coupled with darker and more homogeneous maps. A comparison of the normalised mean rat tumour R_2* response for DMXAA, CA4P and ZD6126 is shown in (**g**), highlighting differing mechanisms of action and temporal response between these VDAs. (Robinson et al. 2005; McPhail et al. 2007)

increases in R_2*, where as DMXAA induced a sharp significant increase in R_2* at 7 min post-treatment, which quickly recovered. However, by 24 h post-treatment the VDA R_2* response was more similar. Comparable to ZD6126, CA4P showed a significant reduction in tumour R_2*. DXMAA also showed a reduction in R_2* at 24 h post-treatment, although it did not reach significance. Histological assessment of tumour perfusion revealed that the degree of Hoechst 33342 uptake was associated with the degree of R_2* reduction at 24 h for both agents.

Taken together, these studies demonstrate that the interpretation of changes in tumour R_2* in response to VDA therapy is complex, as there can be both significant increases and decreases in R_2* depending on what time-point after drug administration is interrogated. ZD6126, CA4P and DMXAA each showed a different acute tumour R_2* response pattern. As mentioned previously, the mechanism of action of DMXAA is very different to that of the other VDAs. Unlike the tubulin-binding agents, DMXAA has been classified as a cytokine inducer (Siemann et al. 2005), but its molecular target remains to be elucidated. So it is perhaps not surprising that the tumour R_2* response to DMXAA is different. However, even between the two tubulin-binding agents ZD6126 and CA4P, tumour R_2* response differed over the hyperacute timecourse, although ultimately by 24 h both ZD6126 and CA4P did show similar reductions in R_2*.

6 Diffusion-Weighted MRI

Diffusion-weighted MRI (DW-MRI) is a non-contrast MR method that can measure the Brownian motion of water protons in tissue and can thus determine intra and extracellular volume ratios (Evelhoch et al. 2000; Stephen and Gillies 2007). This measurement is referred to as the apparent diffusion coefficient (ADC) of water and it is sensitive to aspects of tissue structure, such as cell membrane integrity and other protein barriers (Evelhoch et al. 2000). Hence, ADC measurements can be used to assess tumour cellularity. Apoptosis, necrosis and mitotic catastrophe are processes that decrease cellularity and should therefore increase movement of water and give higher ADC values (Morse et al. 2007). A number of non-targeted cytotoxic therapies, such as cyclophosphamide, BCNU, ganciclovir, paclitaxel, docetaxel and 5-fluorouracil have all been shown to increase ADC in rodent tumour models (Zhao et al. 1996; Chenevert et al., 1997; Hakumäki et al., 1998; Poptani et al. 1998; Galons et al. 1999; Jennings et al. 2002). Moreover, the drug-induced changes in ADC were associated with increased cell death and found to occur earlier than changes in tumour volume (Evelhoch et al. 2000). DW-MRI has since been used for the assessment of targeted therapies, including VDAs.

6.1 Preclinical Assessment of VDAs Using DW-MRI

CA4P has been the most extensively studied VDA using diffusion-weighted MRI. Thoeny et al. used DW-MRI to measure changes in ADC after a single dose of CA4P in a rhabdomyosarcoma tumour model grown subcutaneously in rats (Thoeny et al. 2005a). At both 1 and 6 h post-CA4P, a reduction in ADC was found, yet histology revealed no necrosis. An increase in ADC was found 2 days post-CA4P, which was consistent with reduced cellularity, and this result was confirmed by the presence of tumour necrosis detected by histology. Nine days post-treatment ADC had decreased again but by this time-point the tumour had started to re-grow. DCE-MRI performed on the same tumours corroborated these findings, revealing reduced perfusion at the early time-points but increased perfusion 9 days post-treatment when tumour re-growth was evident.

A continuation of this study aimed to investigate the time-course of ADC changes in necrotic compared to viable tumour tissue after three equally spaced doses of CA4P (Thoeny et al. 2005b). In agreement with the previous results, 6 h post-CA4P there was a significant reduction in ADC, followed by a significant increase in ADC 2 days post-CA4P which coincided with the onset of necrosis. By 9 days post-treatment there was tumour re-growth. A similar efficacy pattern was seen after each sequential dose of CA4P.

Chen et al. performed a comparative DW-MRI study of CA4P and DMXAA in a mouse C3H mammary carcinoma, which also used DCE-MRI to assess tumour perfusion (Chen et al. 2008). Perfusion was significantly decreased over the whole tumour, including the highly-perfused areas, within the first hour after CA4P administration, and remained so for the duration of the experiment (6 h). However, an increase in ADC was only seen 5 h post-CA4P, and this was restricted to the lowest perfused tumour segments. In contrast, DMXAA significantly increased tumour ADC over the whole tumour. However, this increase only occurred after 5 h in the highly-perfused tumour regions. The authors concluded that there are spatial differences in the effects of VDAs on tumours. This study once more highlights the differential response between two VDAs that have distinct mechanisms of action.

The effects of ZD6126 have been investigated using DW-MRI in a DU145 prostate xenograft model in mice (Vogel-Claussen et al. 2007). In this study ADC was determined prior to and 24, 48 and 72 h after a single 200 mg/kg dose of ZD6126. Changes in vascular volume and permeability surface area product (PSP) were also assessed via DCE-MRI using MMCM, and the MRI data was related to histology. Reductions in vascular volume and PSP were detected 24 h post-ZD6126, which were followed by an increase in ADC at 48 and 72 h. Histology showed necrosis was evident by 48 h. These results reflect a logical progression of events caused by ZD6126 treatment, which start with (1) early changes in the vasculature which can be detected by DCE-MRI and demonstrate reduced vascular volume, (2) the loss of cellular integrity which can be detected by DW-MRI and is indicative of necrosis, and (3) the histologically visible onset of necrosis, which is a result of prolonged tumour ischemia. All of these drug-induced effects were detectable before any changes in tumour volume. Similar to the findings of the previous DW-MRI studies discussed earlier, Vogel Claussen et al. also found heterogeneity in the spatial as well as temporal tumour response. Another consistency between studies is that ADC actually decreased 24 h post-treatment, which is a time-point were evidence of drug-induced necrosis has been shown, and an increase in diffusion predicted. Both Theony et al. and Vogel Claussen et al. suggest this decrease in ADC is likely to be due to initial swelling and oedema caused by acute ischemia, which would restrict the movement of water in the tumour tissue.

7 Magnetic Resonance Spectroscopy

In addition to MR imaging, MR spectroscopy (MRS) has also proved a powerful tool in oncology. In vivo MRS can be used as a non-invasive method for the assessment of tumour biochemistry and physiology, and their response to therapy. The most common type of nuclei used for MRS in oncology are ^{31}P and ^{1}H. The metabolites detected by ^{31}P-MRS are inorganic phosphate (Pi), γ-phosphate, α-phosphate, β-phosphate, phosphomonoesters (PME), phosphodiesters (PDE), and phosphocreatine (PCr) (Gillies and Morse 2005).

The metabolic state of a tumour can be measured by ^{31}P-MRS using a high to low energy phosphate ratio, for example β-NTP/Pi. Additionally, ^{31}P-MRS can provide information on membrane turn-over using the PME/PDE ratio, because the PME resonance principally comprises the membrane synthesis substrates phosphoethanolamine and phosphocholine (PE and PC), and the PDE resonance is comprised of the membrane degradation products glycerophosphoethanolamine and glycerophosphocholine (GPE and GPC). The intracellular pH of the tumour can also be derived using the chemical shift of the Pi signal.

The most prominent tumour metabolites observed by in vivo ^{1}H-MRS are N-acetyl aspartate (NAA), lipids, lactate, total choline (tCho) and total creatines (tCr) (Howe et al. 1993; Gillies and Morse 2005). Choline containing metabolites in tumour tissue are of particular interest because they are involved in phospholipid metabolism (i.e. cell membrane metabolism) (Podo 1999). In vivo ^{1}H-MRS can be used to detect all choline containing compounds, although in the MR spectra they appear as one broad resonance, assigned as total choline (tCho). High resolution ^{1}H-MRS of tumour extracts has revealed that the tCho resonance is comprised of signals from free choline, PC and GPC.

Several early clinical ^{31}P-MRS studies demonstrated that PME levels are elevated in lymphomas and head and neck tumours (Negendank 1992), and since then, elevated choline levels have been confirmed for breast, prostate, colon, cervical and brain cancers using ^{1}H-MRS, confirming choline as an important metabolic biomarker of malignancy and grade (Gillies and Morse 2005). However, more recent work has shown that absolute quantification of choline, rather than a ratio measurement, is required to discriminate malignant from benign tissues (Bolan et al. 2003). A study performed by Smith et al. demonstrated that the choline content of tumours is indicative of cell proliferation, as PC levels in rat mammary tumour model (measured by high resolution ^{31}P-MRS of tumour extracts) correlated with tumour growth rate and proliferation (measured by bromodeoxyuridine labelling) (Smith et al. 1991).

7.1 Preclinical Assessment of VDAs Using Magnetic Resonance Spectroscopy

Both ^{31}P and ^{1}H-MRS have been used to assess changes in tumour metabolism and membrane turnover with respect to VDA treatment. In vivo ^{31}P-MRS was first used to assess the effects of CA4P on tumour metabolism (Beauregard et al. 1998). CA4P caused a reduction in the β-NTP/Pi, and therefore tumour energetics, 80 min post-treatment. This coincided with a reduction in tumour pH, and also perfusion as measured by DCE-MRI. A later study by Beauregard et al. used ^{31}P-MRS to assess the effects of both CA4P and DMXAA against HT29 and LS174T colon carcinoma xenografts grown in mice (Beauregard et al. 2002). Both VDAs induced a decrease in tumour energetics 3 h post-treatment in LS174T tumours, but only DMXAA elicited a response in HT29 tumours. Maxwell et al. used a combination of ^{31}P-MRS, ^{1}H-MRS and ^{1}H-MRI to assess the anti-tumour effects of CA4P against a C3H murine mammary carcinoma model (Maxwell et al. 1998). ^{31}P-MRS demonstrated a reduction in tumour energetics using the β-NTP/Pi ratio. However, no necrosis was evident at the same-time point, suggesting that ^{31}P-MRS could provide an early indicator of tumour response.

DMXAA demonstrated a dose-dependent reduction in the β-NTP/Pi ratio, and thus tumour energetics, 6 h post-treatment in a human HT29 xenograft model in mice (McPhail et al. 2005) (Fig. 3). In the same study, total choline levels revealed that there was a significant reduction in cell membrane turnover at the later time-point of 24 h, but only with the highest dose used. The results of this study are of particular interest as ^{31}P-MRS demonstrates tumour dose–response to DMXAA, which both the preclinical and clinical DCE-MRI studies failed to do.

In vivo and ex vivo ^{1}H-MRS were used to assess the anti-tumour effects of ZD6126 in a murine RIF-1 fibrosarcoma model (Madhu et al. 2006). Quantification of tCho in the tumour tissue using in vivo ^{1}H-MRS showed that 200 mg/kg ZD6126 caused a significant reduction in cell membrane turnover 24 h post-treatment. A significant increase in tCho was seen in the control cohort, which is consistent with undisrupted cell proliferation and tumour growth. Ex vivo high-resolution magic angle spinning (HR-MAS) and ^{1}H-MRS of tumour extracts confirmed the in vivo response as they revealed a significant reduction in PC and GPC in the ZD6126-treated cohort. The reduction in choline compounds seen after treatment is indicative of the anti-proliferative effects induced by ZD6126 that are associated with vascular disruption.

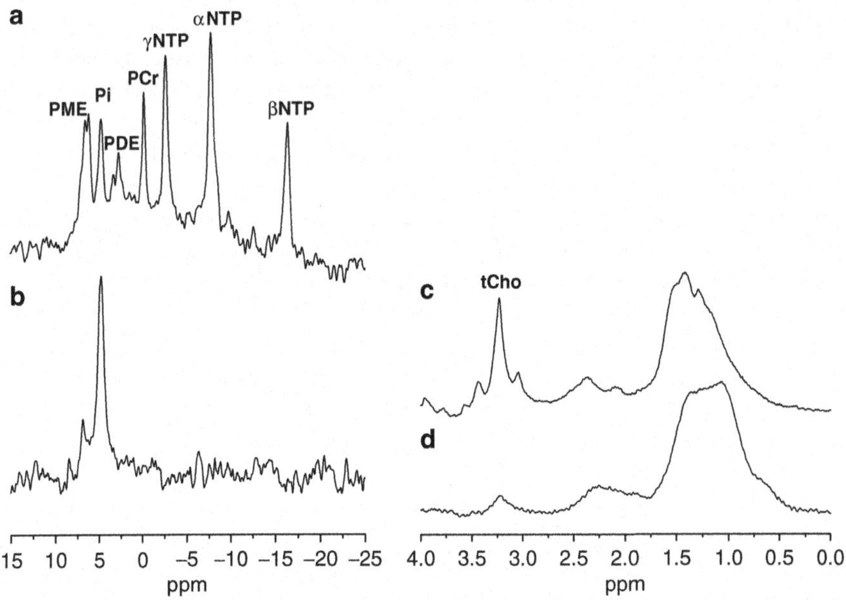

Fig. 3 ^{31}P-MR spectra acquired from a murine HT29 xenograft in vivo (**a**) prior to and (**b**) 6 h after treatment with 21 mg/kg DMXAA. Resonances are identified for γ, α and β nucleoside triphosphates (NTP), inorganic phosphate (Pi), phosphocreatine (PCr), and the resonances of the phospholipid metabolites phosphomonoesters (PME) and phosphodiesters (PDE). Treatment resulted in a dramatic increase in Pi and a depletion of the high-energy phosphates. In vivo localised ^{1}H MRS spectra acquired from a RIF-1 fibrosarcoma (**c**) prior to and (**d**) 24 h after treatment with 200 mg/kg ZD6126. Note the reduction in the resonance from the choline containing metabolites (tCho) at 3.2 ppm following treatment with the VDA (McPhail et al. 2005; Madhu et al. 2006)

8 Non-MR Imaging Modalities

MR has by far been the most extensively used imaging modality to investigate VDA therapy in preclinical studies. However, there are preclinical studies that have employed alternative imaging methods to evaluate VDAs.

8.1 Fluorine-18 Fluorodeoxyglucose-Positron Emission Tomography ([^{18}F]-FDG-PET)

Positron emission tomography (PET) is a form of radiological imaging that detects gamma-rays emitted indirectly by radioactive nuclei attached to a tracer molecule (radiotracer). The nuclei used are typically isotopes with short half-lives, such as ^{15}O, ^{13}N, ^{13}C and ^{18}F (Stephen and Gillies 2007). The most popular PET radiotracer is fluorine-18 fluorodeoxyglucose ([^{18}F]-FDG), an ^{18}F isotope tagged to a glucose analogue that is taken up by metabolically active cancer cells. [^{18}F]-FDG then undergoes phosphorylation by hexokinase, but the resulting FDG-6-phosphate remains effectively trapped within the intracellular compartment (Stephen and Gillies 2007). Thus, [^{18}F]-FDG trapping detected by PET can be used to evaluate glucose metabolism, a factor that is up-regulated in tumour tissue, and especially so in aggressive, metastatic disease (Gatenby and Gillies 2004; Kunkel et al. 2003).

To date there has only been one published preclinical study in which VDA effectiveness was assessed using PET. Zhao et al. used PET to test whether CA4P induced any changes in [^{18}F]-FDG uptake that could be quantitatively related to necrosis in a mouse liver metastasis model (Zhao et al. 1999). PET and histology showed that a single dose of CA4P caused on average a 30% volume destruction of liver metastases by 24 h. In vivo analysis of [^{18}F]-FDG uptake was subsequently validated by ex vivo quantification of [^{18}F]-FDG in the excised tissue, and a strong correlation was found between the in vivo and ex vivo measurements. These findings are consistent with a reduction in tumour metabolism caused by CA4P-induced vascular collapse restricting blood flow to the tumour.

Compared to MR, PET is not such a widely accessible technique. This is due to the need of an expensive on-site cyclotron to generate short-lived radionuclides for the tracers. This may explain why so few preclinical VDA studies have been performed using PET. The longer half-life of ^{18}F makes this radionuclide an exception, as it can be purchased and transported from outside sources. In the CA4P study, [^{18}F]-FDG revealed important information on the effects of CA4P on tumour metabolism. Nevertheless, the authors note that [^{18}F]-FDG is not specific for vascular damage. Hence, [^{18}F]-FDG uptake could reflect areas of the tumour that are no longer perfused, but it could also reflect areas of tumour with abnormal FDG metabolism.

Tumour blood volume can be directly measured via PET by labelling red blood cells with ^{11}C or ^{15}O to create blood pool tracers (Perini et al. 2008). In particular, [^{15}O]–H_2O has proved to be a very sensitive and reproducible tracer to assess perfusion (Taniguchi et al. 2003; Wells et al. 2003). Preclinical studies using [^{15}O]–H_2O PET would provide a more direct and accurate measurement of VDA efficacy, but the short half-life of ^{15}O again is the limiting factor as these studies could only be performed at a site with a cyclotron.

8.2 *Scintigraphic Imaging*

^{99m}Tc-labelled HL-91 (Prognox) is a non-nitromidazole that localises to hypoxic areas of tumour tissue through an unknown mechanism. VDAs induce vascular collapse, and should in theory increase tumour hypoxia as a consequence. Siim et al. performed a study with Prognox to investigate its use to provide a biomarker for tumour blood flow (Siim et al. 2000). Both CA4P and DMXAA were found to inhibit tumour blood flow 3 h post-treatment, as measured by ^{86}RbCl uptake, and they also selectively increased Prognox levels, and thus hypoxia, in tumour tissue. These results confirmed that CA4P and DMXAA caused a reduction in tumour blood flow, which subsequently increased intratumoural hypoxia, and also showed that scintigraphic imaging of Prognox could be used as an indirect measurement of blood flow.

8.3 *High-Frequency Doppler Ultrasound*

Doppler ultrasound (US) employs the Doppler effect to assess blood flow velocity and direction (i.e. whether the flow is towards or away from the ultrasound probe). High-frequency Doppler US (HFD US) was used in a study to assess changes in tumour blood flow after ZD6126 treatment (20 mg/kg) using a human melanoma model grown orthotopically in the skin of nude mice (Goertz et al. 2002). A significant reduction in tumour blood flow was detected 4 h post-treatment, which recovered by 24 h, and these results were histologically validated by Hoechst 33342 uptake. This study successfully demonstrates the use of HFD US as a technique to assess the anti-vascular effects of VDA therapy. However, there are major limitations to the technique, the main one being the restrictions on depth of the tissue being interrogated. Another factor is motion present in the area of interest. This means than HFD US imaging will probably be limited to tumours near the surface of the body, not so much an issue for preclinical experiments, but much more so for the majority of human tumour types.

9 Chapter Summary

It is clear from the review of preclinical literature that MR has been the main imaging modality used to investigate efficacy of VDAs in vivo. DCE-MRI has been the most extensively used method and although it has proved successful in providing biomarkers of tumour perfusion, it is a complex technique and there are still issues of standardising data acquisition and analysis. If MMCM is approved for use in humans perhaps this will help simplify DCE-MRI data interpretation.

VDAs do not only cause a reduction in tumour perfusion, they ultimately induce tumour necrosis, and thus the development of DW-MRI is exciting as it has the potential to provide non-invasive biomarkers of tumour necrosis. Non-MR imaging modalities such as PET have not been as widely used in preclinical VDA studies. The lack of preclinical PET data may be due to the need for an on-site cyclotron to generate radiotracers other than [^{18}F]-FDG and not a reflection on its potential. If an on-site cyclotron is available, then PET is a very powerful tool in drug development, as it can be used to monitor any compound providing it can be radiolabelled with a tracer.

Each one of the imaging modalities discussed has demonstrated the potential to provide non-invasive biomarkers of response to VDA therapy. Therefore, in vivo assessment of VDAs would be strengthened if these imaging methods were combined and multiple biomarkers measured. The future of in vivo imaging is not to use single modalities but instead to combine our knowledge and employ a multimodality imaging strategy. This would provide a number of biomarkers that compliment each other and create the best possible means to robustly measure all facets of VDA tumour response.

References

Barrett T, Kobayashi H, Brechbiel M et al (2006) Macromolecular MRI contrast agents for imaging tumor angiogenesis. Eur J Radiol 60:353–366.

Beauregard DA, Thelwall PE, Chaplin DJ et al (1998) Magnetic resonance imaging and spectroscopy of combretastatin A4 prodrug-induced disruption of tumour perfusion and energetic status. Br J Cancer 77:1761–1767.

Beauregard DA, Pedley RB, Hill SA et al (2002) Differential sensitivity of two adenocarcinoma xenografts to the anti-vascular drugs combretastatin A4 phosphate and 5,6-dimethylxanthenone-4-acetic acid, assessed using MRI and MRS. NMR Biomed 15:99–105.

Bentzen L, Vestergaard-Poulsen P, Nielsen T et al (2005) Intravascular contrast agent-enhanced MRI measuring contrast clearance and tumor blood volume and the effects of vascular modifiers in an experimental tumor. Int J Radiat Oncol Biol Phys 61:1208–1215.

Bolan PJ, Meisamy S, Baker EH et al (2003) In vivo quantification of choline compounds in the breast with ^{1}H MR spectroscopy. Magn Reson Med 50:1134–1143.

Bradley DP, Tessier JJ, Ashton SE et al (2007) Correlation of MRI biomarkers with tumor necrosis in Hras5 tumor xenograft in athymic rats. Neoplasia 9:382–391.

Brasch R and Turetschek K (2000) MRI characterization of tumors and grading angiogenesis using macromolecular contrast media: status report. Eur J Radiol 34:148–155.

Carmeliet P (2003) Blood vessels and nerves: common signals, pathways and diseases. Nat Rev Genet 4:710–720.

Carmeliet P, Jain RK (2000) Angiogenesis in cancer and other diseases. Nature 407:249–257.

Chen G, Horsman MR, Pedersen M et al (2008) The effect of combretastatin A4 disodium phosphate and 5,6-dimethylxanthenone-4-acetic acid on water diffusion and blood perfusion in tumours. Acta Oncol 47:1071–1076.

Chenevert TL, McKeever PE, Ross BD (1997) Monitoring early response of experimental brain tumors to therapy using diffusion magnetic resonance imaging. Clin Cancer Res 3:1457–1466.
Choyke PL, Dwyer AJ, Knopp MV (2003) Functional tumor imaging with dynamic contrast-enhanced magnetic resonance imaging. J Magn Reson Imag 17:509–520.
Dennie J, Mandeville JB, Boxerman JL et al (1998) NMR imaging of changes in vascular morphology due to tumor angiogenesis. Magn Reson Med 40:793–799.
Evelhoch JL, Gillies RJ, Karczmar GS et al (2000) Applications of magnetic resonance in model systems: cancer therapeutics. Neoplasia 2:152–165.
Evelhoch JL, LoRusso PM, He Z et al (2004) Magnetic resonance imaging measurements of the response of murine and human tumors to the vascular-targeting agent ZD6126. Clin Cancer Res 10:3650–3657.
Ferrero E, Villa A, Ferrero ME et al (1996) Tumor necrosis factor alpha-induced vascular leakage involves PECAM1 phosphorylation. Cancer Res 56:3211–3215.
Galbraith SM, Lodge MA, Taylor NJ et al (2002a) Reproducibility of dynamic contrast-enhanced MRI in human muscle and tumours: comparison of quantitative and semi-quantitative analysis. NMR Biomed 15:132–142.
Galbraith SM, Rustin GJ, Lodge MA et al (2002b) Effects of 5,6-dimethylxanthenone-4-acetic acid on human tumor microcirculation assessed by dynamic contrast-enhanced magnetic resonance imaging. J Clin Oncol 20:3826–3840.
Galbraith SM, Maxwell RJ, Lodge MA et al (2003) Combretastatin A4 phosphate has tumor antivascular activity in rat and man as demonstrated by dynamic magnetic resonance imaging. J Clin Oncol 21:2831–2842.
Galons JP, Altbach MI, Paine-Murrieta GD et al (1999) Early increases in breast tumor xenograft water mobility in response to paclitaxel therapy detected by non-invasive diffusion magnetic resonance imaging. Neoplasia 1:113–117.
Gatenby RA, Gillies RJ (2004) Why do cancers have high aerobic glycolysis? Nat Rev Cancer 4:891–899.
Gillies RJ, Morse DL (2005) In vivo magnetic resonance spectroscopy in cancer. Ann Rev Biomed Eng 7:287–326.
Gillies RJ, Bhujwalla ZM, Evelhoch J et al (2000) Applications of magnetic resonance in model systems: tumor biology and physiology. Neoplasia 2:139–151.
Gillies RJ, Raghunand N, Karczmar GS et al (2002) MRI of the tumor microenvironment. J Magn Reson Imag 16:430–450.
Goertz DE, Yu JL, Kerbel RS et al (2002) High-frequency Doppler ultrasound monitors the effects of antivascular therapy on tumor blood flow. Cancer Res 62:6371–6375.
Hakumäki JM, Poptani H, Puumalainen AM et al (1998) Quantitative ^{1}H nuclear magnetic resonance diffusion spectroscopy of BT4C rat glioma during thymidine kinase-mediated gene therapy in vivo: identification of apoptotic response. Cancer Res 58:3791–3799.
Howe FA, Maxwell RJ, Saunders DE et al (1993) Proton spectroscopy in vivo. Magn Reson Quart 9:31–59.
Howe FA, McPhail LD, Griffiths JR et al (2008) Vessel size index magnetic resonance imaging to monitor the effect of antivascular treatment in a rodent tumor model. Int J Radiat Oncol Biol Phys 71:1470–1476.
Jennings D, Hatton BN, Guo J et al (2002) Early response of prostate carcinoma xenografts to docetaxel chemotherapy monitored with diffusion MRI. Neoplasia 4:255–262.
Kallinowski F, Schaefer C, Tyler G et al (1989) In vivo targets of recombinant human tumour necrosis factor-alpha: blood flow, oxygen consumption and growth of isotransplanted rat tumours. Br J Cancer 60:555–560.
Kerkar S, Williams M, Blocksom J et al (2006) TNF-alpha and IL-1beta increase pericyte/endothelial cell co-culture permeability. J Surg Res 132:40–45.
Kestell P, Zhao L, Jameson MB et al (2001) Measurement of plasma 5-hydroxyindoleacetic acid as a possible clinical surrogate marker for the action of antivascular agents. Clin Chim Acta 314:159–166.

Kunkel M, Reichert TE, Benz P et al (2003) Overexpression of Glut-1 and increased glucose metabolism in tumors are associated with a poor prognosis in patients with oral squamous cell carcinoma. Cancer 97:1015–1024.
Lash CJ, Li AE, Rutland M et al (1998) Enhancement of the anti-tumour effects of the antivascular agent 5,6-dimethylxanthenone-4-acetic acid (DMXAA) by combination with 5-hydroxytryptamine and bioreductive drugs. Br J Cancer 78:439–445.
Leach MO, Brindle KM, Evelhoch JL et al (2005) The assessment of antiangiogenic and antivascular therapies in early-stage clinical trials using magnetic resonance imaging: issues and recommendations. Br J Cancer 92:1599–1610.
Lejeune FJ (2002) Clinical use of TNF revisited: improving penetration of anti-cancer agents by increasing vascular permeability. J Clin Invest 110:433–435.
Madhu B, Waterton JC, Griffiths JR et al (2006) The response of RIF-1 fibrosarcomas to the vascular-disrupting agent ZD6126 assessed by in vivo and ex vivo ^{1}H magnetic resonance spectroscopy. Neoplasia 8:560–567.
Maxwell RJ, Nielsen FU, Breidahl T et al (1998) Effects of combretastatin on murine tumours monitored by ^{31}P MRS, ^{1}H MRS and ^{1}H MRI. Int J Radiat Oncol Biol Phys 42:891–894.
Maxwell RJ, Wilson J, Prise VE et al (2002) Evaluation of the anti-vascular effects of combretastatin in rodent tumours by dynamic contrast enhanced MRI. NMR in Biomed 15:89–98.
McIntyre DJ, Robinson SP, Howe FA et al (2004) Single dose of the antivascular agent, ZD6126 (N-acetylcolchinol-O-phosphate), reduces perfusion for at least 96 hours in the GH3 prolactinoma rat tumor model. Neoplasia 6:150–157.
McKeage M, Fong P, Jeffery M et al (2006) 5,6-dimethyxanthenone-4-acetic acid in the treatment of refactory tumours: a phase I safety study of a vascular disrupting agent. Clin Cancer Res 12:1776–1784.
McPhail LD, Chung YL, Basetti M et al (2005) Tumour dose response to the vascular disrupting agent, 5,6-dimethylxanthenone-4-acetic acid, using in vivo magnetic resonance spectroscopy. Clin Cancer Res 11:3705–3713.
McPhail LM, McIntyre DJO, Ludwig C et al (2006) Rat tumour response to the vascular-disrupting agent 5,6-dimethylxanthenone-4-acetic acid as measured by dynamic contrast-enhanced magnetic resonance imaging, plasma 5-hydroxyindoleacetic acid levels, and tumour necrosis. Neoplasia 8:199–206.
McPhail LD, Griffiths JR, Robinson SP (2007) Assessment of tumor response to the vascular disrupting agents 5,6-dimethylxanthenone-4-acetic acid or combretastatin-A4-phosphate by intrinsic susceptibility magnetic resonance imaging. Int J Radiat Oncol Biol Phys 69:1238–1245.
Morse DL, Galons JP, Payne CM et al (2007) MRI-measured water mobility increases in response to chemotherapy via multiple cell-death mechanisms. NMR Biomed 20:602–614.
Negendank W (1992) Studies of human tumors by MRS: a review. NMR Biomed 5:303–324.
O'Connor JP, Jackson A, Parker GJ et al (2007) DCE-MRI biomarkers in the clinical evaluation of anti-angiogenic and vascular disrupting agents. Br J Cancer 96:189–195.
Padhani AR (2003) MRI for assessing antivascular cancer treatments. Br J Radiol 76:S60–S80.
Padhani AR, Choyke PL (2006) New Techniques in Oncologic Imaging. Taylor and Francis. New York.
Padhani AR, Husband JE (2001) Dynamic contrast-enhanced MRI studies in oncology with an emphasis on quantification, validation and human studies. Clin Radiol 56:607–620.
Perini R, Choe R, Yodh AG et al (2008) Non-invasive assessment of tumor neovasculature: techniques and clinical applications. Cancer Metastasis Rev 27:615–630.
Podo F (1999) Tumour phospholipid metabolism. NMR Biomed 12:413–439.
Poptani H, Puumalainen AM, Gröhn OH et al (1998) Monitoring thymidine kinase and ganciclovir -induced changes in rat malignant glioma in vivo by nuclear magnetic resonance imaging. Cancer Gene Ther 5:101–109.
Robinson SP, McIntyre DJ, Checkley D et al (2003a) Tumour dose response to the antivascular agent ZD6126 assessed by magnetic resonance imaging. Br J Cancer 88:1592–1597.

Robinson SP, Rijken PF, Howe FA et al (2003b) Tumor vascular architecture and function evaluated by non-invasive susceptibility MRI methods and immunohistochemistry. J Magn Reson Imag 17:445–454.
Robinson SP, Kalber TL, Howe FA et al (2005) Acute tumor response to ZD6126 assessed by intrinsic susceptibility magnetic resonance imaging. Neoplasia 7:466–474.
Robinson SP, Howe FA, Griffiths JR et al (2007) Susceptibility contrast magnetic resonance imaging determination of fractional tumor blood volume: a noninvasive imaging biomarker of response to the vascular disrupting agent ZD6126. Int J Radiat Oncol Biol Phys 69:872–879.
Salmon HW, Siemann DW (2006) Effect of the second-generation vascular disrupting agent OXi4503 on tumor vascularity. Clin Cancer Res 12:4090–4094.
Seshadri M, Bellnier DA, Cheney RT (2008) Assessment of the early effects of 5,6-dimethylxanthenone-4-acetic acid using macromolecular contrast media-enhanced magnetic resonance imaging: ectopic versus orthotopic tumors. Int J Radiat Oncol Biol Phys 72:1198–1207.
Siemann DW, Chaplin DJ, Horsman MR (2004) Vascular-targeting therapies for treatment of malignant disease. Cancer 100:2491–2499.
Siemann DW, Bibby MC, Dark GG et al (2005) Differentiation and definition of vascular-targeted therapies. Clin Cancer Res 11:416–420.
Siim BG, Laux WT, Rutland MD et al (2000) Scintigraphic imaging of the hypoxia marker 99mTechnetium-labeled 2,2′-(1,4-diaminobutane)bis(2-methyl-3-butanone) dioxime (99mTc-labeled HL-91; Prognox): Noninvasive detection of tumor response to the antivascular agent 5,6-dimethylxanthenone-4-acetic acid. Cancer Res 60:4582–4588.
Smith TA, Eccles S, Ormerod MG et al (1991) The phosphocholine and glycerophosphocholine content of an oestrogen-sensitive rat mammary tumour correlates strongly with growth rate. Br J Cancer 64:821–826.
Stephen RM, Gillies RJ (2007) Promise and progress for functional and molecular imaging of response to targeted therapies. Pharm Res 24:1172–1185.
Taniguchi H, Kunishima S, Koh T (2003) The reproducibility of independently measuring human regional hepatic arterial, portal and total hepatic blood flow using [^{15}O]water and positron emission tomography. Nucl Med Commun 24:497–501.
Thoeny HC, De Keyzer F, Vandecaveye V et al (2005a) Effect of vascular targeting agent in rat tumor model: dynamic contrast-enhanced versus diffusion-weighted MR imaging. Radiology 237:492–499.
Thoeny HC, De Keyzer F, Chen F et al (2005b) Diffusion-weighted magnetic resonance imaging allows noninvasive in vivo monitoring of the effects of combretastatin a-4 phosphate after repeated administration. Neoplasia 7:779–787.
Tofts PS, Brix G, Buckley DL et al (1999) Estimating kinetic parameters from dynamic contrast-enhanced T(1)-weighted MRI of a diffusable tracer: standardized quantities and symbols. J Magn Reson Imag 10:223–232.
Tozer GM, Kanthou C, Baguley BC (2005) Disrupting tumour blood vessels. Nat Rev Cancer 5:423–435.
Tropres I, Grimault S, Vaeth A et al (2001) Vessel size imaging. Magn Reson Med 45:397–408.
Vaupel P, Kallinowski F, Okunieff P (1989) Blood flow, oxygen and nutrient supply, and metabolic microenvironment of human tumors: a review. Cancer Res 49:6449–6465.
Vogel-Claussen J, Gimi B, Artemov D et al (2007) Diffusion-weighted and macromolecular contrast enhanced MRI of tumor response to antivascular therapy with ZD6126. Cancer Biol Ther 6:1469–1475.
Watanabe N, Niitsu Y, Umeno H et al (1988) Toxic effect of tumor necrosis factor on tumor vasculature in mice. Cancer Res 48:2179–2183.
Wells P, Jones T, Price P (2003) Assessment of inter- and intrapatient variability in $C^{15}O_2$ positron emission tomography measurements of blood flow in patients with intra-abdominal cancers. Clin Cancer Res 9:6350–6356.
Wu EX, Tang H, Jensen JH (2004) Applications of ultrasmall superparamagnetic iron oxide contrast agents in the MR study of animal models. NMR Biomed 17:478–483.

Zhao M, Pipe JG, Bonnett J et al (1996) Early detection of treatment response by diffusion-weighted ^{1}H-NMR spectroscopy in a murine tumour in vivo. Br J Cancer 73:61–64.

Zhao S, Moore JV, Waller ML et al (1999) Positron emission tomography of murine liver metastases and the effects of treatment by combretastatin A-4. Eur J Nucl Med 26:231–238.

Zhao L, Ching LM, Kestell P et al (2005) Mechanisms of tumor vascular shutdown induced by 5,6-dimethylxanthenone-4-acetic acid (DMXAA): increased tumor vascular permeability. Int J Cancer 116:322–326.

Zwi LJ, Baguley BC, Gavin JB et al (1994) The morphological effects of the anti-tumor agents flavone acetic acid and 5,6-dimethyl xanthenone acetic acid on the colon 38 mouse tumor. Pathology 26:161–169.

Combining Antiangiogenic Drugs with Vascular Disrupting Agents Rationale and Mechanisms of Action

Yuval Shaked, Paul Nathan, Laura G.M. Daenen, and Robert S. Kerbel

Abstract A highly reproducible characteristic of vascular disrupting agent (VDA) -mediated anti-tumor therapy is the retention of a rim of viable tumor tissue surrounding a much larger central mass of necrotic tissue within days of therapy. Repopulation from the viable rim subsequently compromises much of the striking initial anti-tumor effect frequently caused by the VDA treatment. The repopulation process is driven in part by robust tumor angiogenesis, which therefore constitutes a compelling rationale for combining VDA therapy with an antiangiogenic drug. In this regard, we have found that tumor angiogenesis in the viable rim after VDA therapy can be driven, at least in part, by a rapid systemic host response caused by the VDA treatment itself, namely, induction within hours of the mobilization of bone marrow-derived cells (BMDCs) including circulating endothelial progenitor cells (CEPs). These cells migrate to the drug treated tumor and heavily colonize the remaining viable tumor rim. This systemic host response appears to be driven, at least in part, by rapid induction of high levels of circulating growth factors, including G-CSF and SDF-1. The mobilization and tumor homing of CEPs can be blunted by prior or concurrent administration of an antiangiogenic drug such as anti-VEGF receptor 2 antibodies – which results in enhanced overall anti-tumor activity, e.g. greater levels of tumor necrosis, a much smaller viable tumor rim and increased survival times. In addition to this systemic effect, a more potent 'local' effect may also be obtained by adding an antiangiogenic drug to a VDA as a result of greater levels of apoptosis of endothelial cells in the tumor associated vasculature. Preliminary clinical trial results suggest combination VDA – antiangiogenic drug therapy has promising activity without significant increases in toxicity, and moreover, indicate that some of the preclinical findings, such as rapid VDA-induced elevations of circulating G-CSF and VEGF, are observed in patients as well.

R.S. Kerbel (✉)
Division of Molecular and Cellular Biology Research, Sunnybrook Health, Sciences Centre
2075 Bayview Avenue, Toronto, ON M4N 3M5, Canada
and
Department of Medical Biophysics, University of Toronto, S-217,2075 Bayview Avenue,
Toronto, ON M4N 3M5, Canada
e-mail: Robert.kerbel@sri.utoronto.ca

T. Meyer (ed.), *Vascular Disruptive Agents for the Treatment of Cancer*,
DOI 10.1007/978-1-4419-6609-4_6, © Springer Science+Business Media, LLC 2010

1 Introduction and Background

Vascular disrupting agents (VDAs) have been in development for two decades, i.e. ever since the first studies were published showing apparent vascular disruptive activity of various drugs such as flavone acetic acid (FAA) (Hill et al. 1989) or microtubule inhibiting chemotherapy drugs such as colchicines and vincristine (Baguley et al. 1991). Currently, there are about a dozen such drugs in clinical development, which include several randomized phase III clinical trials (Mckeage and Baguley, 2010). All of these drugs, with one exception, are microtubule inhibiting agents which depolymerize microtubules (Siemann et al. 2005; Tozer et al. 2005, 2008; Siemann et al. 2004; Patterson and Rustin 2007; Horsman and Siemann 2006; Mckeage and Baguley, 2010). The one exception, DMXAA, is thought to function primarily by induction of vascular damaging cytokines such as TNFα (Rehman and Rustin 2008). It is well known that VDAs induce a set of highly reproducible effects which are responsible for their anti-tumor efficacy. They include, first, a rapid targeting of the established but abnormal tumor vasculature, resulting in occlusion of such vessels, and hence acute shutdown of tumor blood flow. Such effects occur within hours of systemic drug administration, and are often followed by massive intratumoral hypoxia and tumor necrosis. However, almost invariably, a viable rim of tumor tissue remains, from which robust tumor regrowth/tumor cell repopulation proceeds (Siemann et al. 2005, 2004; Tozer et al. 2005, 2008; Patterson and Rustin 2007; Horsman and Siemann 2006).

One theory to account for this phenomenon is that tumor cells at the leading edge of expanding tumor mass can co-opt the normal blood vessels present in the host adjacent tissues. Such blood vessels are largely unaffected by the VDA therapy, and begin to sprout new blood vessels, i.e. induce angiogenesis, which contributes to the tumor regrowth/repopulation. As a result, much of the initial striking benefits of the VDA therapy are lost.

The repopulation phenomenon is conceptually similar in some respects to what occurs with other cytotoxic therapies, e.g. after administration of maximum tolerated dose (MTD) chemotherapy, or after radiation therapy (Kim and Tannock 2005). Such treatments are typically associated with objective tumor responses, i.e. some degree of tumor shrinkage, as a result of induction of tumor cell death, but the tumor cell repopulation that follows, which can be rapid, can compromise much of the benefit of this initial tumor cell killing effect (Kim and Tannock 2005; Hudis 2005).

The ability of tumors to repopulate is considered to be a major reason for why such tumor responses frequently only lead to minor clinical benefits in terms of prolongation of overall survival or even progression-free survival times (Kim and Tannock 2005; Hudis 2005). There is also evidence that successive cycles of cytotoxic therapies, e.g. using radiation, can be associated with progressively more rapid rates of repopulation, thus eventually leading to a state which resembles acquired drug/treatment resistance (Kim and Tannock 2005). Elucidating the underlying mechanisms responsible for rapid repopulation following cytotoxic or cytotoxic-like therapies – including VDAs – therefore assumes critical importance in improving the impact and durability of such therapies. From this perspective understanding the mechanisms responsible for repopulation from the viable tumor rim after VDA therapy could have an impact on designing new treatment strategies not only improving the efficacy of VDA therapy, but other cytotoxic therapies as well. By way of example, it is intuitive to assume that repopulation from the viable tumor rim would be driven in part through tumor angiogenesis. If so, combination of a VDA with an antiangiogenic drug would seem to be a rational and ideal effective treatment combination. In this regard, antiangiogenic drugs such as bevacizumab generally have minimal effects on established, mature tumor blood vessels (in contrast to VDAs). Therefore, the combination of an antiangiogenic with a VDA should be complementary in nature, resulting in the concurrent targeting of *both* established as well as newly forming blood vessel capillaries in tumors. This was the rationale proposed by Siemann and colleagues who were the first to report evidence that various combinations involving an antiangiogenic drug with a VDA could cause much more effective and durable anti-tumor responses in various preclinical models than either type of drug used alone (Siemann and Shi 2004, 2008). This was shown, for example, using bevacizumab with the VDA, combretastatin (CA4P) (Siemann and Shi 2008) or the antiangiogenic small molecule drug called ZD6474 (which targets VEGF and EGF receptors) with ZD6126 (a CA4P-like microtubule inhibiting VDA) (Siemann and Shi 2004; Shi and Siemann 2005).

We have extended the findings of Siemann and colleagues by showing what appears to be an additional mechanism to account for the greater anti-tumor effects achieved by combining an antiangiogenic drug with a VDA (Shaked et al. 2006). It involves the rapid induction of the mobilization of bone marrow-derived cells (BMDCs) including circulating endothelial progenitor cells (CEPs) by VDAs, which enter the peripheral blood circulation and selectively home to VDA treated tumors where they can colonize the viable tumor rim in large numbers – a site where they appear to be preferentially retained and contribute to, or amplify, tumor angiogenesis (Shaked et al. 2006). This mobilization effect begins very quickly – within a matter of hours – and appears to be driven, at least in part, by the rapid systemic induction of multiple growth factors, cytokines, and chemokines such as G-CSF, SDF-1, and VEGF (Shaked et al. 2009). The mobilization of CEPs induced by VDAs such as CA4P or a second generation prodrug derivative called OXi-4503 (Salmon and Siemann 2006) can be blocked, at least in part, by certain antiangiogenic drugs such as antibodies to VEGF receptor-2 (Shaked et al. 2006). Blunting this systemic host response therefore leads to reduced tumor angiogenesis at the viable tumor rim, and hence a greater and more durable tumor response. This process may also be accompanied by additional effects that are more 'local' in nature – though we have not studied this in any detail. For example, the vascular damaging effects of a VDA on the tumor vasculature might be amplified by a drug which compromises the pro-survival/anti-apoptotic function of VEGF, e.g. an anti-VEGF antibody, thereby increasing the extent of endothelial cell apoptosis that occurs as a result of the VDA treatment.

One of the main purposes of this review is to summarize the former mechanism in detail, i.e. the rapid mobilization of bone marrow-derived CEPs induced by

VDAs and the blockade of this response that can be brought about by antiangiogenic drugs. First, we give a brief overview of endothelial progenitor cells in tumor angiogenesis.

2 Circulating Endothelial Progenitor Cells in Tumor Angiogenesis

Over the last decade there have been a series of discoveries which have altered considerably the view of how new blood vessel capillaries may be formed, especially in tumors. The prevailing dogma up until about 1989 was that the endothelial cell 'building blocks' of newly forming capillaries were derived exclusively by the division of pre-existing fully differentiated vascular endothelial cells (Kerbel 2008). Thus 'sprouting angiogenesis' in tumors was viewed as a largely local (i.e. intra-tumoral) phenomenon. However, in 1997 Isner's group reported the existence of circulating bone marrow derived endothelial 'progenitor' cells (Asahara et al. 1997). These are cells which normally reside in the bone marrow compartment, can be mobilized quickly by certain stimuli (including pro-angiogenic growth factors such as VEGF) to enter the peripheral blood circulation and subsequently home to sites of existing angiogenesis (Bertolini et al. 2006). Here the cells are thought to adhere to newly forming capillaries and then incorporate themselves into the lumen of a growing vessel, where they differentiate into an endothelial cell (Bertolini et al. 2006). Some early, and then later studies indicated that extremely high percentages of cells (e.g. 20–50%) in a newly forming tumor associated blood vessel capillary were derived from such immigrant bone marrow derived CEPs (Asahara et al. 1997; Garcia-Barros et al. 2003; Spring et al. 2005). These cells are often defined by several markers such as VEGF receptor-2, CD13 (aminopeptidase N) or other vascular endothelial cell markers, minimal or a lack of expression of CD45 (a pan hemapoietic cell marker), and expression of a progenitor cell antigen such as CD133 in humans or CD117 (c-kit) in mice (Bertolini et al. 2006). As a result of these discoveries, there was considerable interest in studying the biology of CEPs not only with respect to their being potential mediators of tumor angiogenesis, but also as targets for antiangiogenic drugs. In addition they might be useful as possible blood-based surrogate biomarkers to help quantitate angiogenesis in vivo, i.e. as pharmacodynamic markers of response to antiangiogenic therapies. Indeed, we reported evidence that in mice, CEPs evaluated in peripheral blood by flow cytometry could indeed be used as a surrogate marker of angiogenesis, and also could be used to determine the optimal biologic dose of certain angiogenic drugs in vivo such as anti-VEGFR-2 antibodies or thrombospondin-1 peptide mimetics (Shaked et al. 2005a).

Nevertheless, the area of endothelial progenitor cell research has been and remains extremely controversial. One of the major sources of this controversy has been a number of reports from different investigators who have failed to detect significant numbers, if any at all, of CEPs in tumor associated vasculature (Peters et al. 2005; Purhonen et al. 2008; Wickersheim et al. 2009). It has been claimed that one source for the discrepancy is the failure to use state-of-the-art microscopy methodologies such as confocal microscopy when trying to detect such cells (Heil et al. 2004). Other standard microscopy methods may not be able to differentiate clearly between a cell which has an intimate perivascular location as opposed to one which has actually insinuated itself in the lumen of blood vessel (Heil et al. 2004). Thus, many cells which have been claimed to be 'CEPs' may in fact be other types of cell which have a perivascular location and can stimulate or amplify angiogenesis – but are not authentic CEPs as they were originally defined (Shaked et al. 2005a). In this regard, the failure to detect significant numbers of CEPs in tumor associated blood vessels is almost always based on various studies analyzing established tumors obtained from *untreated* (therapy-naïve) mice. In contrast, we reported (as discussed below) that administration of certain cytotoxic drugs, including VDAs (Shaked et al. 2006), or maximum tolerated dose chemotherapy using certain drugs such as paclitaxel (Shaked et al. 2008) can cause a rapid and marked increase in putative CEPs which then migrate to the drug treated tumors and appear to incorporate into some of the newly forming blood vessels, as shown in Fig. 1. It is conceivable that this rapid host response may be a consequence of vascular damage inflicted by the therapies on the tumor associated vasculature, and as such represent a manifestation of an 'SOS' host response to repair such damage. In this regard, much of the literature on the

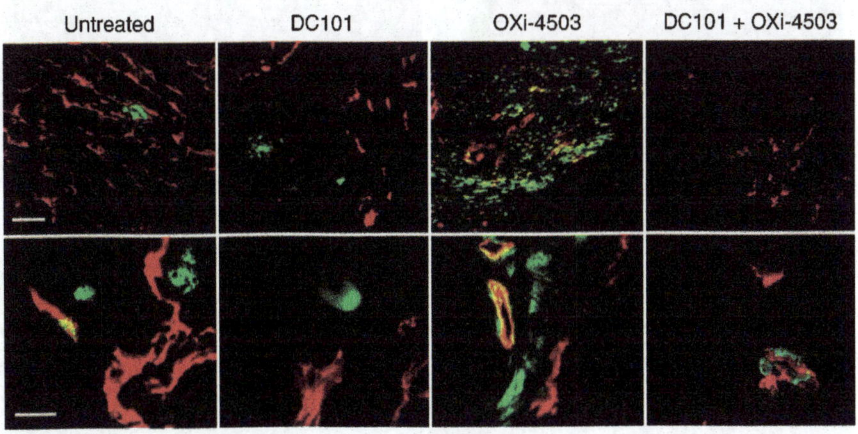

Fig. 1 Colonization of bone marrow derived cells of tumors treated with Oxi-4503. Lewis lung carcinoma grown in lethally irradiated mice that subsequently were transplanted with GFP+bone marrow tagged cells (*green*), were treated with DC101, a VEGFR-2 blocking antibody, Oxi-4503 or the combination of the two drugs. Three days after treatment with Oxi-4503 and/or DC101, tumor were removed, and stained for blood vessels using the CD31 marker (*red*). Untreated mice revealed minimal GFP+bone marrow cell incorporation to tumor blood vessels. In contrast, massive invasion of bone marrow cells to the viable tumor rim was observed in mice treated with Oxi-4503, some of which were incorporated into the tumor blood vessels. The combination of DC101 and Oxi-4503, resulted in the absence of bone marrow cells at the tumor viable rim (scale bar is 50 μm for upper images and 20 μm for lowed images)

biology of CEPs has been reported by cardiovascular researchers, often focusing on the concept that damage to the vasculature, e.g. an infarct or a stroke, can be followed by a rapid mobilization of CEPs and homing of these cells to localized areas of vascular damage which they attempt to repair (Urbich and Dimmeler 2004). This body of work is especially intriguing from the point of view of VDAs since, after all, VDAs are designed to damage the tumor vasculature. Thus if there is any type of anti-cancer drug where one might expect to see a reactive CEP host response induced, it would be VDAs. The addition of an antiangiogenic drug, e.g. anti-VEGF receptor-2 antibodies (DC101) to the VDA, e.g. OXi-4503, results in enhanced tumor necrosis, an obliterated viable tumor rim, reduced tumor blood vessel perfusion, increased hypoxia, and increased survival, as shown in Figs. 2–4.

Another consideration with respect to the rationale of combining an antiangiogenic drug with a VDA, especially one that targets the VEGF pathway such as bevacizumab, stems from the increased local (i.e. intratumoral) anti-vascular effect that such a drug combination would presumably have on tumor associated blood vessels. As

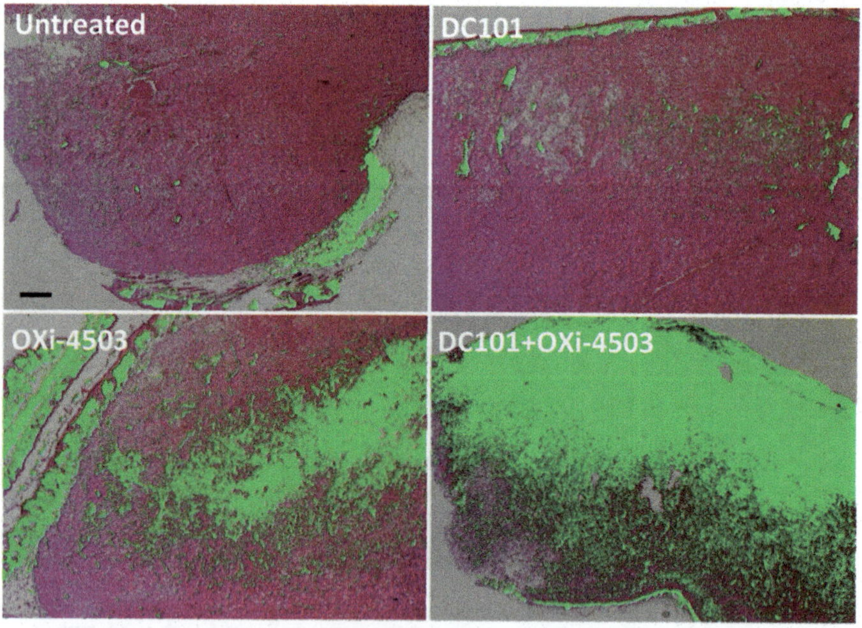

Fig. 2 Necrosis area in MeWo human melanoma tumors following treatment with Oxi-4503 and DC101. MeWo tumors were grown in nude mice that were treated with DC101, Oxi-4503 or the combination of the two drugs. Three days after treatment, tumor were removed, and sections were prepared for the evaluation of necrosis (*green*) by detecting autofluorescent areas of necrotic tissue. Untreated and DC101 treated mice revealed small necrotic areas. Treatment with Oxi-4503 demonstrated necrosis at the tumor center with a thick viable tumor tissue. Treatment with the combination of DC101 and Oxi-4503 revealed almost complete necrotic tissue with minimal residual viable tumor rim (scale bar 100 μm)

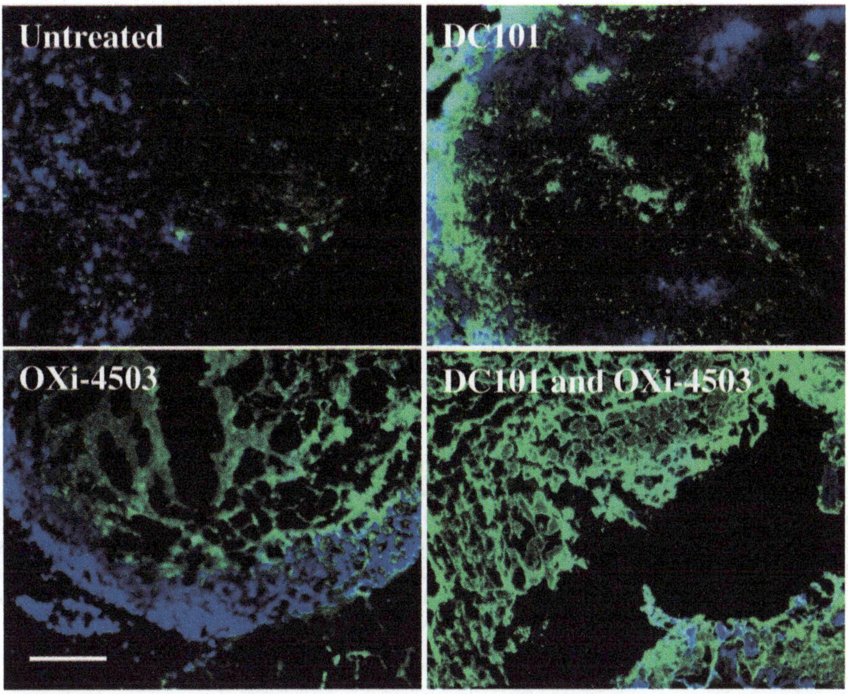

Fig. 3 Hypoxia and perfusion in MeWo tumors following treatment with Oxi-4503 and/or DC101. MeWo human melanoma tumors grown in nude mice that were subsequently treated with Oxi-4503, DC101, or the combination of the two drugs. Hypoxic (*green*) and perfused tumor area (*blue*) were detected by pimonidazole and Hoechst staining methods (respectively). Increases in blood perfusion at the viable tumor rim can be detected 3 days after treatment with Oxi-4503. The combination of DC101 and Oxi-4503 revealed a decrease in perfusion and an increase in hypoxic areas (scale bar 50 μm)

mentioned above, one of the major functions of VEGF as an angiogenesis promoting factor is to function as a pro-survival/anti-apoptotic mediator for vascular endothelial cells (Gerber et al. 1998; Nor et al. 1999). For example, VEGF can activate through VEGFR-2 the PI3 kinase – Akt survival signalling pathway in vascular endothelial cells resulting in upregulation of anti-apoptotic factors such as Bcl-2 and survivin (Gerber et al. 1998; Tran et al. 2002; Krestow et al. 1999). Consequently potential damage or cell death caused by a variety of cytotoxic drugs including VDAs, chemotherapy and radiation, may be minimized by high local concentrations of VEGF in the tumor microenvironment. Furthermore, some of these aforementioned therapies may themselves increase in a rapid manner the levels of circulating VEGF. Indeed, because of the ability of VDAs to rapidly increase tumor hypoxia and the fact that hypoxia is a major driver of VEGF expression (Semenza 2003), one might expect to detect elevated levels of VEGF in tumor tissue as well as systemically after VDA treatment. This has been observed (Shaked et al. 2009) and will also be discussed below. Consequently neutralization of the function of VEGF would appear

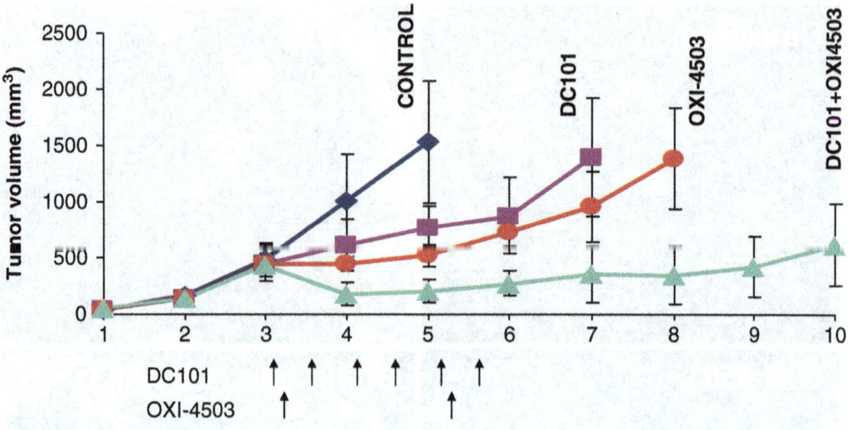

Fig. 4 Treatment efficacy of MeWo tumor-bearing nude mice following therapy with DC101 and/or Oxi-4503. Nude mice were recipients of MeWo human melanoma cells injected subdermally. When tumors reached 500 mm3, treatment was initiated with DC101 (for 3 week-period, twice weekly), 50 mg/kg OXi-4503 (only twice, every other week) or the combination of the two drugs. Tumor volumes were assessed weekly by Vernier scale calipers. The combination of DC101 and Oxi-4503 administered for a total of 3 week period resulted in enhanced treatment efficacy (error bars ± SD) Horizantal axis refers to weeks following tumor and injection

to be a logical strategy when using a VDA for the treatment of cancer. In short, one might expect to obtain an overall increased anti-vascular effect associated with abnormal, established blood vessels in tumors that are sensitive to the action of a VDA. However, this more potent anti-vascular effect might be expected to increase the aforementioned reactive bone marrow-derived cell response, but this would be prevented or minimized by the VEGF pathway targeting antiangiogenic agent (Shaked et al. 2006, 2008). Thus, the overall effect would be to increase the local intratumoral anti-vascular effect using such a two drug combination treatment strategy. The impact of VDAs on rapidly inducing increased systemic levels of VEGF is a part of a larger and emerging story not only with respect to VDAs but with other cytotoxic agents and possibly other drugs as well, namely, rapid host (as well as tumor associated) induction of multiple cytokines, chemokines, and growth factors which may act to stimulate tumor regrowth/repopulation.

In addition to the ability of antiangiogenic drugs to inhibit the host response mediated by EPC mobilization following VDA treatment, we have also investigated the potential of chemotherapy drugs administered at lower doses than the maximum tolerated dose with no extended drug free breaks (termed metronomic chemotherapy) to inhibit host bone marrow response when they are co-administered in combination with VDAs. Our previous studies indicated that metronomic chemotherapy regimens can suppress the number of EPCs in peripheral blood within 1 week of treatment (Bertolini et al. 2003; Shaked et al. 2005b). Therefore, we assumed that metronomic chemotherapy treatment combined with VDAs may inhibit the rapid spikes of EPCs following VDA treatment. Using several tumor models in mice, we showed that in

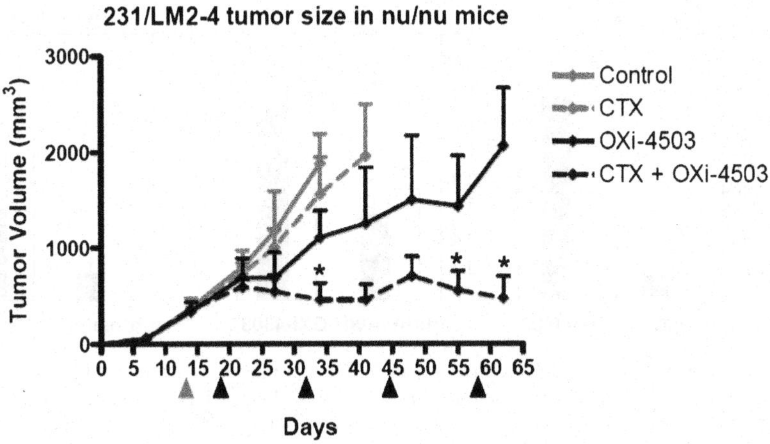

Fig. 5 The assessment of anti-tumor effect in mice treated with metronomic cyclophosphamide, OXi-4503 or a combination of both drugs. Six-to-eight-week old nude mice were implanted othotopically with 2×106 231/LM2-4 cells in their mammary fat pads. When tumor volumes reached ~400 mm³, continuous daily treatment with cyclophosphamide (CTX) and subsequently OXi-4503 every 2 weeks were initiated. Tumor sizes were assessed twice weekly by Vernier caliper measurements and tumor volumes were calculated according to the formula length×width2×0.5. *Grey arrow*, start continuous cyclophosphamide administration; *black arrows*, OXi-4503 administration. Error bars+SD. Cyclophosphamide+OXi-4503 values are compared to OXi-4503 treated mice. * $0.01 < p < 0.05$ using student's *t*-test two-tailed unpaired

both MeWo (human melanoma) and 231/LM2-4 (human breast cancer), the combination of cyclophosphamide administered orally (daily) in a metronomic chemotherapy regimen (20 mg/kg/day) and OXi-4503 can eliminate the spikes of EPCs, which subsequently resulted in decreased viable tumor rim and suppressed overall tumor growth (Fig. 5) (Daenen et al. 2009). These results suggest that both antiangiogenic drug or antiangiogenic treatment strategies when they are administered in combination with a VDA, can prolong tumor growth control and expand survival in various preclinical models.

2.1 Induction of Multiple Growth Factors, Cytokines, and Chemokines by Cytotoxic Agents, Including VDAs

A recurring finding, based on recent studies, which has implications for a number of different anti-cancer therapies is the rapid induction of multiple growth factors which can potentially act to promote tumor growth by mechanisms which may include augmenting tumor angiogenesis. Some examples from our own studies include induction of SDF-1 by maximum tolerated dose taxane therapy (Shaked et al. 2008) and a similarly rapid induction of G-CSF by VDAs such as CA4P and OXi-4503 (Shaked et al. 2009). In the case of OXi-4503, increases of up to 10–20-fold

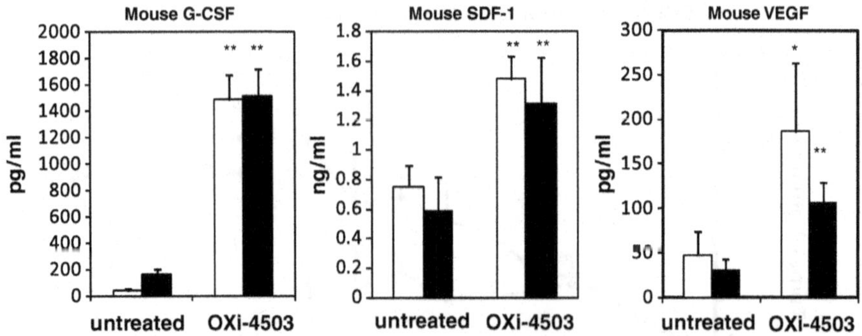

Fig. 6 Circulating mouse G-CSF, SDF-1 and VEGF plasma levels in tumor-free and MeWo tumor-bearing nude mice 4 h after treatment with OXi-4503. Plasma levels of mouse G-CSF, SDF-1, and VEGF were obtained from tumor-free (*open bars*), or tumor-bearing mice (*filled bars*), 4 h after treatment with OXi-4503. Mice treated with Oxi-4503 revealed a tenfold increase in G-CSF plasma levels, as well as increases in both SDF-1 and VEGF plasma levels. $P<0.01$ (**) or $0.05<P<0.01$ (*)

of circulating G-CSF in the plasma of normal mice treated with a single dose of the drug can be observed within 4 h of treatment (Shaked et al. 2009), as shown in Fig. 6. The source of the G-CSF has not been determined. Other growth factors including VEGF, as mentioned above, can be induced as well, and some of this VEGF increase may be independent of VDA induction of elevated tumor hypoxia. For example, VEGF or other growth factor inductions can be observed in VDA treated tumor free mice (Shaked et al. 2009), and can occur very rapidly, before any evidence of elevated tumor hypoxia. In the case of OXi-4503-induced G-CSF, evidence has also been obtained preclinically that this effect contributes to the rapid mobilization of bone marrow derived CEPs. Thus, OXi-4503 treatment of G-CSF receptor deficient tumor-bearing mice results in significant increases in necrotic tumor area probably due to the lack of CEP spikes (Shaked et al. 2009), as shown in Fig. 7. In this regard, G-CSF has been shown to mobilize proangiogenic bone marrow derived circulating cells of various types, including endothelial progenitor cells (Powell et al. 2005) as well as CD11bGr1+ myeloid suppressor-type cells (Shojaei and Ferrara 2008). We would note that G-CSF may be only a 'secondary' molecular mediator accounting for VDA-induced CEP mobilization, since we found that SDF-1 is downregulated in G-CSF–/– mice that were treated with Oxi-4503. In addition we have already reported that in the case of MTD chemotherapy treatment, taxane-induced CEP mobilization is mainly driven by induction of SDF-1 plasma levels. Thus, when SDF-1 was neutralized, we could not detect a spike following treatment with taxanes. There is also clinical evidence for induction in CEP levels following treatment with VDAs, as patients treated with CA4P showed a twofold increases in SDF-1, as well as G-CSF and VEGF plasma levels (see below, next section). In summary, the induction of factors such as VEGF, SDF-1, and G-CSF may promote a more rapid recovery/repopulation of tumor bearing hosts treated with agents such as CA4P, OXi-4503, or other VDAs. Part of

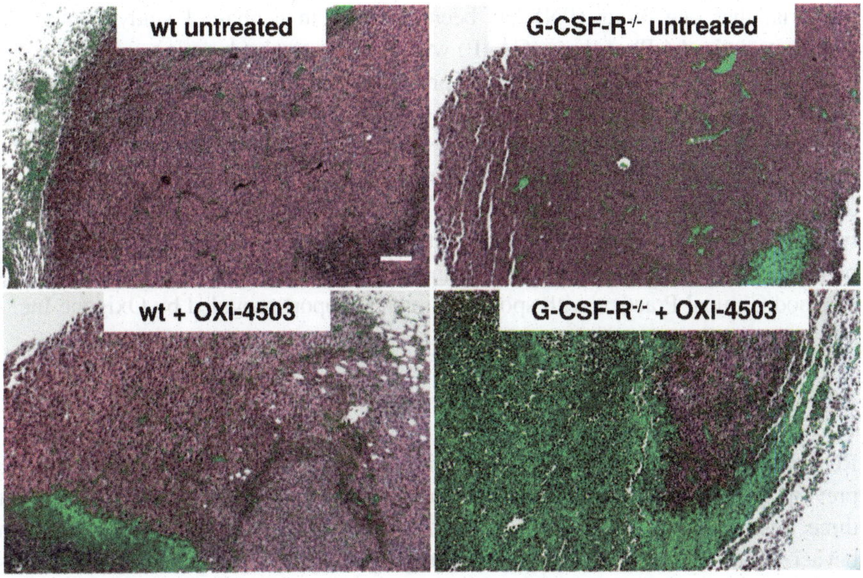

Fig. 7 Relative tumor necrosis detected in G-CSF-R–/– mice following treatment with OXi-4503. Lewis Lung carcinoma grown in either G-CSF-R–/– or wildtype (wt) control mice were removed 3 days following treatment with Oxi-4503. Tumor sections were evaluated for necrosis determined by autofluorescence of necrotic tissue. Significant increases in necrotic areas were observed in tumors grown in G-CSF-R–/– mice 3 days after treatment with Oxi-4503 (bar = 100 μm)

this effect may be due to the increased mobilization of bone marrow derived circulating proangiogenic cells induced by such growth factor alterations. Some of these preclinical observations can be easily verified in clinical studies. For example, patients treated with a VDA can have blood drawn at baseline/pre-treatment times, or within 4 or 24 h after treatment and evaluated for similar changes. This type of analysis has been done and is discussed in the next and final section.

2.2 *Clinical Studies of Combination Vascular Disruptive Agent and Antiangiogenics*

As described above, preclinical data demonstrated a rationale for combining VDA and antiangiogenic therapy. Experimental data also supported the hypothesis that the surviving rim of VDA treated tumors became populated with bone marrow derived endothelial precursor cells, which contributed to the post-treatment angiogenesis seen in this region. VEGF receptor neutralizing antibody in mouse models reduced the influx of bone marrow derived progenitors.

There are at least three ongoing or completed trials involving an antiangiogenic drug combined with a VDA, sometimes with chemotherapy (www.clinicaltrials.gov).

One trial that one of us (PN) has been involved in a phase I study combining Combretastatin A4 Phosphate (CA4P) with Bevacizumab (Avastin).

We aimed to assess the toxicity and preliminary clinical activity of the combination whilst also performing a variety of translational studies designed to (a) interrogate the in vivo effect of the two drugs in combination on the tumor vascular bed using functional imaging and (b) gather information regarding the effects of the two drug combination on other biomarkers of angiogenesis. The study was conducted at two UK centres – Mount Vernon Hospital and The Royal Marsden Hospital. All patients gave written informed consent and the study was conducted to the standards of Good Clinical Practice with sponsorship and support provided by Oxigene Inc.

2.2.1 Study Design

Recommended doses of both CA4P (63 mg/m^2) and bevacizumab (10 mg/m^2) were previously defined. We therefore performed a limited dose escalation of CA4P at three dose levels of 45 mg/m^2, 54 mg/m^2 and 63 mg/m^2 in combination with bevacizumab at a constant dose of 10 mg/kg every 2 weeks. Bevacizumab was administered 4 h after CA4P. Patients with advanced solid malignancies refractory to standard treatment were recruited in cohorts of three to each dose level. If no dose limiting toxicity (DLT) was seen, the next dose level was opened. In the event of a DLT being seen, the cohort was expanded to six patients. The final cohort of CA4P 63 mg/m^2 and bevacizumab 10 mg/kg contained six patients.

The study schema is outlined in Fig. 8. Two baseline DCE-MRI scans were performed during the week before any therapy commenced. This was to allow interscan variability to be assessed. One week before combination treatment was initiated patients received a single dose of CA4P. DCE-MRI scans were performed pre-treatment and 3 h post treatment. Translational cellular and biochemical assays were also performed. The schedule was repeated the following week when combination

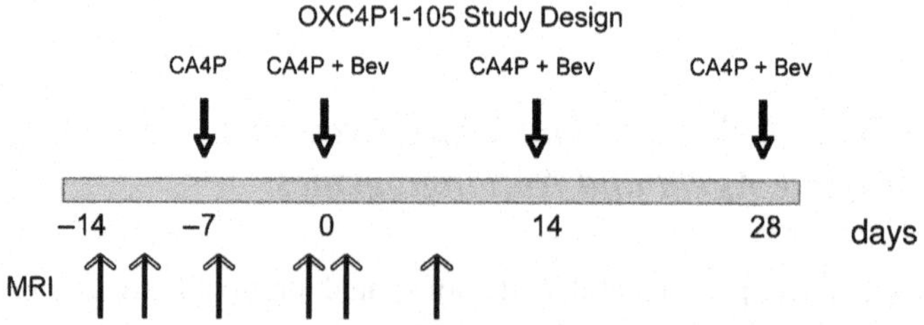

Fig. 8 OXC4P1-105 Study design. Treatment and MRI schedule. Patients received a single dose of CA4P followed 1 week later by combination therapy with CA4P and bevacizumab. CA4P was administered first, followed by bevacizumab 4 h later. This schedule was repeated every 2 weeks. Two baseline DCE-MRI scans were performed in the week before treatment started, 3 h after first CA4P dose, 6 days later and then 3 h after second CA4P dose (1 h before bevacizumab) and 6 days later. Treatment continued fortnightly until evidence of disease progression or development of dose limiting toxicity

treatment commenced. DCE-MRI scans were performed pre-treatment, 3 h after CA4P (this was followed by bevacizumab treatment at 4 h) and 6 days post treatment. This allowed a comparison of the pharmacodynamic effects of single agent VDA and combination treatment with VDA plus antiangiogenic agent.

2.2.2 Patient Population

Fifteen patients gave informed consent and went on to receive treatment. The demographics, diagnosis and cohort allocation are shown in Table 1. Principal inclusion criteria were standard for Phase I studies and stipulated good end organ function. Study specific exclusion criteria were history of ischemic heart disease, radical radiotherapy to thorax or abdomen, squamous cell lung cancer, anti-coagulation and therapeutic use of drugs which prolonged QTc interval.

2.2.3 Results

Adverse event profile, translational endpoints and clinical activity will be reported in full elsewhere. No dose limiting toxicities however were seen and the combination of CA4P (63 mg/m^2) followed by bevacizumab (10 mg/m^2) 4 h later on a two weekly cycle was deliverable.

Two major conclusions were drawn from the translational studies. Firstly, DCE-MRI reductions in Ktrans were sustained at 6 days in the presence of bevacizumab whereas they reversed to normal by 6 days when treated with CA4P alone (Table 2). Secondly, a rise in circulating bone marrow-defined progenitor (CD34 or CD133 positive) cells post CA4P exposure was seen which entirely supported the preclinical observations of

Table 1 Study population

Study No	Cohort	Sex	Age	Diagnosis	PS
01-0001	45 mg/m^2	F	49	Ocular melanoma	0
02-0001	45 mg/m^2	F	46	Ovarian neuroendocrine Ca	1
02-0002	45 mg/m^2	F	62	Ovarian papillary adenoca	0
01-0002	54 mg/m^2	M	56	Renal carcinoma	0
02-0003	54 mg/m^2	F	61	Ovarian serous Ca	0
02-0004	54 mg/m^2	M	72	Colon Ca	0
02-0005	54 mg/m^2	F	50	Colon Ca	0
01-0003	63 mg/m^2	F	40	Melanoma	1
02-0006	63 mg/m^2	M	52	Ca rectum	1
01-0004	63 mg/m^2	F	44	Melanoma	1
02-0008	63 mg/m^2	M	80	Ca colon	1
01-0005	63 mg/m^2	F	51	Carcinoma of breast	1
02-0010	63 mg/m^2	M	60	Adenocarcinoma of rectum	1
02-0012	63 mg/m^2	F	63	Ovarian serous cystadenoca	1
02-0009	63 mg/m^2	F	28	Haemangiosarcoma of breast	2

Table 2 Reduction in DCE-MRI Ktrans in patients receiving either CA4P alone or CA4P + Bevacizumab

95% CI for significant reduction	3 h post CA4P	6 days post CA4P	3 h post second CA4P	6 days post CA4P + Bevacizumab
–5.0%	–26.4%	+5.4%	–32.0%	–36.6%

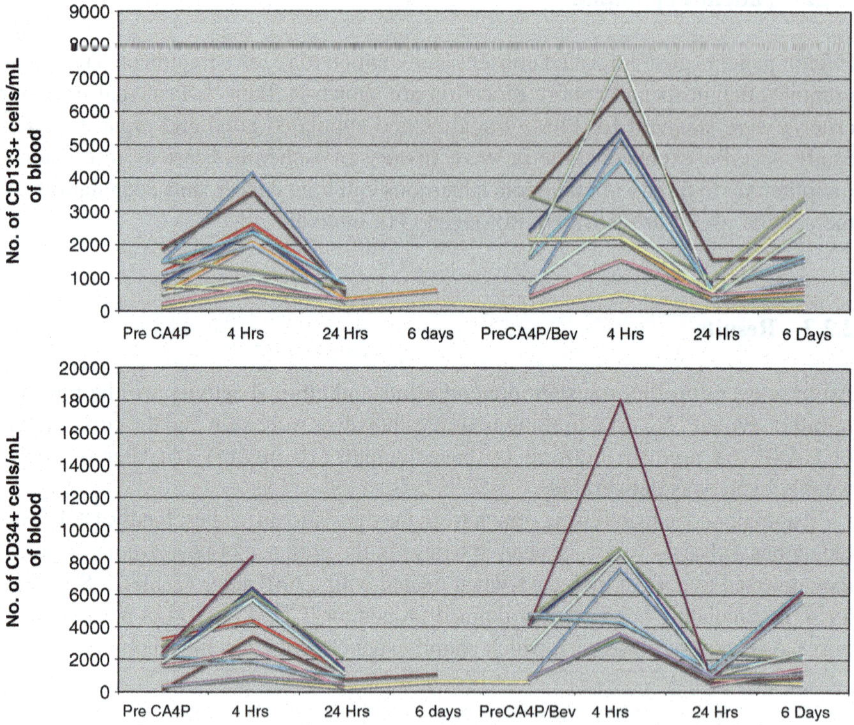

Fig. 9 Circulating CD34 and CD133 expressing bone marrow progenitor cells levels following CA4P or CA4P ± bevacizumab exposure. Individual patient curves for circulating CD34+ and CD133+ bone marrow derived progenitors. An increase in circulating cells was seen at 4 h after each exposure to CA4P

Shaked et al. (Shaked et al. 2006) as shown in Fig. 9. This was associated with a rise in plasma VEGF and G-CSF, again mirroring preclinical observations (Fig. 10).

DCE-MRI data is summarized in Table 2. Ninety-five percent confidence intervals for a significant reduction were calculated for the group as a whole with data from the two pre-treatment baseline scans. A reduction in Ktrans of greater than 5% for the group was statistically significant. After exposure to single agent CA4P, a significant reduction in Ktrans of 26.4% was seen which resolved to baseline by day 6. An equivalent reduction of 32% was seen after second exposure to CA4P following which patients received bevacizumab. At 6 days the reduction in Ktrans was still 36.6%, implying the reduction in Ktrans induced by CA4P was maintained by bevacizumab.

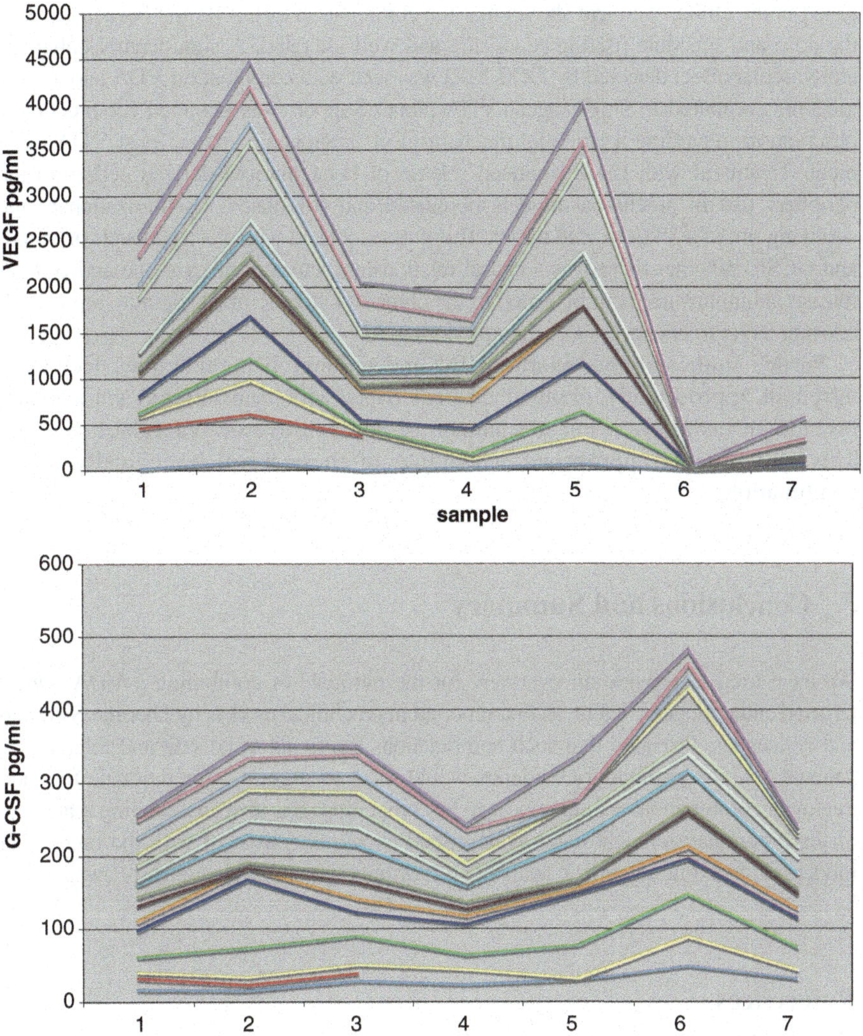

Fig. 10 Plasma VEGF and GCSF following CA4P or CA4P ± bevacizumab. Individual patient curves for Plasma VEGF and GCSF levels following CA4P and CA4P + bevacizumab exposure. The levels of both growth factors increased following VDA exposure

Changes in circulating CD34 and CD133 expressing bone marrow progenitors are shown in Fig. 9. The peak in circulating progenitors was an acute event and had resolved by 24 h post treatment. A rise in both populations was seen after exposure to CA4P. An equivalent rise was seen after exposure to the second dose of CA4P. This was associated with a rise in plasma VEGF and GCSF (Fig. 10) which paralleled the changes seen in these cytokines in preclinical models.

The strong rationale and preclinical supportive evidence for combination therapy with vascular disruptive agents and antiangiogenics require the combination to be actively tested in the clinic. We have shown that the combination of CA4P and bevacizumab at the dose and schedule used appears safe and well tolerated. A significantly enhanced anti-vascular effect detected by DCE-MRI was seen with combination VDA and antiangiogenic compared to single agent VDA alone. Support was obtained for preclinical observations regarding a potential mechanism of 'angiogenic escape' post VDA treatment. Treatment with CA4P induced release of bone marrow derived cells into the periphery that in preclinical models populated and stimulated vascularization of the surviving rim of a VDA treated tumor. This was associated with elevated levels of VEGF and GCSF. Whether there was a causal relationship between the cytokine and cellular release in humans needs to be tested in the clinic as cytokine blockade may represent a relevant target to enhance VDA therapy.

Further studies of combination VDA and antiangiogenic therapies need to be tested in appropriately planned clinical trials with translational studies that provide an insight into the mechanism of any additive or synergistic activity. This will instruct appropriate scheduling of these novel biologically active combinations.

3 Conclusions and Summary

We have tried to provide an overview for the rationale of combining a VDA with a targeted antiangiogenic agent, as first reported in preclinical models by Dietmar Siemann and colleagues. Provided that such combinations are found to be safe and tolerable in patients – which preliminary evidence would seem to suggest – the rationale for such treatment combinations would appear to be compelling. It is also encouraging that some of the preliminary clinical data, as described above, is consistent with the preclinical model findings. Future clinical trials of such drug combinations are eagerly awaited.

References

Asahara T, Murohara T, Sullivan A, Silver M, van der Zee R, Li T, et al. Isolation of putative progenitor endothelial cells for angiogenesis. Science 1997;275:964–7.

Baguley BC, Holdaway KM, Thomsen LL, Zhuang L, Zwi LJ. Inhibition of growth of colon 38 adenocarcinoma by vinblastine and colchicine: evidence for a vascular mechanism. Eur J Cancer 1991;27:482–7.

Bertolini F, Paul S, Mancuso P, Monestiroli S, Gobbi A, Shaked Y, et al. Maximum tolerable dose and low-dose metronomic chemotherapy have opposite effects on the mobilization and viability of circulating endothelial progenitor cells. Cancer Res 2003;63:4342–6.

Bertolini F, Shaked Y, Mancuso P, Kerbel RS. The multifaceted circulating endothelial cell in cancer: from promiscuity to surrogate marker and target identification. Nature Rev Cancer 2006;6:835–45.

Daenen LG, Shaked Y, Man S, Xu P, Voest EE, Hoffman RM, et al. Low-dose metronomic cyclophosphamide combined with vascular disrupting therapy induces potent anti-tumor activity in preclinical human tumor xenograft models. Mol Cancer Ther 2009;8:2872–81.

Garcia-Barros M, Paris F, Cordon-Cardo C, Lyden D, Rafii S, Haimovitz-Friedman A, et al. Tumor response to radiotherapy regulated by endothelial cell apoptosis. Science 2003;300:1155–9.

Gerber HP, McMurtrey A, Kowalski J, Yan M, Keyt BA, Dixit V, et al. Vascular endothelial growth factor regulates endothelial cell survival through the phosphatidylinositol 3 -kinase/Akt signal transduction pathway. Requirement for Flk-1/KDR activation. J Biol Chem 1998;273:30336–43.

Heil M, Ziegelhoeffer T, Mees B, Schaper W. A different outlook on the role of bone marrow stem cells in vascular growth: bone marrow delivers software not hardware. Circ Res 2004;94:573–4.

Hill S, Williams KB, Denekamp J. Vascular collapse after flavone acetic acid: a possible mechanism of its anti-tumour action. Eur J Cancer Clin Oncol 1989;25:1419–24.

Horsman MR, Siemann DW. Pathophysiologic effects of vascular-targeting agents and the implications for combination with conventional therapies. Cancer Res 2006;66:11520–39.

Hudis CA. Clinical implications of antiangiogenic therapies. Oncology 2005;19:26–31.

Kerbel RS. Tumor angiogenesis. New Engl J Med 2008;358:2039–49.

Kim JJ, Tannock IF. Repopulation of cancer cells during therapy: an important cause of treatment failure. Nat Rev Cancer 2005;5:516–25.

Krestow JK, Rak J, Filmus J, Kerbel RS. Functional dissociation of anoikis-like cell death and activity of stress activated protein kinase. Biochem Biophys Res Commun 1999;260:48–53.

McKeague MJ, Baguley BC. Disrupting established tumor blood vessels. Cancer 2010;116: 1859–71.

Nor JE, Christensen J, Mooney DJ, Polverini PJ. Vascular endothelial growth factor (VEGF)-mediated angiogenesis is associated with enhanced endothelial cell survival and induction of Bcl-2 expression. Am J Pathol 1999;154:375–81.

Patterson DM, Rustin GJ. Vascular damaging agents. Clin Oncol (R Coll Radiol) 2007;19:443–56.

Peters BA, Diaz LA, Polyak K, Meszler L, Romans K, Guinan EC, et al. Contribution of bone marrow-derived endothelial cells to human tumor vasculature. Nat Med 2005;11:261–2.

Powell TM, Paul JD, Hill JM, Thompson M, Benjamin M, Rodrigo M, et al. Granulocyte colony-stimulating factor mobilizes functional endothelial progenitor cells in patients with coronary artery disease. Arterioscler Thromb Vasc Biol 2005;25:296–301.

Purhonen S, Palm J, Rossi D, Kaskenpaa N, Rajantie I, Yla-Herttuala S, et al. Bone marrow-derived circulating endothelial precursors do not contribute to vascular endothelium and are not needed for tumor growth. Proc Natl Acad Sci U S A 2008;105:6620–5.

Rehman F, Rustin G. ASA404: update on drug development. Expert Opin Investig Drugs 2008;17:1547–51.

Salmon HW, Siemann DW. Effect of the second-generation vascular disrupting agent OXi4503 on tumor vascularity. Clin Cancer Res 2006;12:4090–4.

Semenza GL. Targeting HIF-1 for cancer therapy. Nat Rev Cancer 2003;3:721–32.

Shaked Y, Bertolini F, Man S, Rogers MS, Cervi D, Foutz T, et al. Genetic heterogeneity of the vasculogenic phenotype parallels angiogenesis: implications for cellular surrogate marker analysis of antiangiogenesis. Cancer Cell 2005;7:101–11.

Shaked Y, Emmengger U, Man S, Cervi D, Bertolini F, Ben-David Y, et al. The optimal biological dose of metronomic chemotherapy regimens is associated with maximum antiangiogenic activity. Blood 2005;106:3058–61.

Shaked Y, Ciarrocchi A, Franco M, Lee CR, Man S, Cheung AM, et al. Therapy-induced acute recruitment of circulating endothelial progenitor cells to tumors. Science 2006;313:1785–7.

Shaked Y, Henke E, Roodhart J, Mancuso P, Langenberg M, Colleoni M, et al. Rapid chemotherapy-induced surge in endothelial progenitor cells: implications for antiangiogenic drugs as chemosensitizing agents. Cancer Cell 2008;14:263–73.

Shaked Y, Tang T, Woloszynek J, Daenen L, Man S, Xu P, et al. Contribution of G-CSF to the acute mobilization of endothelial precursor cells by vascular disrupting agents. Cancer Res 2009;69:7524–8.

Shi W, Siemann DW. Targeting the tumor vasculature: enhancing antitumor efficacy through combination treatment with ZD6126 and ZD6474. In Vivo 2005;19:1045–50.

Shojaei F, Ferrara N. Refractoriness to antivascular endothelial growth factor treatment: role of myeloid cells. Cancer Res 2008;68:5501–4.

Siemann DW, Shi W. Efficacy of combined antiangiogenic and vascular disrupting agents in treatment of solid tumors. Int J Radiat Oncol Biol Phys 2004;60:1233–40.

Siemann DW, Shi W. Dual targeting of tumor vasculature: combining Avastin and vascular disrupting agents (CA4P or OXi4503). Anticancer Res 2008;28:2027–31.

Siemann DW, Chaplin DJ, Horsman MR. Vascular-targeting therapies for treatment of malignant disease. Cancer 2004;100:2491–9.

Siemann DW, Bibby MC, Dark GG, Dicker AP, Eskens FA, Horsman MR, et al. Differentiation and definition of vascular-targeted therapies. Clin Cancer Res 2005;11:416–20.

Spring H, Schuler T, Arnold B, Hammerling GJ, Ganss R. Chemokines direct endothelial progenitors into tumor neovessels. Proc Natl Acad Sci U S A 2005;102:18111–6.

Tozer GM, Kanthou C, Baguley BC. Disrupting tumour blood vessels. Nat Rev Cancer 2005;5:423–35.

Tozer GM, Kanthou C, Lewis G, Prise VE, Vojnovic B, Hill SA. Tumour vascular disrupting agents: combating treatment resistance. Br J Radiol 2008;81:S12–S20.

Tran J, Master Z, Yu J, Rak J, Dumont DJ, Kerbel RS. A role for survivin in chemoresistance of endothelial cells mediated by VEGF. Proc Natl Acad Sci U S A 2002;99:4349–54.

Urbich C, Dimmeler S. Endothelial progenitor cells: characterization and role in vascular biology. Circ Res 2004;95:343–53.

Wickersheim A, Kerber M, de Miguel LS, Plate KH, Machein MR. Endothelial progenitor cells do not contribute to tumor endothelium in primary and metastatic tumors. Int J Cancer 2009;125:1771–7.

Part II
Imaging in the Development of Vascular Disruptive Agents

MRI to Assess Vascular Disruptive Agents

Martin Zweifel and Anwar R. Padhani

Abstract A number of clinically applicable imaging techniques are able to assess the antivascular effects of antiangiogenic drugs and vascular disruptive agents (VDAs) via changes induced in functional kinetic parameters. These techniques include dynamic contrast enhanced magnetic resonance imaging (DCE-MRI), dynamic susceptibility enhanced MRI, diffusion MRI, positron emission tomography (PET) with oxygen labelled water, perfusion/functional computed tomography (CT) and microbubble enhanced ultrasound. Each of these techniques yield quantitative or semi-quantitative kinetic parameters which can be related to blood flow, blood volume, extraction fraction, and vessel permeability. Changes in some of these imaging biomarkers can be used during the drug development process because they can serve as pharmacodynamic indicators of vascular activity in vivo. In this chapter, we discuss imaging techniques for the assessment of tumour vascularity that have been used to assess VDAs in clinical studies, with an emphasis on magnetic resonance imaging (MRI) methods.

1 Introduction

The clinical development of drugs in oncology traditionally involves the assessment of dose-limiting toxicity (DLT) and maximum tolerated dose (MTD) in phase I trials by dose escalation, based on the paradigm that the highest applicable dose will result in the greatest anti-tumour effect. MTD is then taken forward into single-arm phase II trials with response rate as primary endpoint. This paradigm appears outdated for drugs with novel anticancer therapies such as vascular disruptive agents (VDAs) for a number of reasons including: (1) in experimental tumours it has been shown that most VDAs are active at doses well below the MTD, (2) some dose limiting toxicities (DLTs) may not be related to vascular disruptive

M. Zweifel (✉)
Department of Oncology, Mount Vernon Cancer Centre, Rickmansworth Road, Northwood, Middlesex, HA6 2RN, UK
e-mail: martin.zweifel@doctors.org.uk

T. Meyer (ed.), *Vascular Disruptive Agents for the Treatment of Cancer*,
DOI 10.1007/978-1-4419-6609-4_7,

activity, (3) vascular disruptive activity as single agents might not readily translate into anti-tumour efficacy when used in combination therapy, (4) efficacy of VDA treatment appears to vary between tumour types, stage and between patients and, (5) clinical experience shows that VDAs have significant toxicity including tumour pain, fistula formation and neuropathy with a narrow safety window. Thus, optimal treatment with VDAs requires information on the biology and functional status of the tumour vasculature before and during therapy. Non-invasive, imaging characterization of the angiogenic status of specific tumours may allow rational selection of VDAs treatments in terms of appropriateness, for dose selection and scheduling.

A number of clinically applicable imaging techniques are able to assess the antivascular effects of VDAs via changes induced in functional kinetic parameters. These techniques include dynamic contrast enhanced MRI (DCE-MRI), dynamic susceptibility enhanced MRI (DSC-MRI), diffusion MRI, PET with oxygen labelled water, perfusion/functional CT and microbubble enhanced ultrasound. Each of these techniques yield quantitative or semi-quantitative kinetic parameters which can be related to blood flow, blood volume, extraction fraction, and vessel permeability. Changes in some of these imaging biomarkers can be used during the drug development process because they can serve as pharmacodynamic indicators of vascular activity in vivo. Such functional imaging techniques have found roles in early drug development (pre-clinical and phase I) whereas morphological imaging methods have maintained their dominance for later phase clinical studies. Thus, in the twenty-first century, phase I studies now go beyond defining pharmacokinetics (PK) and MTD, with hypothesis testing on mode of action of drugs becoming normal. The information gained using PD biomarkers can be used for internal decision making on compound development, either to drop failing compounds or to accelerate development of promising agents. In order to achieve these aims it is first necessary to understand clearly clinical/pharmaceutical goals and to define corresponding objectives to be met by PD biomarkers. Thus, objectives in pre-clinical and early clinical studies that deploy imaging biomarkers could include:

1. To demonstrate mechanism of action in vivo usually via modulation of kinetic parameters when the drug is given.
2. To show drug dose–vascular response relationships which can in turn enable the definition of a biologically active dose.
3. To identify the therapeutic dose window, which lies between the MTD (clinically defined) and biologically active dose (imaging defined). If in vivo studies are well conducted then it may also be possible to define a dosing schedule to be taken into phase II.
4. To demonstrate drug exposure-tumour efficacy relationships by correlating pharmacokinetics (blood concentration of the drug) with pharmacodynamic measurements.

In this chapter, we discuss imaging techniques for the assessment of tumour vascularity that have been used to assess VDAs in clinical studies. A review of the literature shows that the majority of clinical studies have used MRI methods; this will therefore be the major focus of this chapter. We begin by describing the biological basis for the most commonly used in vivo MRI technique (i.e. DCE-MRI). We show how imaging data are acquired, give a brief outline of the quantification process, lay out an understanding of the physiological meaning of biomarkers that can be obtained and finally discuss the results obtained from their use in the early clinical development of VDAs. The observations made on MRI are compared to those seen on functional CT and with perfusion PET imaging where appropriate. As we look to the future, readers will also be introduced to new opportunities brought on by the improved ability of MRI to acquire multiple, biologically relevant parameters, quantitatively, in a spatial and time resolved way. These multiparametric MRI can then be used to explore secondary effects of VDAs on the tumour microenvironment (pH, oxygenation, interstitial fluid pressure) or on cellular metabolic disruption (changes in energetics, proliferation rates, cell death).

2 Imaging the Vascularity of Tissues: Comparison of Methods

Various modalities can be used to demonstrate the physiology of tumour angiogenesis, each technique bringing its own advantages and disadvantages. Both CT and MRI have the advantage of good spatial resolution, they are minimally invasive, and are more widely available than PET scanners. CT, PET and SPECT all expose patients to ionising radiation, which can be problematic when repeat serial follow-up studies are needed to monitor treatment response.

CT has the advantage of producing images in which the attenuation (measured in Hounsfield units) is directly proportional to the iodine concentration of the contrast medium, which allows accurate quantification and facilitates comparisons between centres. Dynamic CT can be used for imaging the functionality of microvessel and has basic principles in common with DCE-MRI. It sequentially images an anatomical region as contrast media passes through it, and information on blood flow/volume, mean transit time and capillary permeability are derived from the enhancement patterns observed. To date there has only been limited research involving dynamic CT to study VDAs, in part due to the concerns over radiation exposure related to repeated imaging.

Ultrasound, depending on the technique used, can image vascular structures down to sizes of 40 μm in diameter (Ferrara et al. 2000). Contrast-enhanced ultrasound is becoming more widely used and makes use of microbubbles which are generally several microns in diameter. Their relatively large size compared to conventional CT or MR contrast media means that they remain confined within the vascular space, allowing measurement of perfusion and blood volume. Additionally, the microbubbles can be destroyed by ultrasound energy, enabling vessel re-fill rates to be assessed. However, there are certain anatomical regions such as the lung and brain that are poorly accessible by ultrasound, and the technique, which appears very promising, remains operator-dependent.

PET has many highly desirable properties including high sensitivity. PET studies require cyclotron-produced radioisotopes, which decay by positron emission.

Isotopes used for PET imaging have short half-lives, i.e. oxygen-15 (^{15}O; ~2 min), nitrogen-13 (^{13}N; 10 min), carbon-11 (^{11}C; 20 min), and Fluorine-18 (^{18}F; 110 min). These isotopes act as tracers, which are incorporated into biomolecules. Examples relevant to angiogenesis imaging include ^{15}O-water and ^{11}C-carbon monoxide for estimating bulk tumour blood flow and red cell blood volume, respectively. ^{15}O is particularly difficult to use because of its short half-life, which necessitates an onsite cyclotron with a radiopharmaceutical laboratory for its production. Both ^{15}O-water and ^{11}C-carbon monoxide PET are performed in dynamic mode, so limiting the volume of tissue that can be evaluated. ^{18}F, due to its prolonged half-life, is more widely used, particularly linked to deoxy-glucose (^{18}FDG) to assess glucose metabolism within tumours. Recent research has centred on the use of ^{18}F labelled targets of angiogenic markers such as ^{18}F-labelled RGD (i.e. arginine-glycine-aspartic acid) glycopeptides to target endothelial cells expressing the $\alpha_v\beta_3$ integrin (Zhang et al. 2006); this is a static whole body technique. The fact that PET tracers have the ability to measure picomolar concentrations of molecules makes them suitably sensitive to detect markers of angiogenesis within tumours. However, the poorer spatial resolution, expense, limited availability of radiochemistry, cyclotrons and scanners, and radiation dose are significant barriers to the routine clinical use of PET techniques for angiogenesis imaging.

Combining more than one modality in the same imaging session may help to overcome the disadvantages of the individual techniques by maximizing information content. The most pertinent current example of such a hybrid technology is PET-CT, which combines the sensitive, functional imaging of PET with the anatomical information and spatial resolution of CT. The problem of aligning datasets from separate PET and CT scans is overcome by dual PET-CT scanners; additionally, CT can be used for attenuation correction of the PET data. Recently, a number of studies have begun to explore the relationship between tumour blood flow (measured by the CT component of PET-CT scanners) and glucose metabolism [reviewed in Miles and Williams (2008)]. These studies show high variability in the coupling of blood flow and metabolism depending in part on spatial location with tumours, tumour type, size and stage. The biological meaning and patient significance of the decoupling between perfusion and glucose metabolism is not completely understood but it has been noted that the adaptive response (low flow and high glucose uptake) is associated with poorer therapy outcomes for some patient groups such as those with breast cancer and non-small cell lung cancer, presumably because the tumours are hypoxic. Such flow metabolic relationships have not yet been studied in the clinic in response to therapy with VDAs.

3 MRI for Assessing Tissue Vascularity

There are numerous MRI ways of assessing the functional properties tissue vasculature including techniques that make use of exogenously administered contrast agents. A full discussion of these techniques is outside the scope of this chapter and interested readers are directed to a recent review of these methods (Oostendorp et al. 2009). In this chapter, we focus on contrast enhanced MRI methods that use low-molecular weight contrast agents because this is the most commonly used clinical imaging technique.

3.1 Biological Basis for Observations of Dynamic MRI

Dynamic MRI involves the acquisition of serial images before, during, and after the intravenous injection of a contrast agent. MR contrast agents leak at variable rates through the vasculature, with leakage rates being dependent on the charge and size of the contrast medium molecules relative to the size of vascular pores. The temporal resolution requirements of dynamic MRI techniques are related to how quickly the contrast medium leaves the vascular compartment. Thus, temporal resolutions for small molecular weight contrast media are relatively fast (in the order of 5–20 s), whereas for larger contrast agents, temporal resolutions in the order of 1–2 min maybe adequate.

Clinical dynamic MRI is usually performed using low molecular weight gadolinium-chelate-based contrast agents (molecular weight [MW] < 1,000 Da). When these contrast agents are used, two distinct phenomena can be observed, depending on the experimental set-up. Dynamic relaxivity-based contrast techniques use a rapid series of T1-weighted images to observe the passage of contrast media, usually resulting in tissue 'brightening'; by default, this technique is referred to as DCE-MRI. This technique is sensitive to the presence of contrast medium both within vessels and in the extravascular, extracellular space – the latter predominates due to the low blood volumes in tissues and tumours (approximately 5–10%). Conversely, if very fast (every 1–2 s) susceptibility weighted or T2*-weighted sequences are used to monitor the effects of contrast medium passage, transient 'darkening' of tissue is observed during the first and second pass of contrast media through tissues, because the technique is sensitive to the presence of concentrated contrast medium within the vascular space. This technique is usually referred to as dynamic susceptibility weighted MRI (DSC-MRI).

For full data quantification (see below), it is usually necessary to obtain, or to estimate, an arterial input function (AIF) (Fig. 1). This can be achieved by measuring signal changes in arteries near to the anatomical location of the organ/tissue or tumour being studied. This can be performed before or at the same time as the dynamic data acquisitions. If accurately measured, the AIF helps to compensate for changes related to the rate of injection and the cardiac output of patients. To enable quantification of signal changes, it is necessary to incorporate methods that allow concentration of contrast agent to be obtained at each time point during the measurement period (as already noted, this is intrinsic for dynamic CT). For DCE-MRI, this is often done by obtaining 'T1 maps' prior to contrast medium injection, which effectively allows conversion of the MR signal intensity into contrast agent concentration. For DSC-MRI, conversion of signal changes into contrast agent

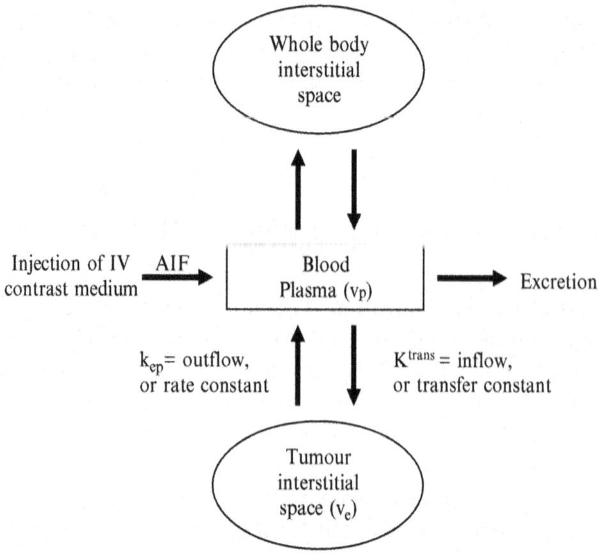

Fig. 1 Body compartments accessed by low-molecular weight, gadolinium containing contrast media injected intravenously. *AIF* arterial input function

concentration is more problematic and it is for this reason that measurements of blood flow and blood volume are prefaced with the term 'relative': relative blood flow (rBF) and relative blood volume (rBV).

3.2 *Quantification of DCE-MRI*

Dynamic contrast images can be analysed by quantitative or semi-quantitative means; these parameters providing information on blood flow, blood volume, microvessel permeability, extraction fraction, and on plasma and interstitial volumes. Pharmacokinetic analysis of DCE-MRI is the most widely used method of measuring vessel permeability changes, analyses typically being derived from variations of the Tofts' two-compartment kinetic model (Fig. 1) which, in turn, has its roots in Kety's dynamic model (Kety 1960a, b). In this model, an injected contrast agent leaks into the extravascular-extracellular space (EES) and assessments of tissue perfusion and permeability can be derived from the shape of the tumour wash-in and wash-out curves. Immature blood vessels would be expected to be very leaky and thus have a rapid forward leakage rate (Fig. 1). The transfer constant K^{trans} (unit: min^{-1}) describes this forward leakage rate of the contrast medium. For blood vessels where leakage is rapid (that is when extraction fraction is high; typically found in tumours), perfusion will determine contrast agent distribution and K^{trans} approximates to tissue blood flow per unit volume (Tofts et al. 1999).

There are other circumstances where transport out of the vasculature does not deplete intravascular contrast medium concentration (i.e. a lower first pass extraction fraction), a situation found in some brain tumours which have a largely intact blood-brain barrier, but also in extracranial tumours after treatment with chemotherapy and/or late after radiotherapy, and in fibrotic lesions and in some normal tissues, then K^{trans} approximates to the product of permeability times surface area (permeability surface area product, PS) (Wilkinson et al. 2006). After a variable time, the contrast agent diffuses back into the vasculature (described by the rate constant or k_{ep}; unit: min^{-1}) and is excreted usually by the kidneys. Washout of contrast medium is faster as plasma contrast agent concentrations fall when capillary permeability is very high, due to a typically rapid return of contrast medium. Other quantitative kinetic parameters that can be derived from pharmacokinetic modelling of DCE-MRI data include the fraction plasma volume (v_p; unit: %) and the fractional extravascular, extracellular space (v_e – or simply leakage space; unit: %).

Quantitative parameters such as K^{trans} are complicated to derive, which can deter their use at the workbench. Difficulties arise from more complex data acquisition requirements and from the fact that kinetic models may not exactly fit the DCE-MRI data obtained because all models make assumptions that may not be valid for every tissue or tumour type. One the other hand, semi-quantitative parameters are simple to acquire, but tend to be more dependent on the exact injection and acquisition protocol used in the study. The initial area under the gadolinium concentration curve (IAUGC) is a relatively robust and simple kinetic parameter to derive and is able to characterize all enhancing regions without the problems associated with model fitting failures. IAUGC has been recommended as a practical substitute for K^{trans} in clinical studies by several authors (Lankester et al. 2005, 2007a, b; Leach et al. 2005; Thukral et al. 2007). If IAUGC is to be used then it needs to be validated for this purpose. The strength of correlations against K^{trans} depends on the exact cut-off time use for calculation, with 60 s recommended by international consensus panels (Leach et al. 2005). However, readers should remember that IAUGC, as a semi-quantitative parameter does not have a simple relationship to the physiological parameters of interest (perfusion, permeability and leakage space) (Walker-Samuel et al. 2007), being dependent on both transfer constant and leakage space to varying degrees. On the other hand, transfer constant provides a more direct insight into underlying tissue pathophysiological processes.

Another semi-quantitative parameter that appears to be helpful for monitoring the effects of antivascular drugs is the percentage of non-enhancing (NE) pixels. This parameter is analogous to the CT density parameter incorporated into the Choi criteria (Benjamin et al. 2007) for the evaluation of imatinib mesylate on gastrointestinal stromal tumours (GIST). Recent analyses by us have shown that increasing numbers of NE pixels is a specific measure of effectiveness of drugs that target directly the tumour microvasculature but not of drugs that cause vascular shutdown via indirect mechanisms such as chemotherapy induced tumour cell death (Taylor et al. 2009). These NE pixels represent non-vascularised tissues and anatomically

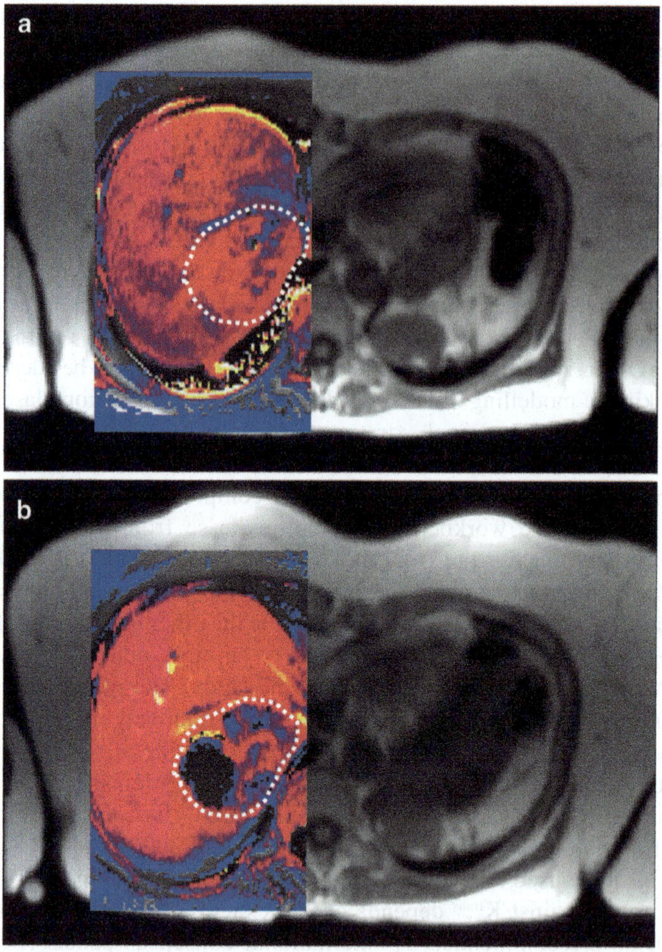

Fig. 2 K^{trans} map (coloured overlay on T1 weighed MRI image) of a 57-year old female patient with colon cancer and liver metastasis (white dotted area) before (**a**) and 4 h after (**b**) first treatment with CA1P (OXi4503). Part of the liver metastasis shows reduced perfusion (*dark blue region*) or complete vascular shutdown (*black region*) after 4 h

represent cystic degeneration and necrosis (Fig. 2). Our experience shows that the tubulin binding VDA combretastatin A4 phosphate CA4P and bevacizumab both cause such profound vascular shutdown that results in increased numbers of NE pixels but these effects are not seen with chemotherapy of breast cancer.

There are uncertainties in the accuracy of kinetic parameter estimates derived from the application of tracer kinetic models in clinical DCE-MRI experiments. These derive from model-based assumptions and from assumptions made for the determination of tissue Gd-DTPA concentrations. For example, in the original implementation of Tofts' model, population based AIFs were used (although this is not a strict requirement) (Weinmann et al. 1984) and it was assumed that tissue blood volume contributes negligible signal compared with that arising from contrast medium in the interstitial space (Tofts 1997). Buckley suggested that the application of these model-based assumptions leads to systematic overestimation of the transfer constant in tumours (Buckley 2002b). Modern two compartment model implementations leave AIF choice to investigators and allow derivation of plasma volume fraction provided that AIF choice and temporal data sampling rates are appropriate. An important point for readers to remember is that the presence of gadolinium containing contrast medium is detected only indirectly, by its effect on tissue water (i.e. the contrast medium itself is not detected unlike in perfusion CT). In tissues, contrast medium is confined to the extracellular space, whereas the bulk of water is intracellular. As a result, transmembrane water exchange can affect the accuracy of the tissue contrast agent concentration estimates (Landis et al. 2000; Buckley 2002a) which additionally needs to be taken into account.

3.3 Validation of DCE-MRI as a Vascular Biomarker

DCE-MRI has been widely validated in the last decade in a number of ways, including direct correlative studies against immuno-histochemical microvessel density measurements, and tissue expressions of pro-angiogenic growth factors including vascular endothelial growth factor (broad correlations in some studies and no correlations in others) (Padhani and Dzik-Jurasz 2004; Schlemmer et al. 2004). Tissue validation studies have also come from correlative studies against widely accepted surrogates of tissue perfusion including ^{14}C-aminoisobutyric acid quantitative autoradiography (Ferrier et al. 2007). More recently, in vivo correlative imaging studies have been performed. Thus, transfer constant as a marker of tumour blood flow has now been validated against blood volume/blood flow derived from DSC-MRI studies (Lankester et al. 2007b), ^{15}O-water PET (Eby et al. 2008) and microbubble ultrasound (Niermann et al. 2007). These cross imaging validation studies have shown that the relationship is not upheld in every tumour type (e.g. in gliomas, because a variably intact blood brain barrier reduces the first pass extraction of the contrast agent (Wilkinson et al. 2006)). Similarly, the strength of correlations also decreases when therapies that reduce microvessel permeability are used, again because the first pass extraction fraction of small molecular weight contrast agents is reduced.

3.4 DCE-MRI in the Clinical Assessment of Antiangiogenic Agents

From an imaging perspective, drugs targeting the tumour vasculature can be broadly divided into antiangiogenic drugs and vascular disruptive agents. The effects of these drugs on kinetic imaging parameters have been found to be similar regardless of the mechanism of drug action, with the dominant effect of successful therapy being reductions in blood flow and permeability. Importantly, it is the timing of the onset and duration of vascular changes that enables these two therapeutic strategies to be distinguished on imaging. Both xenograft and human imaging studies of antiangiogenic drugs show that antivascular effects are not immediate, arising at least 1–2 days post drug administration. In contrast vascular disruptive agents cause rapid shutdown of the vasculature within minutes to hours of drug administration and reversibility of effects being visible in the short term (usually seen within 24–48 h). 'Normalisation' of the vasculature induced by antiangiogenic drugs as described originally by Jain (Jain 2001) can be detected on DCE-MRI and is evidenced by regional increases in non-enhancing pixels (that is vascular pruning) with reductions in permeability and leakage space. Improved flow in non-pruned vessels can also be detected in other regions. So it is the combination of vascular pruning, reductions in vascular permeability and leakage space, and regional increases in flow that suggest that 'normalisation' is occurring (Batchelor et al. 2007; Kamoun et al. 2009).

At the time this manuscript is written, 36 phase I and II studies have been published as papers or abstracts that have evaluated the DCE-MRI effects of antiangiogenic and vascular disruptive drugs on tumour vascularity, including data on more than 600 patients. Studies have been done in different clinical settings including (1) phase I clinical trials in heavily pre-treated patients, (2) studies where antiangiogenic agents are administered as monotherapy and (3) studies where antiangiogenic agents are administered with conventional therapies (usually cytotoxic chemotherapy). In the latter category, a few studies can be found where the first cycle of therapy is the antiangiogenic agent alone, with subsequent cycles having combination treatment.

3.4.1 Phase I Studies

Both, anti-VEGF antibodies, and receptor tyrosine kinase inhibitors (TKIs) demonstrate changes in DCE-MRI parameters in phase I studies. The most convincing DCE-MRI data has come from studies where tyrosine kinase receptor inhibitors that target multiple mechanisms (multitarget tyrosine kinase inhibitors [MTKIs]) were used. Effective MTKIs all appear to inhibit KIT, platelet-derived growth factor, and vascular endothelial growth factor receptor 2 (VEGFR-2). Most also inhibit VEGFR-1, some inhibit VEGFR-3, and other additional receptor tyrosine kinases, introducing distinct but subtle differences between the agents (Morgan et al. 2003; Conrad et al. 2004; O'Donnell et al. 2005; Liu et al. 2005; Rosen et al. 2006; Rosen et al. 2007; Jonker et al. 2007; Xiong, Herbst et al. 2004; Mross et al. 2005a,b; Padhani et al. 2006; Drevs et al. 2005; Thomas et al. 2005).

One of the first MTKI to be evaluated was PTK787/ZK222584 (PTK/ZK, vatalanib succinate), an oral angiogenesis inhibitor targeting all known vascular endothelial growth factor (VEGF) receptor tyrosine kinases, the platelet-derived growth factor receptor tyrosine kinase, and the c-kit protein tyrosine kinase. Phase I studies showed a 40–58% reduction of K_i (equivalent to K^{trans}) after 2 days of the first treatment. These studies concluded that both DCE-MRI and pharmacokinetic data were helpful for defining the biologically active dose. Interestingly, changes in K_i also appear to predict responses and disease progression in patients with metastatic colorectal cancer to the liver (Morgan et al. 2003). Patients with a best response of stable disease had significantly greater reductions in K_i at both day 2 and at the end of cycle 1 compared with progressors. They confirmed significant negative correlations between changes in tumour K_i and increases in PTK/ZK oral dose and plasma levels, indicating a relationship between drug exposure and changes in tumour pharmacodynamics. Regrettably these early promising results did not ultimately translate into patient benefit in two phase III clinical trails when PTK/ZK was used in combination with chemotherapy.

AG013736 (axitinib) is another orally bioavailable MTKI. Mechanistically, AG013736 inhibits the tyrosine kinase activities of all known VEGF receptors, platelet-derived growth factor receptor-ß, and c-Kit in low nanomolar concentrations. Rapid decreases in K^{trans} and $IAUC_{90}$, were observed on day 2 (>40% reductions in K^{trans} in 11 or 17 evaluable patients) (Liu et al. 2005). Interestingly, statistically significant decreases were noted for both mean K^{trans} and $IAUC_{90}$ for increasing values of log-transformed drug AUC and C_{max}. It was evident that higher exposures of AG-013736 were associated with a greater decrease in mean K^{trans} with similar correlations between mean $IAUC_{90}$ with respect to plasma AG013736 $AUC_{0\text{-}24}$ concentrations.

However, not all phase I studies have shown reductions in DCE-MRI kinetic parameters or clear relationships between plasma drug exposure and tumour DCE-MRI changes. For example, studies with SU5416 (semaxanib) showed mixed results, with progressive disease despite reduced IAUC (Medved et al. 2004); with two other studies not documenting consistent changes in DCE-MRI parameters (Dowlati et al. 2005; O'Donnell et al. 2005). Negative results were seen in a small study with SU6668, a PDGFR-, VEGFR-2-, and FGFR-1 TKI inhibitor (Xiong et al. 2004). Another orally bioavailable MTKI is AMG-706 (moesanib), which targets VEGFR-1, -2, -3, and PDGFR. In a phase I study incorporating DCE-MRI, Rosen et al showed decreases in K^{trans} or IAUC ranged from –52% to +62%, but there was no significant correlation of either K^{trans} or IAUC with AMG-706 AUC at either day 3 or 21 (Rosen et al. 2007). The anti-VEGF antibody HuMV833 reduced rate constant (k_{ep}) in tumours; however, no dose relationship was observed. This was ascribed by the authors to the heterogeneous antibody distribution and clearance between and within patients and between and within individual tumours (Jayson et al. 2002).

3.4.2 Antiangiogenic Agents as Monotherapy

BAY 43-9006 (sorafenib), a tumour proliferation and angiogenesis inhibitor which works through blockade of the Raf/MEK/ERK pathway at the level of Raf kinase and the receptor tyrosine kinases VEGFR-2 and PDGFR-β, has been tested in 17 renal cell carcinoma patients. Seven partial responses and seven minor responses according to WHO criteria have been observed. DCE-MRI data from 12 evaluable patients demonstrated declines in K^{trans} and v_e. Both high K^{trans} at baseline, and percent decline in K^{trans}, correlated with time to progression (O'Dwyer et al. 2005).

However, in another, larger prospective study with sorafenib (n=56), Hahn et al. conducted a randomized trial to investigate DCE-MRI changes in renal cancer patients who were randomly assigned to placebo or 200 or 400 mg twice per day of sorafenib. DCE-MRI was performed at baseline and after 4 weeks (Hahn et al. 2008). DCE-MRI parameters included K^{trans} and $IAUGC_{90}$. Dose response relationships in both K^{trans} and $IAUGC_{90}$ were observed with greater effects at higher doses. As noted also by O'Dwyer et al., patients with tumours with high baseline K^{trans} and $IAUGC_{90}$ had a better progression free survival. However, unlike O'Dwyer et al. changes in DCE-MRI parameters after 4 weeks of sorafenib are not predictive of PFS, suggesting that DCE-MRI biomarkers are not surrogate end points for efficacy in renal cancer patients treated with sorafenib.

3.4.3 Antiangiogenic Agents with Conventional Therapies

A few studies have evaluated the antiangiogenic effects of a single cycle of bevacizumab, an anti-VEGF monoclonal antibody in patient with newly diagnosed locally advanced and inflammatory breast cancer (Overmoyer et al. 2004; Wedam et al. 2006; Thukral et al. 2007). All studies show that after a single dose of bevacizumab, K^{trans} and k_{ep} and $IAUGC_{180}$ were significantly reduced from baseline values. In subsequent cycles, patients received combination bevacizumab therapy and chemotherapy, and DCE-MRI parameters all decreased substantially. Thukral et al. noted that parameter values measured between cycles 1 and 4 showed greater differences than did those measured between cycles 4 and 7, suggesting that the greatest effect on tumour microvascularity occurred early in the course of therapy. Importantly, DCE-MRI parameter changes after the first cycle 1 were not reflective of the eventual success of combination therapy (Wedam et al. 2006; Thukral et al. 2007).

An interesting new study has attempted to separate the antiangiogenic effects of chemotherapy from those due to angiogenesis inhibitors. Baar et al. performed a randomised phase II trial designed to evaluate the additional biomarker effect on angiogenesis when bevacizumab is added to docetaxel (Baar et al. 2009). Forty-nine patients were randomised and no differences in overall clinical response, progression-free survival, or overall survival were observed. $IAUGC_{90}$ showed greater decreases in the bevacizumab+docetaxel arm with overall greater decreases in tumour volume suggesting a greater antiangiogenic effect for the combination therapy.

3.5 DCE-MRI in Pre-clinical Development of VDAs

DCE-MRI has been used in the pre-clinical development of the vascular disruptive agents' combretastatin A4 phosphate (CA4P; fosbretabulin), and ZD6126, ASA404 (DMXAA). Several studies in rodent models demonstrated that CA4P induces acute, reversible reductions in tumour blood flow that leads to central necrosis within tumours. Chaplin et al. studied the effects of CA4P on perfusion in tumours in mice. Blood flow measurements using a diffusible tracer, 86RbCl, demonstrated that 6 h after treatment with 100 mg/kg intraperitoneal CA4P, perfusion is reduced by 50–60% with an associated 90% of vessels rendered non-functional. The discrepancy between these percentages was ascribed to increased blood flow in the normal tissue vasculature supplying the tumour rim, caused by the ischemia-induced release of vasoactive mediators. Consequently, vascular shutdown resulted in extensive cell loss 24 h following treatment, but this effect did not have any significant effect on tumour growth, probably due to an actively proliferating population of cells at the periphery of tumours (Chaplin et al. 1999).

Maxwell et al. used DCE-MRI to evaluate CA4P in the rat P22 carcinosarcoma model. Changes in K^{trans} 4 and 24 h after CA4P infusion were comparable with those obtained using radiolabelled ^{125}iodoantipyrine (IAP), which is considered the gold standard for the assessment of tumour perfusion (Maxwell et al. 2002). The study also showed a decrease in leakage space (v_e), which is counter-intuitive, as one would expect oedema to occur after the administration of CA4P (Kanthou and Tozer 2002). Maxwell et al. hypothesized that vascular shutdown of tumour regions will lead to falls in v_e which measures the proportion of EES that Gd-DTPA has access to rather than the whole EES. In keeping with this assertion is the findings recently made by Batchelor et al. who evaluated the action of the MTKI AZD-2171 in recurrent glioblastoma patients showing rapid and persistence of reductions of v_e which as coincident the re-establishment of the blood brain barrier (Batchelor et al. 2007). Using P22 tumours in rats, Galbratih et al. (Galbraith et al. 2003) also demonstrated reductions in IAUC of 90% and 95%, and in K^{trans} of 73% and 64%, respectively, at 1 and 6 h after the infusion of CA4P at 30 mg/kg, which was comparable with blood flow changes previously using ^{125}iodoantipyrine (IAP) (Prise et al. 2002).

Using different murine tumours, Beauregard et al. also showed reductions in contrast medium inflow 3 h after CA4P injection, corresponding histologically with haemorrhagic tumour necrosis (Beauregard et al. 1998, 2001). Interestingly, there was a differential response with the greatest changes seen in two tumour types (LoVo and RIF-1).

A good pre-clinical example of the multifunctional imaging approach to evaluate vascular disruptive activity can be found in the study on the effects of CA4P and DMXAA on two human colon cancer xenograft models (HT29 and LS174T) in mice. Beauregard et al. evaluated antitumour effects of the two VDAs, noting changes in perfusion (the anticipated primary target) and in tumour energy status (secondary effects resulting from vascular disruption) (Beauregard et al. 2002). To assess the antivascular effects, DCE-MRI (with both macromolecular and small molecular weight gadolinium chelates) and phosphorus spectroscopy were used, noting changes in perfusion and macromolecular permeability and tumour cell energy status via changes in the ratio of the integrals of the signals from inorganic phosphate and nucleoside triphosphates. Using these techniques, Beauregard et al. found that there was close concordance between vascular disruption and subsequent changes in energy status. Heterogeneity in response to these drugs was observed in different tumour models and they noted that differential susceptibility to drug action was related at least in part to greater tumour macromolecular vascular permeability (Beauregard et al. 2002).

Inconsistent results were seen by McPhail et al. in the assessment of DMXAA on rat GH3 prolactinomas, where there was no dose response relationship with DCE-MRI parameters despite evidence of vascular damage with increased plasma 5-hydroxyindoleacetic acid (5-HIAA) levels (McPhail et al. 2006). In murine C38colonic adenocarcinomas, Evelhoch et al. demonstrated dose-dependent decreases in IAUC in 13 mice treated with ZD6126 (Evelhoch et al. 2004). Robinson et al. have also shown significantly reduced IAUC 24 h after ZD6126 in both rat GH3 prolactinomas and murine RIF-1 fibrosarcomas, with an increase in intrinsic susceptibility rate ($R_2^* = 1/T_2^*$), indicating increased tumour hypoxia as a result of therapy (Robinson et al. 2003).

4 DCE-MRI in the Clinical Development of VDAs

At the time the manuscript is written, data from ten studies including a total of 100 patients were published as papers or abstracts (Table 1).

4.1 DMXAA

In the phase I trial of DMXAA, Galbraith et al. demonstrated significant reductions in median $IAUC_{90}$ in the majority of 16 patients at various time points after treatment (Galbraith et al. 2002). There was no evidence of a dose response reduction in tumour $IAUC_{90}$ after the administration of DMXAA to patients. However in a further safety phase I study performed in New Zealand, no reductions in DCE-MRI parameters were seen at 26 h post DMXAA but an increase in v_e was seen (McKeage et al. 2006). It has been speculated that the acute antivascular effects disappeared by 26 h but this contradicts the results of the Galbraith et al. study (Galbraith et al. 2002). Increases in v_e may be explained by DMXAA mechanisms of action, which include induction of cytokines (particularly tumour necrosis factor (TNF-alpha), serotonin and nitric oxide (NO)) as well as its antivascular and antiangiogenic effects. Several studies have shown that cytokines, TNF-α in particular, can increase vascular permeability but also decreases tumour blood flow by inducing vascular collapse and haemorrhage. Since changes in K^{trans} and IAUGC are related to both tumour blood flow and vessel permeability; the two physiological parameters cannot be decoupled so the net effect may be inconsistent.

4.2 ZD6126

The classic description of vascular targeting activity on DCE-MRI (rapid shutdown of the vasculature and reversibility of effects) has been noted in a limited phase I trial of ZD6126 where significant decreases in $IAUC_{60}$ were seen in six patients

Table 1 Studies using DCE-MRI for the evaluation of vascular disruptive agents (VDAs)

Agent	*n*	Phase	Tumour type	Did imaging support the purported mechanism of action?	Was there a drug dose–vascular response relationship?	Did DCE-MRI parameters correlate with the clinical course?	Was DCE-MRI helpful in defining dose schedule to take into phase II?	Comments	Study
Flavonoid									
ASA404 (DMXAA)	16	I	Mixed	Yes 9/16 patients with significant AUC reductions 24 h after first dose, and 8/11 had AUC reductions >66% 24 h after last dose	No No dose–response relationship found	No	No	–	Galbraith et al. (2002)
	15	I	Mixed	No No significant K^{trans} or k_{ep} changes found, but counter-intuitive significant K^{trans} increase seen in one dose group	No Counter-intuitive blood flow changes (v_e increase)	No	No	v_e increase due to cytokine release, or wrong time point for DCE-MRI assessment (24 h post-infusion)?	McKeage et al. (2006)

(continued)

Table 1 (continued)

Agent	*n*	Phase	Tumour type	Did imaging support the purported mechanism of action?	Was there a drug dose–vascular response relationship?	Did DCE-MRI parameters correlate with the clinical course?	Was DCE-MRI helpful in defining dose schedule to take into phase II?	Comments	Study
Combretastatin analogues (tubulin binding VDAs)									
CA4P	7	I	Mixed	No	No	–	–		Dowlati et al. (2002)
(fosbretabulin)	18	I	Mixed	Yes	Yes K^{trans} 37% reduced in 6/16 patients at ≥52 mg/m^2, no changes at 20 and 40 mg/m^2	–	Yes. Biologically active dose (≥52 mg/m^2) assessed by DCE-MRI	Time course of changes in rat and human tumours similar	Galbraith et al. (2003)
	10	I	Mixed	Yes Reduction in K^{trans} in 8/10 patients	No No dose-relationship observed.	No	–	Lack of dose-response relationship due to segmental vascular shutdown?	Stevenson et al. (2003)
CA4P (fosbretabulin) +bevacizumab	15	I	Mixed	Yes Significant reductions in tumour perfusion/ vascular permeability, sustained following bevacizumab	–	No	No	Combination of VDA and bevacizumab demonstrated additive effect	Nathan et al. (2008)

CA4P (fosbretabulin) +^{131}I-A5B7 (anti-CEA antibody)	12	I	Mixed	Yes K^{trans} and IAUGC reductions in 9/12 patients	Partly Trend for greater reductions in all kinetic parameters at higher doses of CA4P (54 mg/m^2)	No	–	–	Meyer et al. (2009)
CA4P (fosbretabulin) +paclitaxel +carboplatin	13	II	Mixed	Yes Reduction in blood flow in both dose groups	–	Yes Two patients with thyroid cancer showing SD and PD had also greatest reduction in blood flow	–	–	Akerley et al. (2007)
CA1P (OXi4503)	17	I	Mixed	Yes K^{trans} reductions seen.	Yes K^{trans} reductions more frequently at higher dose levels	–	–	(Study ongoing at the time of publication of the manuscript)	Patterson et al. (2008)
Colchicin analogue (tubulin binding VDA)									
ZD6126	9	I	Mixed, liver meta-stasis	Yes Reduced IAUC in all tumours (range: 1% to 72%)	Yes Dose-dependent reductions of 36% to 72% in 6/9 patients at 6 h	–	Yes Biologically active dose at ≥80 mg/m^2	–	Evelhoch et al. (2004); LoRusso et al. (2008)

(eight lesions) treated at doses of 80 mg/m^2 and above, at 6 h post infusion which was then maintained at 24 h with partial recovery at 18–21 days (Evelhoch et al. 2002; LoRusso et al. 2008). There was also a significant trend of greater antivascular effect with increasing drug exposure ($P<0.01$).

4.3 CA4P

Changes in tumour blood flow following CA4P have been assessed in nine Phase I and II oncology clinical studies where considerable variations in dosing ranged from 27 to 114 mg/m^2. A number of techniques have been used to evaluate antivascular effects in vivo including perfusion CT, DCE-MRI and PET. A broad spectrum of tumour types has been imaged at various stages of disease progression with heterogeneity in size, age, type and/or level of vascularity. The numbers of subjects imagined in each study was small, limiting the power of sub-analyses. The interval between CA4P infusion and the imaging study has also been variable. Nonetheless, in all of these studies, decreases in tumour perfusion following CA4P administration have been observed, and in most studies these achieved statistical significance.

Tumour antivascular activity was demonstrated in the first phase I trial (Rustin et al. 2003) using DCE-MRI in 18 patients, measuring transfer constant (K^{trans}) and IAUGC over the first 24 h after initial treatment with CA4P (Galbraith et al. 2003). Significant reductions in tumour K^{trans} were seen in six of 16 patients treated at ≥52 mg/m^2 (Fig. 3), with significant group mean reductions of 37% and 29% at 4 and 24 h, respectively, after treatment. The mean reduction in tumour

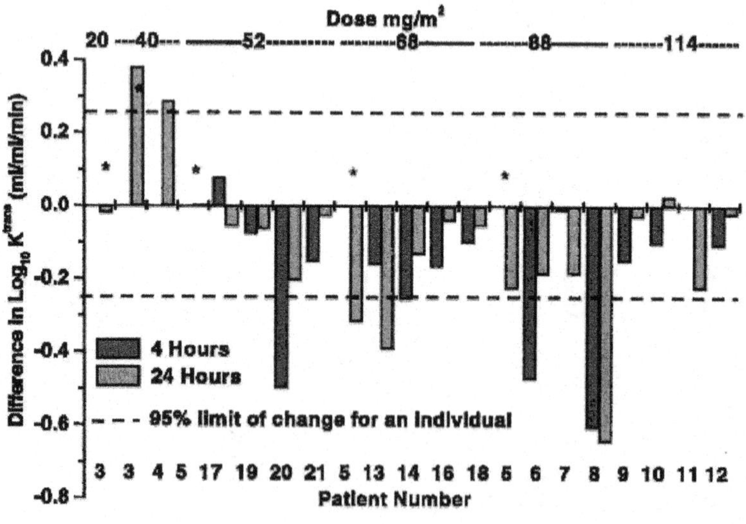

Fig. 3 K^{trans} differences (in Log_{10}) at 4 and 24 h versus baseline in patients receiving different doses of CA4P (Reprinted with kind permission from Galbraith et al. 2003)

IAUGC was 33% and 18%, respectively, at these times. No reduction was seen in muscle K^{trans} or in kidney IAUGC.

Interestingly, in a patient who was responding and receiving eight cycles of CA4P over 10 months, a gradual decrease of K^{trans} response was noted with every cycle, indicating loss of efficacy of CA4P treatment over time, although tumour response was maintained for a couple of months (Fig. 4). These DCE-MRI data confirmed that CA4P has antivascular activity in tumours at doses at and below the maximum tolerated dose (68 mg/m^2). No significant changes were seen in patients treated at 20–40 mg/m^2, indicating a threshold dose level below which effects on the microvasculature are not seen at the 4 h time point. DCE-MRI data indicate a relatively selective effect on tumour, with no significant reduction in mean kinetic parameters in muscle or kidney.

In the Dowlati et al. study, a reduction in tumour contrast agent enhancement was measured in six of seven patients treated at 60 mg/m^2 in the once-every-3-weeks study (Dowlati et al. 2002). In another study using a different schedule (weekly for 3 weeks followed by 1 week of rest), CA4P was shown to reduce K^{trans} in 6 of 16 patients treated at ≥52 mg/m^2, with a significant mean reduction of 37% and 29% at 4 and 24 h, respectively (Galbraith et al. 2003).

DCE-MRI data were obtained from ten patients in the Stevenson et al. study (Stevenson et al. 2003). K^{trans} decreased in eight of ten patients. v_e decreased by ≥10% in seven patients and significantly in the entire group. The higher the apparent perfusion at baseline, the larger the change observed after CA4P administration ($p<0.001$). Thus, highly vascular tumours like thyroid cancer showed larger decreases after CA4P administration, similar to the finding observed by Galbraith et al. (Galbraith et al. 2003).

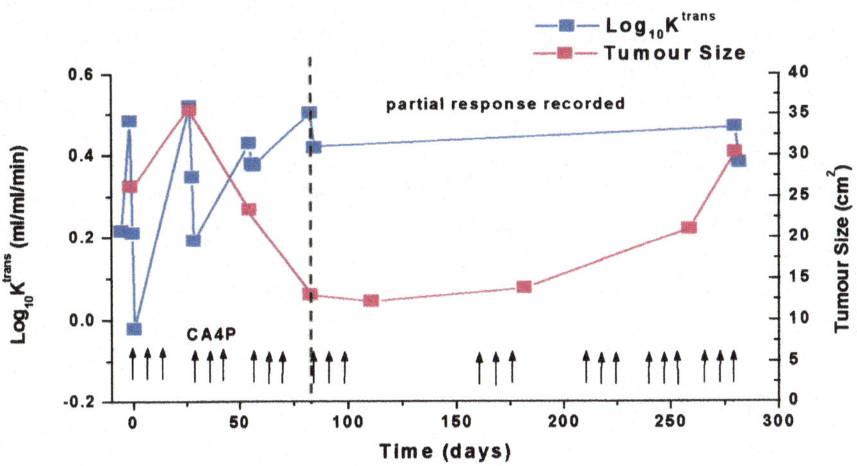

Fig. 4 Serial changes in K^{trans} in a patient who received a total of eight cycles (24 infusions) of CA4P in the Rustin et al. study (Rustin et al. 2003). DCE-MRI investigations were not performed with every cycle. A gradual decrease in K^{trans} response is seen with each cycle, indicating a loss of efficacy of CA4P over time. This patient had >50% reduction in tumour size after the third cycle, although one lesion increased in size by the fourth cycle. At the final DCE-MRI examination, a new lesion was seen

Blood flow changes were assessed by DCE-MRI following combined treatment with carboplatin and CA4P in study CA4P-103 (Bilenker et al. 2005). The highest CA4P dose in this study, 36 mg/m^2, was below the threshold for reproducible blood flow change determined in the CA4P-066 trial (Galbraith et al. 2003). Nonetheless, decreased K^{trans} was observed in three of five valuable patients: pancreatic cancer (29.1%), anaplastic thyroid cancer (46.4%), and renal cell cancer (63.7%). Changes were consistent with observations in monotherapy studies.

In a unique study, combination treatment of CA4P with bevacizumab (Nathan et al. 2008) was evaluated by DCE-MRI. Pre-clinical models have demonstrated that the addition of an anti-VEGF antibody to a VDA significantly increases anti-tumour activity, possibly by inhibiting neo-vascularization of the surviving rim (Shaked et al. 2006). The first clinical study combining a VDA with an antiangiogenic drug was to establish the safety of the CA4P/bevacizumab combination and to demonstrate synergy of action in vivo using DCE-MRI. The study showed statistically significant reductions in K^{trans} after one dose of CA4P, which as anticipated, reversed on drug wash-out. However, there was a failure of tumour vasculature to recover when CA4P was given with bevacizumab.

In a combination trial of CA4P with paclitaxel and carboplatin in patients with advanced imageable malignancies, a mean reduction in tumour blood flow was observed for both dose groups (46% versus 19% respectively) randomized to one of two dose levels of CA4P (45 or 63 mg/m^2) administered weekly on days 1, 8 and 15. Remarkably, the two patients showing clinical response (thyroid cancer with stable disease, and partial remission, respectively) had also the greatest reduction in blood flow. K^{trans} was reduced by 73% and 79% 24 h after CA4P infusion (Akerley et al. 2007).

Lastly, in a combination trial of CA4P with radioimmunotherapy with the ^{131}iodine labeled A5B7 anti-CEA antibody in patients with advanced gastrointestinal carcinoma, DCE-MRI confirmed falls in kinetic parameters (K^{trans}/$IAUGC_{60}$) in 9/12 patients (Meyer et al. 2009). Uniquely in this study, cardiac output was measured at the same time as the DCE-MRI study to rule out the possibility that tumour VDA activity was mediated via decreases in cardiac output (CO). CO and DCE-MRI measurements were performed before and 4 h following CA4P alone on 12 patients. Increases in CO occurred after CA4P whilst statistically significant falls in tumour K^{trans} values were seen, thus indicating that there is no evidence for reductions in CO as a cause for reduced tumour K^{trans} after CA4P.

4.4 CA1P (OXi-4503)

The first phase I study of OXi-4503, a combretastatin analogue with higher potency than CA4P, is still ongoing at the time the manuscript is published. Out of 23 patients treated in escalating doses (0.06–15.4 mg/m^2), tumours from two patients showed significant K^{trans} reductions so far (Fig. 4). There is preliminary evidence for a dose–vascular response relationship (Patterson et al. 2007).

5 VDA Experience with Positron Emission Tomography (PET)

Out of 34 patients enrolled in the first phase I trial (Rustin et al. 2003), 13 patients underwent PET scanning, measuring tumour perfusion using ^{15}O-labelled water, and tumour blood volume using ^{15}O-labelled carbon monoxide (C^{15}O) (Anderson et al. 2003). The first PET measurement after CA4P was at 30 min, whilst most DCE-MRI measurements were performed at 4 h. Tumour perfusion measurements indicated a dose-threshold effect for doses ≥52 mg/m^2. Twenty-four hours after CA4P administration tumour perfusion increased, but at doses ≥52 mg/m^2 remained significantly reduced compared with pre-treatment values (Fig. 5). Blood volume changes in tumours were not dose dependent with rapid reductions at 30 min, and 24 h later, there were no longer significantly different from pre-treatment data. This study included also data on perfusion changes in normal tissue. Splenic perfusion and blood volume were significantly reduced 30 min after CA4P administration by 35%, and 18%, respectively, and returned to baseline after 24 h. Kidney perfusion and blood volume were both significantly reduced by 6%, and returned to baseline after 24 h. Systemic haemodynamic data 30 min after CA4P administration revealed a significant

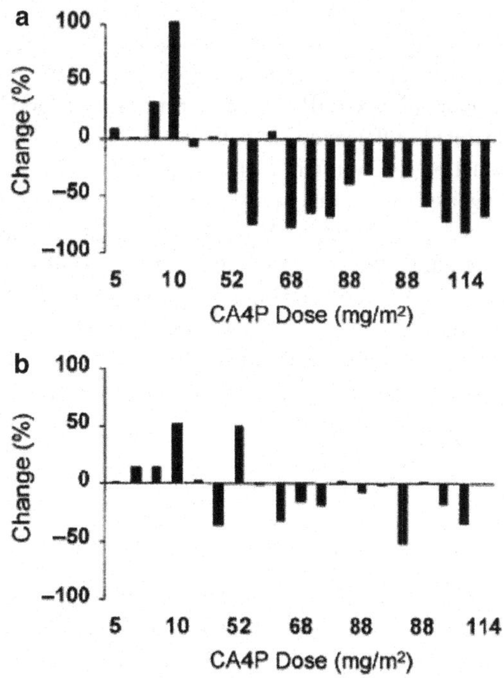

Fig. 5 Tumor perfusion measurements using positron emission tomography (PET) with oxygen-15 (^{15}O)-labeled water indicated a dose-threshold effect for doses ≥52 mg/m^2 (**a**). Twenty-four hours after CA4P administration tumor perfusion increased, but at doses ≥52 mg/m^2 remained significantly reduced compared with pre-treatment values (**b**) (Reprinted with kind permission from Anderson et al. 2003)

increase in systolic and diastolic blood pressure of 9%, and 12%, respectively, and a significant decrease in heart rate and cardiac output of 10%, which was no longer detected after 24 h. However, cardiac stroke volume was not affected, indicating that CA4P treatment has no direct clinical effect on the heart. Decreased perfusion of kidney and spleen was consistent with decreased cardiac output, although the greater decrease in spleen might indicate some tissue specific differences in CA4P response, an observation which already has been made in animal models (Tozer et al. 1999; Murata et al. 2001). The fact that tumour tissue recovered more slowly from vascular effects of CA4P than normal tissue indicates some tumour specificity, and raised the question, if a dose schedule involving greater than once-a-week dosing might confer a benefit in terms of therapeutic gain.

6 VDA Experience with Perfusion Computed Tomography (CT)

Volumetric dynamic contrast-enhanced CT has been used to evaluate the antivascular effects of CA4P and palliative radiotherapy in patients with advanced non-small-cell lung cancer. CA4P was given after the second fraction of radiotherapy (Ng et al. 2007; Mandeville et al. 2008). Six of the eight patients showed increases in tumour permeability surface area product (PS) by 23.6% after the second fraction of radiotherapy. Four hours after CA4P, a reduction in tumour blood volume (BV) by 22.9% was demonstrated in the same six patients. Increase in PS after radiotherapy correlated with reduction in BV after CA4P particularly at the tumour rim. One of the most interesting aspects of this study was the demonstration that following radiotherapy the reduction in tumour BV was sustained at 72 h after CA4P.

When different radiotherapy and CA4P administration schedules were compared, decreases in blood volume were only observed in groups receiving single dose CA4P after two fractions RT, and weekly CA4P after two, four and six fractions RT, respectively, but not in the one receiving twice weekly CA4P after every fraction RT, indicating a schedule dependent synergistic interaction between CA4P and RT (Mandeville et al. 2008).

7 Conclusions

Perfusion imaging provides unique information on the vascular properties of tissues and tumours and their responses to antiangiogenic and vascular disruptive agents in pre-clinical and clinical phase I studies. Their successful use is dependent on the need to clearly define trials objectives, which can be achieved provided that studies are well planned & conducted with appropriate QA/QC steps. If done well, observations from such imaging studies do improve our biological understanding of mechanisms of drug action, interactions, and on their magnitude and duration of effects. Many studies show that in general there is good concordance with pre-clinical data and with other angiogenesis biomarkers. Such studies also show considerable heterogeneity in responsiveness between and within lesion responses and between and within patients (even primary and secondary lesions differ in their responses). It is clear from imaging observations that not all antiangiogenic and vascular disruptive agents have the same effects in terms of onset times and duration of effects. Future challenges for imaging include correlation with clinical measures of efficacy and determining the relationship with blood and serum biomarkers.

References

Akerley, W. L., M. Schabel, et al. (2007). A randomized phase 2 trial of combretatstatin A4 phosphate (CA4P) in combination with paclitaxel and carboplatin to evaluate safety and efficacy in subjects with advanced imageable malignancies." *J Clin Oncol, ASCO Annual Meeting Proceedings Part I* **25**(18S): 14060.

Anderson, H. L., J. T. Yap, et al. (2003). "Assessment of pharmacodynamic vascular response in a phase I trial of combretastatin A4 phosphate." *J Clin Oncol* **21**(15): 2823–30.

Baar, J., P. Silverman, et al. (2009). "A vasculature-targeting regimen of preoperative docetaxel with or without bevacizumab for locally advanced breast cancer: impact on angiogenic biomarkers." *Clin Cancer Res* **15**(10): 3583–90.

Batchelor, T. T., A. G. Sorensen, et al. (2007). "AZD2171, a pan-VEGF receptor tyrosine kinase inhibitor, normalizes tumor vasculature and alleviates edema in glioblastoma patients." *Cancer Cell* **11**(1): 83–95.

Beauregard, D. A., S. A. Hill, et al. (2001). "The susceptibility of tumors to the antivascular drug combretastatin A4 phosphate correlates with vascular permeability." *Cancer Res* **61**(18): 6811–5.

Beauregard, D. A., R. B. Pedley, et al. (2002). "Differential sensitivity of two adenocarcinoma xenografts to the anti-vascular drugs combretastatin A4 phosphate and 5,6-dimethylxanthenone-4-acetic acid, assessed using MRI and MRS." *NMR Biomed* **15**(2): 99–105.

Beauregard, D. A., P. E. Thelwall, et al. (1998). "Magnetic resonance imaging and spectroscopy of combretastatin A4 prodrug-induced disruption of tumour perfusion and energetic status." *Br J Cancer* **77**: 1761–7.

Benjamin, R. S., H. Choi, et al. (2007). "We should desist using RECIST, at least in GIST." *J Clin Oncol* **25**(13): 1760–4.

Bilenker, J. H., K. T. Flaherty, et al. (2005). "Phase I trial of combretastatin a-4 phosphate with carboplatin." *Clin Cancer Res* **11**(4): 1527–33.

Buckley, D. L. (2002a). "Transcytolemmal water exchange and its affect on the determination of contrast agent concentration in vivo." *Magn Reson Med* **47**(2): 420–4.

Buckley, D. L. (2002b). "Uncertainty in the analysis of tracer kinetics using dynamic contrast-enhanced T1-weighted MRI." *Magn Reson Med* **47**(3): 601–6.

Chaplin, D. J., G. R. Pettit, et al. (1999). "Anti-vascular approaches to solid tumour therapy: evaluation of combretastatin A4 phosphate." *Anticancer Res* **19**(1A): 189–95.

Conrad, C., H. Friedman, et al. (2004). "A phase I/II trial of single-agent PTK 787/ZK 222584 (PTK/ZK), a novel, oral angiogenesis inhibitor, in patients with recurrent glioblastoma multiforme (GBM)." *J Clin Oncol (Meeting Abstracts)* **22**(14 (suppl)): 1512.

Dowlati, A., K. Robertson, et al. (2002). "A phase I pharmacokinetic and translational study of the novel vascular targeting agent combretastatin A-4 phosphate on a single-dose intravenous schedule in patients with advanced cancer." Cancer Res **62**(June 15): 3408–16.

Dowlati, A., K. Robertson, et al. (2005). "Novel Phase I dose de-escalation design trial to determine the biological modulatory dose of the antiangiogenic agent SU5416." *Clin Cancer Res* **11**(21): 7938–44.

Drevs, J., M. Medinger, et al. (2005). "Phase I clinical evaluation of AZD2171, a highly potent VEGF receptor tyrosine kinase inhibitor, in patients with advanced tumors." *J Clin Oncol, 2005 ASCO Annual Meeting Proceedings* **23**(16S): 3002.

Eby, P. R., S. C. Partridge, et al. (2008). "Metabolic and vascular features of dynamic contrast-enhanced breast magnetic resonance imaging and (15)O-water positron emission tomography blood flow in breast cancer." *Acad Radiol* **15**(10): 1246–54.

Evelhoch, J., P. LoRusso, et al. (2002). *Dynamic contrast-enhanced MRI evaluation of the effects of ZD6126 on tumor vasculature in a phase I clinical trial.* Proc. ISMRM, Honolulu, Hawaii.

Evelhoch, J. L., P. M. LoRusso, et al. (2004). "Magnetic resonance imaging measurements of the response of murine and human tumors to the vascular-targeting agent ZD6126." *Clin Cancer Res* **10**(11): 3650–7.

Ferrara, K. W., C. R. Merritt, et al. (2000). "Evaluation of tumor angiogenesis with US: imaging, Doppler, and contrast agents." *Acad Radiol* **7**(10): 824–39.

Ferrier, M. C., H. Sarin, et al. (2007). "Validation of dynamic contrast-enhanced magnetic resonance imaging-derived vascular permeability measurements using quantitative autoradiography in the RG2 rat brain tumor model." *Neoplasia* **9**(7): 546–55.

Galbraith, S. M., R. J. Maxwell, et al. (2003). "Combretastatin A4 phosphate has tumor antivascular activity in rat and man as demonstrated by dynamic magnetic resonance imaging." *J Clin Oncol* **21**(15): 2831–42.

Galbraith, S. M., G. J. Rustin, et al. (2002). "Effects of 5,6-dimethylxanthenone-4-acetic acid on human tumor microcirculation assessed by dynamic contrast-enhanced magnetic resonance imaging." *J Clin Oncol* **20**(18): 3826–40.

Hahn, O. M., C. Yang, et al. (2008). "Dynamic contrast-enhanced magnetic resonance imaging pharmacodynamic biomarker study of sorafenib in metastatic renal carcinoma." *J Clin Oncol* **26**(28): 4572–8.

Jain, R. K. (2001). "Normalizing tumor vasculature with anti-angiogenic therapy: a new paradigm for combination therapy." *Nat Med* **7**(9): 987–9.

Jayson, G. C., J. Zweit, et al. (2002). "Molecular imaging and biological evaluation of HuMV833 anti-VEGF antibody: implications for trial design of antiangiogenic antibodies." *J Natl Cancer Inst* **94**(19): 1484–93.

Jonker, D. J., L. S. Rosen, et al. (2007). "A phase I study of BMS-582664 (brivanib alaninate), an oral dual inhibitor of VEGFR and FGFR tyrosine kinases, in patients (pts) with advanced/metastatic solid tumors: Safety, pharmacokinetic (PK), and pharmacodynamic (PD) findings." Journal of Clinical Oncology, 2007 ASCO Annual Meeting Proceedings Part I 25(18S (June 20 Supplement)): Abstract 3559.

Kamoun, W. S., C. D. Ley, et al. (2009). "Edema control by cediranib, a vascular endothelial growth factor receptor-targeted kinase inhibitor, prolongs survival despite persistent brain tumor growth in mice." *J Clin Oncol* **27**(15): 2542–52.

Kanthou, C. and G. M. Tozer (2002). "The tumor vascular targeting agent combretastatin A-4-phosphate induces reorganization of the actin cytoskeleton and early membrane blebbing in human endothelial cells." *Blood* **99**(6): 2060–69.

Kety, S. (1960a). "Blood-tissue exchange methods. Theory of blood-tissue exchange and its application to measurement of blood flow." *Meth Med Res* **8**: 223–27.

Kety, S. (1960b). "Measurement of local blood flow by the exchange of an inert, diffusible substance." *Methods Med Res* **8**: 228–36.

Landis, C. S., X. Li, et al. (2000). "Determination of the MRI contrast agent concentration time course in vivo following bolus injection: effect of equilibrium transcytolemmal water exchange." *Magn Reson Med* **44**(4): 563–74.

Lankester, K. J., R. J. Maxwell, et al. (2007a). "Combretastatin A-4-phosphate effectively increases tumor retention of the therapeutic antibody, 131I-A5B7, even at doses that are sub-optimal for vascular shut-down." *Int J Oncol* **30**(2): 453–60.

Lankester, K. J., J. N. Taylor, et al. (2007b). "Dynamic MRI for imaging tumor microvasculature: comparison of susceptibility and relaxivity techniques in pelvic tumors." *J Magn Reson Imaging* **25**(4): 796–805.

Lankester, K. J., N. J. Taylor, et al. (2005). "Effects of platinum/taxane based chemotherapy on acute perfusion in human pelvic tumours measured by dynamic MRI." *Br J Cancer* **93**(9): 979–85.

Leach MO, Brindle KM, et al. (2005). "The assessment of antiangiogenic and antivascular therapies in early-stage clinical trials using magnetic resonance imaging: issues and recommendations." *Br J Cancer* **92**: 1599–1610.

Liu G, Rugo HS, et al. (2005). "Dynamic contrast-enhanced magnetic resonance imaging as a pharmacodynamic measure of response after acute dosing of AG-013736, an oral angiogenesis inhibitor, in patients with advanced solid tumors: results from a phase I study." *J Clin Oncol* **23**(24): 5464–73.

LoRusso, P. M., S. M. Gadgeel, et al. (2008). "Phase I clinical evaluation of ZD6126, a novel vascular-targeting agent, in patients with solid tumors." *Invest New Drugs* **26**(2): 159–67.

Mandeville, H. C., V. Goh, et al. (2008). "Volumetric perfusion CT assessment of concurrent combretastatin-A4-phosphate (CA4P) and radiotherapy (RT) in non-small cell lung cancer." *J Clin Oncol* **26**(May 20 suppl): abstr 14517.

Maxwell, R. J., J. Wilson, et al. (2002). "Evaluation of the anti-vascular effects of combretastatin in rodent tumours by dynamic contrast enhanced MRI." *NMR Biomed* **15**(2): 89–98.

McKeage, M. J., P. Fong, et al. (2006). "5,6-Dimethylxanthenone-4-acetic acid in the treatment of refractory tumors: a phase I safety study of a vascular disrupting agent." *Clin Cancer Res* **12**(6): 1776–84.

McPhail, L. D., D. J. McIntyre, et al. (2006). "Rat tumor response to the vascular-disrupting agent 5,6-dimethylxanthenone-4-acetic acid as measured by dynamic contrast-enhanced magnetic resonance imaging, plasma 5-hydroxyindoleacetic acid levels, and tumor necrosis." *Neoplasia* **8**(3): 199–206.

Medved, M., G. Karczmar, et al. (2004). "Semiquantitative analysis of dynamic contrast enhanced MRI in cancer patients: variability and changes in tumor tissue over time." *J Magn Reson Imaging* **20**(1): 122–8.

Meyer, T., A. M. Gaya, et al. (2009). "A phase I trial of radioimmunotherapy with 131I-A5B7 anti-CEA antibody in combination with combretastatin-A4-phosphate in advanced gastrointestinal carcinomas." *Clin Cancer Res* **15**(13): 4484–92.

Miles, K. A. and R. E. Williams (2008). "Warburg revisited: imaging tumour blood flow and metabolism." *Cancer Imaging* **8**: 81–6.

Morgan, B., A. L. Thomas, et al. (2003). "Dynamic contrast-enhanced magnetic resonance imaging as a biomarker for the pharmacological response of PTK787/ZK 222584, an inhibitor of the vascular endothelial growth factor receptor tyrosine kinases, in patients with advanced colorectal cancer and liver metastases: results from two phase I studies." *J Clin Oncol* **21**(21): 3955–64.

Mross, K., J. Drevs, et al. (2005a). "Phase I clinical and pharmacokinetic study of PTK/ZK, a multiple VEGF receptor inhibitor, in patients with liver metastases from solid tumours." *Eur J Cancer* **41**(9): 1291–9.

Mross, K. B., D. Gmehling, et al. (2005b). A clinical phase I, pharmacokinetic (PK), and pharmacodynamic study of twice daily BIBF 1120 in advanced cancer patients. *J Clin Oncol* (Meeting Abstracts).

Murata, R., J. Overgaard, et al. (2001). "Comparative effects of combretastatin A-4 disodium phosphate and 5,6- dimethylxanthenone-4-acetic acid on blood perfusion in a murine tumour and normal tissues." *Int J Radiat Biol* **77**(2): 195–204.

Nathan, P., I. Judson, et al. (2008). "A phase I study of combretastatin A4 phosphate (CA4P) and bevacizumab in subjects with advanced solid tumors." *J Clin Oncol* **26**(May 20 suppl): 3550.

Ng, Q. S., V. Goh, et al. (2007). "Tumor antivascular effects of radiotherapy combined with combretastatin a4 phosphate in human non-small-cell lung cancer." *Int J Radiat Oncol Biol Phys* **67**(5): 1375–80.

Niermann, K. J., A. C. Fleischer, et al. (2007). "Measuring tumor perfusion in control and treated murine tumors: correlation of microbubble contrast-enhanced sonography to dynamic contrast-enhanced magnetic resonance imaging and fluorodeoxyglucose positron emission tomography." *J Ultrasound Med* **26**(6): 749–56.

O'Donnell, A., A. Padhani, et al. (2005). "A Phase I study of the angiogenesis inhibitor SU5416 (semaxanib) in solid tumours, incorporating dynamic contrast MR pharmacodynamic end points." *Br J Cancer* **93**(8): 876–83.

O'Dwyer, P. J., M. Rosen, et al. (2005). "Pharmacodynamic study of BAY 43-9006 in patients with metastatic renal cell carcinoma." *J Clin Oncol (Meeting Abstracts)* **23**(16 (suppl)): 3005.

Oostendorp, M., M. J. Post, et al. (2009). "Vessel growth and function: depiction with contrast-enhanced MR imaging." *Radiology* **251**(2): 317–35.

Overmoyer, B., P. Silverman, et al. (2004). "Phase II trial of neoadjuvant docetaxel with or without bevacizumab in patients with locally advanced breast cancer." *J Clin Oncol, 2004 ASCO Annual Meeting Proceedings (Post-Meeting Edition)* **22**(14S (supplement)): Abstract 727.

Padhani, A. R. and A. Dzik-Jurasz (2004). "Perfusion MR imaging of extracranial tumor angiogenesis." *Top Magn Reson Imaging* **15**(1): 41–57.

Padhani, A. R., N. J. Taylor, et al. (2006). "Dynamic MRI evaluation of the triple receptor tyrosine kinase inhibitor BIBF 1120 in patients with advanced solid tumours." *Proc Intl Soc Magn Reson Med* 14: 765.

Patterson, D. M., N. Charnley, et al. (2008). "Phase I evaluation of vascular disrupting agent OXi4503." *J Clin Oncol* **26**(May 20 suppl): abstract 3551.

Patterson, D. M., P. Ross, et al. (2007). "Phase I evaluation of OXi4503, a vascular disrupting agent, in patients with advanced solid tumours." *J Clin Oncol (Meeting Abstracts)* **25**(18 suppl): 14146.

Prise, V. E., D. J. Honess, et al. (2002). "The vascular response of tumor and normal tissues in the rat to the vascular targeting agent, combretastatin A-4-phosphate, at clinically relevant doses." *Int J Oncol* **21**(4): 717–26.

Robinson, S. P., D. J. McIntyre, et al. (2003). "Tumour dose response to the antivascular agent ZD6126 assessed by magnetic resonance imaging." *Br J Cancer* **88**(10): 1592–7.

Rosen, L. S., R. Kurzrock, et al. (2007). "Safety, pharmacokinetics, and efficacy of AMG 706, an oral multikinase inhibitor, in patients with advanced solid tumors." *J Clin Oncol* **25**(17): 2369–76.

Rosen, L. S., G. Wilding, et al. (2006). "Phase I dose escalation study to determine the safety, pharmacokinetics and pharmacodynamics of BMS-582664, a VEGFR/FGFR inhibitor in patients with advanced/metastatic solid tumors." *J Clin Oncol* (Meeting Abstracts) 24(18 (suppl)): 3051.

Rustin, G. J., S. M. Galbraith, et al. (2003). "Phase I clinical trial of weekly combretastatin A4 phosphate: clinical and pharmacokinetic results." *J Clin Oncol* **21**(15): 2815–22.

Schlemmer, H. P., J. Merkle, et al. (2004). "Can pre-operative contrast-enhanced dynamic MR imaging for prostate cancer predict microvessel density in prostatectomy specimens?" *Eur Radiol* **14**(2): 309–17.

Shaked, Y., A. Ciarrocchi, et al. (2006). "Therapy-induced acute recruitment of circulating endothelial progenitor cells to tumors." *Science* **313**(5794): 1785–87.

Stevenson, J. P., M. Rosen, et al. (2003). "Phase I trial of the antivascular agent combretastatin A4 phosphate on a 5-day schedule to patients with cancer: magnetic resonance imaging evidence for altered tumor blood flow." *J Clin Oncol* **21**(23): 4428–38.

Taylor, N. J., N. Tunariu, et al. (2009). "Non-enhancing pixels: a specific additional DCE-MRI kinetic parameter for assessing antivascular effects of anti-angiogenic and vascular disruptive agents." *Proceedings of the joint meeting of International Society of Magnetic Resonance in Medicine, 16th Scientific Meeting and Exhibition, Honolulu*: 2262.

Thomas, A. L., B. Morgan, et al. (2005). "Phase I study of the safety, tolerability, pharmacokinetics, and pharmacodynamics of PTK787/ZK 222584 administered twice daily in patients with advanced cancer." *J Clin Oncol* **23**(18): 4162–71.

Thukral, A., D. M. Thomasson, et al. (2007). "Inflammatory breast cancer: dynamic contrast-enhanced MR in patients receiving bevacizumab – initial experience." *Radiology* **244**(3): 727–35.

Tofts, P., G. Brix, et al. (1999). "Estimating kinetic parameters from dynamic contrast-enhanced T(1)-weighted MRI of a diffusable tracer: standardized quantities and symbols." *J Magn Reson Imaging* **10**(3): 223–32.

Tofts, P. S. (1997). "Modeling tracer kinetics in dynamic Gd-DTPA MR imaging." *J Magn Reson Imaging* **7**: 91–101.

Tozer, G. M., V. E. Prise, et al. (1999). "Combretastatin A-4 phosphate as a tumor vascular-targeting agent: early effects in tumors and normal tissues." *Cancer Res* **59**(7): 1626–34.

Walker-Samuel, S., C. C. Parker, et al. (2007). "Reproducibility of reference tissue quantification of dynamic contrast-enhanced data: comparison with a fixed vascular input function." *Phys Med Biol* **52**(1): 75–89.

Wedam, S. B., J. A. Low, et al. (2006). "Antiangiogenic and antitumor effects of bevacizumab in patients with inflammatory and locally advanced breast cancer." *J Clin Oncol* **24**(5): 769–77.

Weinmann, H. J., M. Laniado, et al. (1984). "Pharmacokinetics of GdDTPA/dimeglumine after intravenous injection into healthy volunteers." *Physiol Chem Phys Med NMR* **16**(2): 167–72.

Wilkinson, I. D., D. A. Jellineck, et al. (2006). "Dexamethasone and enhancing solitary cerebral mass lesions: alterations in perfusion and blood-tumor barrier kinetics shown by magnetic resonance imaging." *Neurosurgery* **58**(4): 640–6; discussion 640–6.

Xiong, H. Q., R. Herbst, et al. (2004). "A phase I surrogate endpoint study of SU6668 in patients with solid tumors." *Invest New Drugs* **22**(4): 459–66.

Zhang, X., Z. Xiong, et al. (2006). "Quantitative PET imaging of tumor integrin alphavbeta3 expression with 18F-FRGD2." *J Nucl Med* **47**(1): 113–21.

Contrast Ultrasound in Imaging Tumor Angiogenesis

Grzegorz Korpanty and Rolf A. Brekken

Abstract New strategies to detect tumor angiogenesis and monitor response of tumor vasculature to therapy are needed. There are a plethora of anti-angiogenic strategies being evaluated pre-clinically and in the clinical setting; however, a significant unmet challenge is following the response of tumors to anti-angiogenic therapy. Herein we review current modalities being investigated for this purpose and highlight the utility of contrast ultrasound imaging using targeted microbubbles (MB). MB are small (1–10 μm) gas-filled intravascular tracers. MB can be targeted via antibodies, peptides or other moieties to virtually any endothelial cell surface marker and thus selectively mark specific vascular beds (e.g., tumor blood vessels). Furthermore targeted MB can be used to non-invasively evaluate the expression level of particular molecular antigens (e.g., CD105, VEGFR2) and monitor the effect of therapy on target expression. We conclude that targeted MB represent a novel and attractive tool for non-invasive, vascular-targeted molecular imaging of tumor angiogenesis and for monitoring vascular effects specific to anti-tumor therapy in vivo.

Abbreviations

APN	aminopeptidase N
BV	blood vessels
EC	endothelial cells
FN	fibronectin
MMP	matrix metalloproteinases
PSMA	prostate specific membrane antigen
SMC	smooth muscle cell
TEM	tumor endothelial marker
VEGF:VEGFR	complex of VEGF and its receptor

R.A. Brekken (✉)
Division of Surgical Oncology, Departments of Surgery and Pharmacology,
The Hamon Center for Therapeutic Oncology Research, UT Southwestern Medical Center,
6000 Harry Hines Blvd, Dallas, TX 75390-8593, USA
e-mail: rolf.brekken@utsouthwestern.edu

T. Meyer (ed.), *Vascular Disruptive Agents for the Treatment of Cancer*,
DOI 10.1007/978-1-4419-6609-4_8,

1 Background

Angiogenesis (formation of new vessels from pre-existing ones) is a crucial early event in the process of tumor development. New vessels supply the tumor with nutrients that are needed for further local growth and enable distant metastases (Folkman 1995). Judah Folkman (1971) highlighted the potential therapeutic implications of tumor angiogenesis. He hypothesized that if tumor angiogenesis is inhibited, then tumor growth and metastasis will be impaired greatly or even impossible. The subsequent quest for endogenous and exogenous inhibitors of angiogenesis has yielded a variety of promising therapeutic agents that block one or more angiogenic pathways, a few of which have been approved by the FDA (e.g., bevacizumab, sorafenib, sunitinib) for use as single agents or in combination with chemotherapy in specific populations of cancer patients (Sessa et al. 2008). There has also been a dramatic expansion in the exploration of novel anti-angiogenic agents pre-clinically and in clinical trials (Ferrara 2002). Some of the most promising data comes from the development of agents that inhibit one of the key growth factors involved in tumor angiogenesis – vascular endothelial growth factor (VEGF) (Ferrara et al. 2003). Bevacizumab is a monoclonal antibody against VEGF that was the first anti-angiogenic agent that improved significantly the overall survival of patients with colorectal and non-squamous non-small cell lung cancer (Ferrara et al. 2005).

Various agents that target tumor angiogenesis are currently under investigation in different cancer types in many clinical trials (Ferrara and Kerbel 2005). While some of these agents show more encouraging results than the others, what seems to be a common clinical problem is the lack of an effective tool to monitor tumor response to these novel therapies (Jubb et al. 2006). It seems that the RECIST (Response Evaluation Criteria in Solid Tumors) criteria that are commonly used clinically to monitor tumor response may not be an effective or even accurate measure of response to anti-angiogenic agents. Very often anti-angiogenic agents enhance the central necrosis of the tumor without changing to a measurable extent the overall tumor size, which is a central parameter in RECIST evaluation (Jaffe 2006).

An area of intense debate is how anti-angiogenic agents actually work in terms of combating cancer (Duda et al. 2007). According to the Folkman hypothesis, interference with the process of tumor angiogenesis results in either inhibition of new vessel formation or progressive loss of already existing vessels supporting tumor growth. An inadequate blood supply caused by denigration of the vascular network as a result of anti-angiogenic therapy, slows and eventually prevents tumor growth and causes the tumor to regress to a "state of dormancy," which can be undetectable clinically (Folkman 1971). Evidence for this paradigm can be found in pre-clinical studies in which fast growing human tumors are treated with anti-VEGF therapy for long periods of time (Asano et al. 1999; Brekken et al. 2000; Gerber et al. 2000). However, clinical experience with anti-VEGF strategies given as a single agent have not provided substantial support for this mechanism of action (Sessa et al. 2008).

An alternative explanation for anti-VEGF activity and possibly anti-angiogenic agents in general has been proposed. Rakesh Jain has suggested that anti-VEGF therapy actually "normalizes" tumor vasculature and transiently improves blood flow within the tumor, thus enhancing the efficiency of the delivery of chemotherapy (Jain 2001, 2005). Tumor vasculature is heterogeneous in structure and function due to the microenvironment of the tumor. A minority of blood vessels are intimately associated with pericytes and as a result are more functional and stable (Baluk et al. 2005). These vessels are not as dependent on VEGF stimulation for survival. In contrast, a large proportion of tumor blood vessels are tortuous, leaky, and immature. These vessels often lack completely or have sparse interaction with pericytes. Furthermore, these vessels are more dependent on survival signals provided by VEGF and other growth factors. When VEGF levels are decreased via therapy, these vessels are regress leaving behind a more stable vascular network. There is also compelling evidence that VEGF actively suppresses pericyte recruitment (Greenberg et al. 2008), thus blocking VEGF activity may also result in active recruitment of pericyte coverage of remaining blood vessels. As a result of pruning and/or suppression of the inhibitory affects of VEGF the vasculature that remains in the face of anti-VEGF therapy consists of a higher percentage of pericyte associated blood vessels that are more efficient in function. This process has been termed "normalization" and reflects chaotic nature of the tumor vasculature and its compartmentalization into VEGF-independent and VEGF-dependent networks within the same tumor. Normalization can result in the transient re-direction of blood flow within the tumor through the more stable and functional vasculature. This can improve the delivery of chemotherapy into the tumor. Additionally, because stable vessels within the tumor are less leaky, interstitial pressure may decrease and thus facilitate improved tissue penetration of chemotherapy. This concept has been supported by pre-clinical studies in tumor-bearing mice (Salnikov et al. 2006; Tong et al. 2004) and in clinical studies (Willett et al. 2004). A supportive corollary to this is that anti-angiogenic therapy has been shown to increase the efficacy of radiation therapy due to transient improvement in tumor oxygenation as a result of anti-angiogenic treatment (Duda et al. 2007).

2 Imaging of Tumor Angiogenesis

The majority of non-invasive techniques used to assess the effects of anti-angiogenic therapy do not directly visualize tumor blood vessels. Rather surrogate markers for vascular function such as blood flow are used commonly. These techniques assume that during the course of treatment blood flow within the tumor changes, either increasing due to "normalization" or decreasing due to diminished blood supply and vessel regression (McDonald and Choyke 2003; Provenzale 2007; Shaked et al. 2005). Clinically relevant imaging techniques include magnetic resonance imaging (MRI), computed tomography (CT), positron emission tomography (PET) and ultrasound (US). Each of these techniques can be used with appropriate contrast media to evaluate hemodynamic function within tissues including solid tumors.

Perfusion (dynamic contrast-enhanced; DCE) MRI has been used successfully in both animal and clinical models to follow hemodynamic function (Padhani and Leach 2005). DCE-MRI makes use of paramagnetic tracers, mostly consisting of a low-molecular-weight gadolinium (Gd) and is the standard method for measurement of vascular function in clinical trials of anti-angiogenic drugs (Barrett et al. 2007). Signal enhancement obtained by DCE-MRI depends on the tissue perfusion and permeability, contrast concentration, and the extravascular space volume (Tofts et al. 1999). DCE-MRI has been especially useful in clinical studies of patients with liver and brain tumors (Gossmann et al. 2002; Leach et al. 2003; Miller et al. 2005; Morgan et al. 2003; Rosen and Schnall 2007; Willett et al. 2004). CT-based perfusion imaging techniques is also used to assess the vascular effects of anti-angiogenic treatments (Broumas et al. 2005; Zhu et al. 2008). Although DCE-MRI gives better spatial resolution and is a superior method for brain imaging studies, CT still remains a preferred method for imaging structures within the thorax, abdomen and pelvis. Thus some clinical studies investigating anti-angiogenic agents have used perfusion CT rather than DCE-MRI to evaluate tumor blood flow (Dugdale et al. 1999; Pollard et al. 2004; Tsushima et al. 2004).

In addition, PET-based imaging techniques are widely used in clinical oncology (Castell and Cook 2008). PET uses positron-emitting tracers, of which $H_2{}^{15}O$ can be used to study tumor blood flow and this method has been used in clinical trials with good results (Lodge et al. 2000). $H_2{}^{15}O$ is a positron-emitting tracer that can diffuse freely into the tissues and its tissue uptake correlates with blood perfusion (de Langen et al. 2008). Both $H_2{}^{15}O$ PET and DCE-MRI are useful for monitoring tumor microvasculature. $H_2{}^{15}O$ PET is particularly useful in the assessment of tissue perfusion while DCE-MRI measures also vascular permeability. A major disadvantage of both methods is their limited availability for patients because they require highly skilled and trained staff that are typically only available in large radiology and/or nuclear medicine departments.

3 Contrast Ultrasound

World-wide, ultrasound (US) is one of the most commonly used non-invasive imaging techniques. It provides not only anatomical information but is also used to assess physiological function (e.g., blood flow with Doppler ultrasound) or serve as a therapeutic tool (e.g., high frequency ultrasound ablation of the tissue) (Franklin et al. 1961; Fry et al. 1954). Because blood is only slightly less echogenic than surrounding tissue, US is not very effective for imaging small blood vessels. However, the introduction of US contrast agents (microbubbles) expanded the clinical and research applications of US especially in the area of vascular imaging. Microbubbles (MB) are small particles (1–10 μm) that are injected intravenously. They are truly intravascular tracers that do not extravasate unless there is structural damage to the vessel wall. MB consist of a gaseous core and a shell that is composed of either protein (e.g., albumin) or lipid mixture (Correas et al. 2001). MB enhance greatly the echogenicity of the blood pool when injected intravenously and enable distinction of vascular structures from the surrounding tissue. MB resonate in an ultrasound field. Furthermore, by contracting and expanding in response to the ultrasound wave MB enhance both grey scale images and flow mediated Doppler signals. Their high echogenic properties are due to the difference of compressibility of the gaseous core within the MB and the surrounding blood components and tissue (Morgan et al. 2000). MB have proven their usefulness in clinical echocardiography, especially in the evaluation of systolic myocardial function, ejection fraction, delineating endocardial border and myocardial blood flow (Cheng et al. 1998; Cohen et al. 1998; Cwajg et al. 2000).

Imaging metastatic deposits or primary liver tumors (e.g., hepatocellular carcinoma) with contrast US is an example of the clinical application for MB-enhanced US imaging (Krix 2005; Krix et al. 2005). The liver is one of the organs that is most commonly affected by distant metastases and early detection of small (subcentimeter) lesions by contrast-enhanced US is of clinical significance (Forsberg et al. 1999; Harvey et al. 2000; Kim et al. 2000b). Comparative studies of the sensitivity and specificity of PET, CT, DCE-MRI, and MB-enhanced US for detection of tumor perfusion showed that contrast US is an effective and correlative method with significant clinical potential (Kim et al. 2006; Niermann et al. 2007; Yankeelov et al. 2006).

3.1 Targeted Imaging with Microbubbles-Enhanced Ultrasound

MB behave hemodynamically like red blood cells, they circulate freely after injection and are small enough to reach the capillary microcirculation (Ismail et al. 1996). The idea of targeted imaging using contrast US is based on the selective accumulation of MB in specific vascular beds that can be reached by US wave and subsequently imaged. MB do not adhere to the normal vascular endothelium. After multiple transfers through the pulmonary microcirculation, gas that is entrapped within the shell is exhaled through the lungs and the remnants of the shell are taken-up by macrophages of the reticulo-endothelial system in the spleen, liver and bone marrow. However, MB with albumin-containing shell can adhere to endothelial cells that are activated by inflammatory cytokines, or activated leukocytes, which enables MB to be targeted passively to the areas of vascular inflammation (Lindner et al. 2000a, b; Villanueva et al. 1997). MB can be also targeted actively to specific vascular beds by conjugation of targeting moieties (e.g., antibodies or peptides) to the MB shell (Dayton and Ferrara 2002; Korpanty et al. 2005; Lanza and Wickline 2001). In pre-clinical studies, MB have been targeted to various endothelial markers expressed on inflamed or ischaemic tissues such as the myocardium or kidney (Lindner et al. 2001; Villanueva et al. 1998; Villanueva and Wagner 2008). Tumor endothelial cells also express a variety of molecules that can serve as potential ligands for targeted MB (St Croix et al. 2000).

3.2 Imaging Tumor Angiogenesis with Targeted MB and Ultrasound

Endothelial cells lining tumor blood vessels express specific molecules that are absent or expressed a much lower levels on endothelium in normal non-cancerous tissue. Thus tumor vasculature is an attractive subject for imaging with targeted MB and US (Eberhard et al. 2000). The list of potential target molecules selective for tumor vasculature is growing and includes growth factor receptors, integrins, ephrins, endoglin, TEMs (tumor endothelial markers), and markers of cell stress (Table 1). It became even more relevant clinically to image tumor vasculature after anti-angiogenic agents became more commonly used in cancer therapy (Cherrington et al. 2000). The development of surrogate markers of pathological angiogenesis to monitor the response of patients to anti-angiogenic therapy is of critical importance if anti-angiogenic strategies are to be a viable modality for cancer therapy. Contrast US using targeted MB can be an efficient tool to monitor the expression of surface markers that are known to be expressed by tumor endothelial cells. This strategy can be used to visualize tumor blood vessels and in addition can follow the expression level of markers that are known to be altered by anti-angiogenic therapy (e.g., VEGFR2 levels in the face of anti-VEGF therapy) (McDonald and Choyke 2003).

One of the first studies exploiting the concept of contrast US with ligand specific MB used $\alpha_v\beta_3$ integrin as a target (Brooks et al. 1994). $\alpha_v\beta_3$ integrin-specific MB bound specifically to tumor blood vessels and accumulated within vascular areas in the tumor. Furthermore, signal enhancement from the targeted MB correlated with immunohistochemical staining of $\alpha_v\beta_3$ integrin in the same tumor samples (Ellegala et al. 2003). $\alpha_v\beta_3$ integrin has also been used as a tumor vasculature specific target in studies that using MRI and paramagnetic targeted nanoparticles as contrast agents (Sipkins et al. 1998; Winter et al. 2003).

VEGFR2 (VEGF receptor 2) is a commonly used marker of proliferating vascular endothelial cells and has been used by multiple groups as a molecular target for MB. Animal models of angiosarcoma, glioma, and breast cancer showed that VEGFR2 targeted MB enhanced US imaging in evaluation of tumor angiogenesis (Lee et al. 2008; Lyshchik et al. 2007).

What seems to be a consistent finding in many studies with targeted MB and US imaging is that the intensity of the ultrasound signal obtained due to targeted contrast agent correlates with the level of expression of the target when assessed pathologically by immunohistochemistry. This finding has powerful implications for further clinical studies that evaluate the response of tumor vessels to anti-angiogenic therapies. In many animal models such attempts showed very promising results. Recently, our group evaluated vascular response to anti-angiogenic and chemotherapy in mouse models of pancreatic cancer using MB targeted against VEGFR2, the VEGF:VEGFR complex, and endoglin (Korpanty et al. 2007). Using three different formulations of tumor vessel specific MB and US, we were able to non-invasively monitor vascular function of subcutaneous and orthotopic pancreatic tumors in mice. We found that targeting to VEGFR2, endoglin, or VEGF:VEGFR

Table 1 Potential markers of tumor blood vessels

Targeting moiety	Antigen	Location of marker	References
Multiple	VEGF:VEGFR	Angiogenic BV	Ke et al. (1996), Brekken et al. (1998), Cooke et al. (2001), Molema et al. (1998)
MKID2	$\alpha_3\beta_1$	Angiogenic BV	Gonzalez et al. (2002)
GoH3	$\alpha_6\beta_1$	Angiogenic BV	Gonzalez et al. (2002)
EN7/44	p30.5	Proliferating EC	Hagemeier et al. (1986)
Multiple	CD105 (endoglin)	Proliferating EC	Burrows et al. (1995), Seon et al. (1997), Thorpe and Burrows (1995), Westphal et al. (1993), Wang et al. (1993), Wang et al. (1995)
FB5	Endosialin	Proliferating EC	Rettig et al. (1992)
MK 2.7	VCAM-1	Activated EC	Ran and Thorpe (2002)
	E-selectin, CD62E	Activated EC	Ran and Thorpe (2002)
4A11	H-5-2, Lewis^y-6	Activated EC	Koch et al. (1994)
	CD44	Activated EC	Griffioen et al. (1997)
Metastatin	Hyaluronan	Activated EC	Liu et al. (2001)
Vitaxin; RGD cyclic peptide	$\alpha_V\beta_3$; $\alpha_V\beta_5$	Activated EC	Sipkins et al. (1998), Gasparini et al. (1998), Pasqualini et al. (1997)
Multiple	$\alpha_1\beta_1$; $\alpha_2\beta_1$	Activated EC	Senger et al. (1997, 2002)
Multiple	$\alpha_5\beta_1$	Activated EC	Kim et al. (2000a)
3SB, 3G4, Bavituximab	Phosphatidylserine	Activated EC	Ran and Thorpe (2002)
TV-1	FN	Basement membrane	Epstein et al. (1995)
L19	ED-B isoform of FN	Basement membrane	Nilsson et al. (2001), Carnemolla et al. (1996), Marty et al. (2002), Borsi et al. (2002)
HUIV26, HUI77	Denaturated collagens	Proteolyzed basement membrane	Xu et al. (2000, 2001)
Multiple	NG2 proteoglycan	Pericytes	Burg et al. (1999)
NGR peptide	CD13/APN	Tumor EC	Pasqualini et al. (2000)

complex was specific for tumor vasculature as there was no signal enhancement in non-tumor tumor tissue. Furthermore, we found that anti-VEGF therapy or treatment with gemcitabine reduced the expression of the molecular targets bound by the MB. Our contrast US intensity data correlated with immunohistochemical analysis of tumor samples. This was the first indication that targeted MB could be used to follow expression of a cell surface target. Additionally, these studies also validated that gemcitabine can effect endothelial cells in tumors. Other groups have since confirmed our findings using targeted MB to image the response of tumor vessels to the therapy (Palmowski et al. 2008).

We have also explored the use of antibodies that bind to cell surface markers of cell stress as targeting agents for MB. Bavituximab (Ran et al. 2005; Soares et al. 2008) is a mouse/human chimeric antibody specific for phosphatidylserine (PS), an anionic phospholipid that is typically segregated to the inner leaflet of the cell membrane. However under certain conditions PS is "flipped" to the outer leaflet and accessible to binding proteins such as antibodies. Bavituximab was developed as a vascular targeting agent and is being evaluated clinically as a therapeutic agent in multiple solid tumors (Tomillero and Moral 2008). We constructed MB linked to bavituximab to non-invasively monitor PS exposure on blood vessels of tumors and to determine if anti-angiogenic therapy altered PS exposure. We found that mice-bearing MiaPaCa-2 tumors that were treated with anti-VEGF therapy had an increase in the localization of MB targeted with bavituximab (Fig. 1). This is in contrast to the localization of MB linked to an antibody specific for VEGFR2, which showed a decrease in VEGFR2 similar to previous findings (Korpanty et al. 2007). We also evaluated the localization of bavituximab-MB by immunohistochemistry in tumor tissue and several normal organs (Fig. 1). There was abundant localization of the MB in tumor tissue with the majority of the signal being focused on blood vessels. There was also uptake in the liver, most likely macrophages and a relatively small amount of signal from other organs including the heart. Thus, targeting MB to PS appears to be a relevant marker of tumor vasculature that actually increases in the face of therapy and could therefore be a very useful readout for following response to anti-VEGF in particular and possibly anti-angiogenic therapy in general.

Technically MB can be modified to target more than one ligand as it was previously shown under in vitro conditions (Weller et al. 2005). Using MB that are able to bind selectively to more than one target is an attractive idea and may provide even more specificity to distinguish blood vessels in tumors versus non-tumor tissue. In a mouse model of ovarian cancer, MB that were conjugated with antibodies specific for VEGFR2 and $\alpha_v\beta_3$ integrin enhanced the US signal when compared with MB that were conjugated with a single targeting antibody. Dual targeted MB enhanced US was proven to increase sensitivity and specificity of imaging tumor angiogenesis (Willmann et al. 2008).

4 Conclusions

Anti-angiogenic therapies are an important component of cancer therapy protocols and have already proven to prolong overall survival in many patients with metastatic cancer. After more than a decade of advanced clinical trials with these agents, appropriate selection of patients, reliable and non-invasive monitoring of the effects of the anti-angiogenic agents are still the subjects of extensive research.

Non-invasive imaging of molecular changes on tumor blood vessels that result from anti-angiogenic therapy is still not available clinically. However, contrast US with targeted MB has proven to be an efficient method for monitoring the response of tumor vasculature to therapy in pre-clinical studies. This represents significant progress since the first images of contrast enhanced US were made in the late 1960s

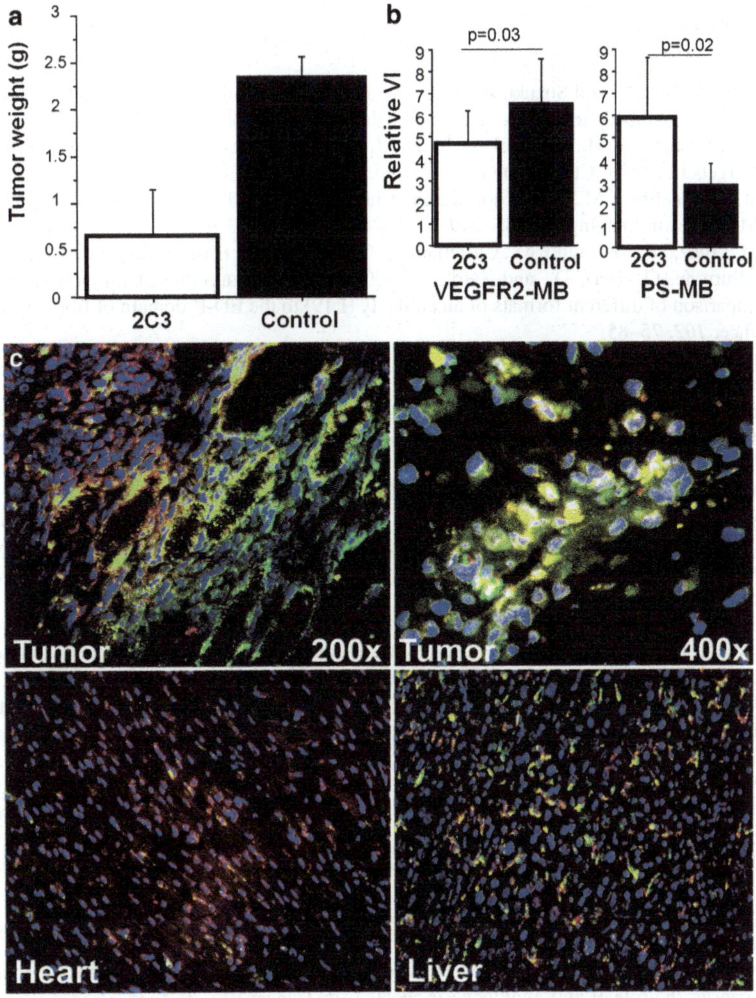

Fig. 1 Anti-VEGF therapy induces exposure of phosphatidylserine on tumor blood vessels. (**a**) Mice bearing MiaPaCa-2 tumors were treated with control or an anti-VEGF antibody (2C3). Mean (± SD) tumor weight at the end of the experiment is shown. (**b**) Before sacrifice, the animals were imaged with contrast US using microbubbles (MB) conjugated to antibodies specific for VEGFR2 (VEGFR2-MB) or phosphatidylserine (PS-MB). Mean relative video intensity (+/–SD) of MB signal is shown. (**c**) A subset of animals were sacrificed 10 min post injection of PS-MB and tumor and other tissues were snap frozen and processed for fluorescence microscopy. MB were constructed with rhodamine-conjugated albumin (*red*) and FITC-conjugated bavituximab (*green*). Representative images of PS-MB localization to tumor tissue and heart and liver are shown

(Gramiak and Shah 1968). Targeted MB enhanced US imaging has become a more widely accepted method in the field of tumor angiogenesis research. The advantages of US over MRI or CT including portability, real-time imaging, and low cost will help this method become a clinical tool that is useful not only in the field of oncology but also in other angiogenesis-related diseases.

References

Asano, M., Yukita, A., and Suzuki, H. (1999). Wide spectrum of antitumor activity of a neutralizing monoclonal antibody to human vascular endothelial growth factor. Jpn J Cancer Res *90*, 93–100.

Baluk, P., Hashizume, H., and McDonald, D. M. (2005). Cellular abnormalities of blood vessels as targets in cancer. Curr Opin Genet Dev *15*, 102–111.

Barrett, T., Brechbiel, M., Bernardo, M., and Choyke, P. L. (2007). MRI of tumor angiogenesis. J Magn Reson Imaging *26*, 235–249.

Borsi, L., Balza, E., Bestagno, M., Castellani, P., Carnemolla, B., Biro, A., Leprini, A., Sepulveda, J., Burrone, O., Neri, D., and Zardi, L. (2002). Selective targeting of tumoral vasculature: comparison of different formats of an antibody (L19) to the ED-B domain of fibronectin. Int J Cancer *102*, 75–85.

Brekken, R. A., Huang, X., King, S. W., and Thorpe, P. E. (1998). Vascular endothelial growth factor as a marker of tumor endothelium. Cancer Res *58*, 1952–1959.

Brekken, R. A., Overholser, J. P., Stastny, V. A., Waltenberger, J., Minna, J. D., and Thorpe, P. E. (2000). Selective inhibition of vascular endothelial growth factor (VEGF) receptor 2 (KDR/Flk-1) activity by a monoclonal anti-VEGF antibody blocks tumor growth in mice. Cancer Res *60*, 5117–5124.

Brooks, P. C., Clark, R. A., and Cheresh, D. A. (1994). Requirement of vascular integrin alpha v beta 3 for angiogenesis. Science *264*, 569–571.

Broumas, A. R., Pollard, R. E., Bloch, S. H., Wisner, E. R., Griffey, S., and Ferrara, K. W. (2005). Contrast-enhanced computed tomography and ultrasound for the evaluation of tumor blood flow. Invest Radiol *40*, 134–147.

Burg, M. A., Pasqualini, R., Arap, W., Ruoslahti, E., and Stallcup, W. B. (1999). NG2 proteoglycan-binding peptides target tumor neovasculature. Cancer Res *59*, 2869–2874.

Burrows, F. J., Derbyshire, E. J., Tazzari, P. L., Amlot, P., Gazdar, A. F., King, S. W., Letarte, M., Vitetta, E. S., and Thorpe, P. E. (1995). Up-regulation of endoglin on vascular endothelial cells in human solid tumors: implications for diagnosis and therapy. Clin Cancer Res *1*, 1623–1634.

Carnemolla, B., Neri, D., Castellani, P., Leprini, A., Neri, G., Pini, A., Winter, G., and Zardi, L. (1996). Phage antibodies with pan-species recognition of the oncofoetal angiogenesis marker fibronectin ED-B domain. Int J Cancer *68*, 397–405.

Castell, F., and Cook, G. J. (2008). Quantitative techniques in 18FDG PET scanning in oncology. Br J Cancer *98*, 1597–1601.

Cheng, S. C., Dy, T. C., and Feinstein, S. B. (1998). Contrast echocardiography: review and future directions. Am J Cardiol *81*, 41G-48G.

Cherrington, J. M., Strawn, L. M., and Shawver, L. K. (2000). New paradigms for the treatment of cancer: the role of anti-angiogenesis agents. Adv Cancer Res *79*, 1–38.

Cohen, J. L., Cheirif, J., Segar, D. S., Gillam, L. D., Gottdiener, J. S., Hausnerova, E., and Bruns, D. E. (1998). Improved left ventricular endocardial border delineation and opacification with OPTISON (FS069), a new echocardiographic contrast agent. Results of a phase III multicenter trial. J Am Coll Cardiol *32*, 746–752.

Cooke, S. P., Boxer, G. M., Lawrence, L., Pedley, R. B., Spencer, D. I., Begent, R. H., and Chester, K. A. (2001). A strategy for antitumor vascular therapy by targeting the vascular endothelial growth factor: receptor complex. Cancer Res *61*, 3653–3659.

Correas, J. M., Bridal, L., Lesavre, A., Mejean, A., Claudon, M., and Helenon, O. (2001). Ultrasound contrast agents: properties, principles of action, tolerance, and artifacts. Eur Radiol *11*, 1316–1328.

Cwajg, J., Xie, F., O'Leary, E., Kricsfeld, D., Dittrich, H., and Porter, T. R. (2000). Detection of angiographically significant coronary artery disease with accelerated intermittent imaging after intravenous administration of ultrasound contrast material. Am Heart J *139*, 675–683.

Dayton, P. A., and Ferrara, K. W. (2002). Targeted imaging using ultrasound. J Magn Reson Imaging *16*, 362–377.

de Langen, A. J., van den Boogaart, V. E., Marcus, J. T., and Lubberink, M. (2008). Use of H2(15) O-PET and DCE-MRI to measure tumor blood flow. Oncologist *13*, 631–644.

Duda, D. G., Jain, R. K., and Willett, C. G. (2007). Antiangiogenics: the potential role of integrating this novel treatment modality with chemoradiation for solid cancers. J Clin Oncol *25*, 4033–4042.

Dugdale, P. E., Miles, K. A., Bunce, I., Kelley, B. B., and Leggett, D. A. (1999). CT measurement of perfusion and permeability within lymphoma masses and its ability to assess grade, activity, and chemotherapeutic response. J Comput Assist Tomogr *23*, 540–547.

Eberhard, A., Kahlert, S., Goede, V., Hemmerlein, B., Plate, K. H., and Augustin, H. G. (2000). Heterogeneity of angiogenesis and blood vessel maturation in human tumors: implications for antiangiogenic tumor therapies. Cancer Res *60*, 1388–1393.

Ellegala, D. B., Leong-Poi, H., Carpenter, J. E., Klibanov, A. L., Kaul, S., Shaffrey, M. E., Sklenar, J., and Lindner, J. R. (2003). Imaging tumor angiogenesis with contrast ultrasound and microbubbles targeted to alpha(v)beta3. Circulation *108*, 336–341.

Epstein, A. L., Khawli, L. A., Hornick, J. L., and Taylor, C. R. (1995). Identification of a monoclonal antibody, TV-1 directed against the basement membrane of tumor vessels, and its use to enhance the delivery of macromolecules to tumors after conjugation with interleukin 2. Cancer Res *55*, 2673–2680.

Ferrara, N. (2002). VEGF and the quest for tumour angiogenesis factors. Nat Rev Cancer *2*, 795–803.

Ferrara, N., and Kerbel, R. S. (2005). Angiogenesis as a therapeutic target. Nature *438*, 967–974.

Ferrara, N., Gerber, H. P., and LeCouter, J. (2003). The biology of VEGF and its receptors. Nat Med *9*, 669–676.

Ferrara, N., Hillan, K. J., and Novotny, W. (2005). Bevacizumab (Avastin), a humanized anti-VEGF monoclonal antibody for cancer therapy. Biochem Biophys Res Commun *333*, 328–335.

Folkman, J. (1971). Tumor angiogenesis: therapeutic implications. N Engl J Med *285*, 1182–1186.

Folkman, J. (1995). Angiogenesis in cancer, vascular, rheumatoid and other disease. Nat Med *1*, 27–31.

Forsberg, F., Goldberg, B. B., Liu, J. B., Merton, D. A., Rawool, N. M., and Shi, W. T. (1999). Tissue-specific US contrast agent for evaluation of hepatic and splenic parenchyma. Radiology *210*, 125–132.

Franklin, D. L., Schlegel, W., and Rushmer, R. F. (1961). Blood flow measured by Doppler frequency shift of back-scattered ultrasound. Science *134*, 564–565.

Fry, W. J., Mosberg, W. H., Jr., Barnard, J. W., and Fry, F. J. (1954). Production of focal destructive lesions in the central nervous system with ultrasound. J Neurosurg *11*, 471–478.

Gasparini, G., Brooks, P. C., Biganzoli, E., Vermeulen, P. B., Bonoldi, E., Dirix, L. Y., Ranieri, G., Miceli, R., and Cheresh, D. A. (1998). Vascular integrin alpha(v)beta3: a new prognostic indicator in breast cancer. Clin Cancer Res *4*, 2625–2634.

Gerber, H.-P., Kowalski, J, Sherman, D, et al. (2000). Complete inhibition of rhabdomyosarcoma xenograft growth and neovascularization requires blockade of both tumor and host vascular endothelial growth factor. Cancer Research *60*, 6253–6258.

Gonzalez, A. M., Gonzales, M., Herron, G. S., Nagavarapu, U., Hopkinson, S. B., Tsuruta, D., and Jones, J. C. (2002). Complex interactions between the laminin alpha 4 subunit and integrins regulate endothelial cell behavior in vitro and angiogenesis in vivo. Proc Natl Acad Sci U S A *99*, 16075–16080.

Gossmann, A., Helbich, T. H., Kuriyama, N., Ostrowitzki, S., Roberts, T. P., Shames, D. M., van Bruggen, N., Wendland, M. F., Israel, M. A., and Brasch, R. C. (2002). Dynamic contrast-enhanced magnetic resonance imaging as a surrogate marker of tumor response to anti-angiogenic therapy in a xenograft model of glioblastoma multiforme. J Magn Reson Imaging *15*, 233–240.

Gramiak, R., and Shah, P. M. (1968). Echocardiography of the aortic root. Invest Radiol *3*, 356–366.

Greenberg, J. I., Shields, D. J., Barillas, S. G., Acevedo, L. M., Murphy, E., Huang, J., Scheppke, L., Stockmann, C., Johnson, R. S., Angle, N., and Cheresh, D. A. (2008). A role for VEGF as a negative regulator of pericyte function and vessel maturation. Nature *456*, 809–813.

Griffioen, A. W., Coenen, M. J., Damen, C. A., Hellwig, S. M., van Weering, D. H., Vooys, W., Blijham, G. H., and Groenewegen, G. (1997). CD44 is involved in tumor angiogenesis; an activation antigen on human endothelial cells. Blood *90*, 1150–1159.

Hagemeier, H.-H., Vollmer, E., Goerdt, S., Schulze-Osthoff, K., and Sorg, C. (1986). A monoclonal antibody reacting with endothelial cells of budding vessels in tumors and inflammatory tissues, and non-reactive with normal adult tissues. Int J Cancer *38*, 481–488.

Harvey, C. J., Blomley, M. J., Eckersley, R. J., Heckemann, R. A., Butler-Barnes, J., and Cosgrove, D. O. (2000). Pulse-inversion mode imaging of liver specific microbubbles: improved detection of subcentimetre metastases. Lancet *355*, 807–808.

Ismail, S., Jayaweera, A. R., Camarano, G., Gimple, L. W., Powers, E. R., and Kaul, S. (1996). Relation between air-filled albumin microbubble and red blood cell rheology in the human myocardium. Influence of echocardiographic systems and chest wall attenuation. Circulation *94*, 445–451.

Jaffe, C. C. (2006). Measures of response: RECIST, WHO, and new alternatives. J Clin Oncol *24*, 3245–3251.

Jain, R. K. (2001). Normalizing tumor vasculature with anti-angiogenic therapy: a new paradigm for combination therapy. Nat Med *7*, 987–989.

Jain, R. K. (2005). Normalization of tumor vasculature: an emerging concept in antiangiogenic therapy. Science *307*, 58–62.

Jubb, A. M., Oates, A. J., Holden, S., and Koeppen, H. (2006). Predicting benefit from anti-angiogenic agents in malignancy. Nat Rev Cancer *6*, 626–635.

Ke, L., Qu, H., Nagy, J. A., Eckelhoefer, I. A., Masse, E. M., Dvorak, A. M., and Dvorak, H. F. (1996). Vascular targeting of solid and ascites tumours with antibodies to vascular endothelial growth factor. Eur J Cancer *32A*, 2467–2473.

Kim, S., Bell, K., Mousa, S. A., and Varner, J. A. (2000a). Regulation of angiogenesis in vivo by ligation of integrin alpha5beta1 with the central cell-binding domain of fibronectin. Am J Pathol *156*, 1345–1362.

Kim, T. K., Choi, B. I., Han, J. K., Hong, H. S., Park, S. H., and Moon, S. G. (2000b). Hepatic tumors: contrast agent-enhancement patterns with pulse-inversion harmonic US. Radiology *216*, 411–417.

Kim, D. W., Huamani, J., Niermann, K. J., Lee, H., Geng, L., Leavitt, L. L., Baheza, R. A., Jones, C. C., Tumkur, S., Yankeelov, T. E., *et al.* (2006). Noninvasive assessment of tumor vasculature response to radiation-mediated, vasculature-targeted therapy using quantified power Doppler sonography: implications for improvement of therapy schedules. J Ultrasound Med *25*, 1507–1517.

Koch, A. E., Nickoloff, B. J., Holgersson, J., Seed, B., Haines, G. K., Burrows, J. C., and Leibovich, S. J. (1994). 4A11, a monoclonal antibody recognizing a novel antigen expressed on aberrant vascular endothelium. Upregulation in an in vivo model of contact dermatitis. Am J Pathol *144*, 244–259.

Korpanty, G., Grayburn, P. A., Shohet, R. V., and Brekken, R. A. (2005). Targeting vascular endothelium with avidin microbubbles. Ultrasound Med Biol *31*, 1279–1283.

Korpanty, G., Carbon, J. G., Grayburn, P. A., Fleming, J. B., and Brekken, R. A. (2007). Monitoring response to anticancer therapy by targeting microbubbles to tumor vasculature. Clin Cancer Res *13*, 323–330.

Krix, M. (2005). Quantification of enhancement in contrast ultrasound: a tool for monitoring of therapies in liver metastases. Eur Radiol *15 Suppl 5*, E104–108.

Krix, M., Plathow, C., Essig, M., Herfarth, K., Debus, J., Kauczor, H. U., and Delorme, S. (2005). Monitoring of liver metastases after stereotactic radiotherapy using low-MI contrast-enhanced ultrasound – initial results. Eur Radiol *15*, 677–684.

Lanza, G. M., and Wickline, S. A. (2001). Targeted ultrasonic contrast agents for molecular imaging and therapy. Prog Cardiovasc Dis *44*, 13–31.

Leach, M. O., Brindle, K. M., Evelhoch, J. L., Griffiths, J. R., Horsman, M. R., Jackson, A., Jayson, G., Judson, I. R., Knopp, M. V., Maxwell, R. J., *et al.* (2003). Assessment of antiangiogenic and antivascular therapeutics using MRI: recommendations for appropriate methodology for clinical trials. Br J Radiol *76 Spec No 1*, S87–91.

Lee, D. J., Lyshchik, A., Huamani, J., Hallahan, D. E., and Fleischer, A. C. (2008). Relationship between retention of a vascular endothelial growth factor receptor 2 (VEGFR2)-targeted ultrasonographic contrast agent and the level of VEGFR2 expression in an in vivo breast cancer model. J Ultrasound Med *27*, 855–866.

Lindner, J. R., Coggins, M. P., Kaul, S., Klibanov, A. L., Brandenburger, G. H., and Ley, K. (2000a). Microbubble persistence in the microcirculation during ischemia/reperfusion and inflammation is caused by integrin- and complement-mediated adherence to activated leukocytes. Circulation *101*, 668–675.

Lindner, J. R., Dayton, P. A., Coggins, M. P., Ley, K., Song, J., Ferrara, K., and Kaul, S. (2000b). Noninvasive imaging of inflammation by ultrasound detection of phagocytosed microbubbles. Circulation *102*, 531–538.

Lindner, J. R., Song, J., Christiansen, J., Klibanov, A. L., Xu, F., and Ley, K. (2001). Ultrasound assessment of inflammation and renal tissue injury with microbubbles targeted to P-selectin. Circulation *104*, 2107–2112.

Liu, N., Lapcevich, R. K., Underhill, C. B., Han, Z., Gao, F., Swartz, G., Plum, S. M., Zhang, L., and Green, S. J. (2001). Metastatin: a hyaluronan-binding complex from cartilage that inhibits tumor growth. Cancer Res *61*, 1022–1028.

Lodge, M. A., Carson, R. E., Carrasquillo, J. A., Whatley, M., Libutti, S. K., and Bacharach, S. L. (2000). Parametric images of blood flow in oncology PET studies using [15O]water. J Nucl Med *41*, 1784–1792.

Lyshchik, A., Fleischer, A. C., Huamani, J., Hallahan, D. E., Brissova, M., and Gore, J. C. (2007). Molecular imaging of vascular endothelial growth factor receptor 2 expression using targeted contrast-enhanced high-frequency ultrasonography. J Ultrasound Med *26*, 1575–1586.

Marty, C., Odermatt, B., Schott, H., Neri, D., Ballmer-Hofer, K., Klemenz, R., and Schwendener, R. A. (2002). Cytotoxic targeting of F9 teratocarcinoma tumours with anti-ED-B fibronectin scFv antibody modified liposomes. Br J Cancer *87*, 106–112.

McDonald, D. M., and Choyke, P. L. (2003). Imaging of angiogenesis: from microscope to clinic. Nat Med *9*, 713–725.

Miller, J. C., Pien, H. H., Sahani, D., Sorensen, A. G., and Thrall, J. H. (2005). Imaging angiogenesis: applications and potential for drug development. J Natl Cancer Inst *97*, 172–187.

Molema, G., Meijer, D. K., and de Leij, L. F. (1998). Tumor vasculature targeted therapies: getting the players organized. Biochem Pharmacol *55*, 1939–1945.

Morgan, K. E., Allen, J. S., Dayton, P. A., Chomas, J. E., Klibaov, A. L., and Ferrara, K. W. (2000). Experimental and theoretical evaluation of microbubble behavior: effect of transmitted phase and bubble size. IEEE Trans Ultrason Ferroelectr Freq Control *47*, 1494–1509.

Morgan, B., Thomas, A. L., Drevs, J., Hennig, J., Buchert, M., Jivan, A., Horsfield, M. A., Mross, K., Ball, H. A., Lee, L., *et al.* (2003). Dynamic contrast-enhanced magnetic resonance imaging as a biomarker for the pharmacological response of PTK787/ZK 222584, an inhibitor of the vascular endothelial growth factor receptor tyrosine kinases, in patients with advanced colorectal cancer and liver metastases: results from two phase I studies. J Clin Oncol *21*, 3955–3964.

Niermann, K. J., Fleischer, A. C., Huamani, J., Yankeelov, T. E., Kim, D. W., Wilson, W. D., and Hallahan, D. E. (2007). Measuring tumor perfusion in control and treated murine tumors: correlation of microbubble contrast-enhanced sonography to dynamic contrast-enhanced magnetic resonance imaging and fluorodeoxyglucose positron emission tomography. J Ultrasound Med *26*, 749–756.

Nilsson, F., Kosmehl, H., Zardi, L., and Neri, D. (2001). Targeted delivery of tissue factor to the ED-B domain of fibronectin, a marker of angiogenesis, mediates the infarction of solid tumors in mice. Cancer Res *61*, 711–716.

Padhani, A. R., and Leach, M. O. (2005). Antivascular cancer treatments: functional assessments by dynamic contrast-enhanced magnetic resonance imaging. Abdom Imaging *30*, 324–341.

Palmowski, M., Huppert, J., Ladewig, G., Hauff, P., Reinhardt, M., Mueller, M. M., Woenne, E. C., Jenne, J. W., Maurer, M., Kauffmann, G. W., *et al.* (2008). Molecular profiling of angiogenesis with targeted ultrasound imaging: early assessment of antiangiogenic therapy effects. Mol Cancer Ther *7*, 101–109.

Pasqualini, R., Koivunen, E., and Ruoslahti, E. (1997). Alpha v integrins as receptors for tumor targeting by circulating ligands. Nat Biotechnol *15*, 542–546.

Pasqualini, R., Koivunen, E., Kain, R., Lahdenranta, J., Sakamoto, M., Stryhn, A., Ashmun, R. A., Shapiro, L. H., Arap, W., and Ruoslahti, E. (2000). Aminopeptidase N is a receptor for tumor-homing peptides and a target for inhibiting angiogenesis. Cancer Res *60*, 722–727.

Pollard, R. E., Garcia, T. C., Stieger, S. M., Ferrara, K. W., Sadlowski, A. R., and Wisner, E. R. (2004). Quantitative evaluation of perfusion and permeability of peripheral tumors using contrast-enhanced computed tomography. Invest Radiol *39*, 340–349.

Provenzale, J. M. (2007). Imaging of angiogenesis: clinical techniques and novel imaging methods. AJR Am J Roentgenol *188*, 11–23.

Ran, S., and Thorpe, P. E. (2002). Phosphatidylserine is a marker of tumor vasculature and a potential target for cancer imaging and therapy. Int J Radiat Oncol Biol Phys *54*, 1479–1484.

Ran, S., He, J., Huang, X., Soares, M., Scothorn, D., and Thorpe, P. E. (2005). Antitumor effects of a monoclonal antibody that binds anionic phospholipids on the surface of tumor blood vessels in mice. Clin Cancer Res *11*, 1551–1562.

Rettig, W. J., Garinchesa, P., Healey, J. H., Su, S. L., Jaffe, E. A., and Old, L. J. (1992). Identification of endosialin, a cell surface glycoprotein of vascular endothelial cells in human cancer. Proc Natl Acad Sci U S A *89*, 10832–10836.

Rosen, M. A., and Schnall, M. D. (2007). Dynamic contrast-enhanced magnetic resonance imaging for assessing tumor vascularity and vascular effects of targeted therapies in renal cell carcinoma. Clin Cancer Res *13*, 770s-776s.

Salnikov, A. V., Heldin, N. E., Stuhr, L. B., Wiig, H., Gerber, H., Reed, R. K., and Rubin, K. (2006). Inhibition of carcinoma cell-derived VEGF reduces inflammatory characteristics in xenograft carcinoma. Int J Cancer *119*, 2795–2802.

Senger, D. R., Claffey, K. P., Benes, J. E., Perruzzi, C. A., Sergiou, A. P., and Detmar, M. (1997). Angiogenesis promoted by vascular endothelial growth factor: regulation through alpha1beta1 and alpha2beta1 integrins. Proc Natl Acad Sci U S A *94*, 13612–13617.

Senger, D. R., Perruzzi, C. A., Streit, M., Koteliansky, V. E., de Fougerolles, A. R., and Detmar, M. (2002). The alpha(1)beta(1) and alpha(2)beta(1) integrins provide critical support for vascular endothelial growth factor signaling, endothelial cell migration, and tumor angiogenesis. Am J Pathol *160*, 195–204.

Seon, B. K., Matsuno, F., Haruta, Y., Kondo, M., and Barcos, M. (1997). Long-lasting complete inhibition of human solid tumors in SCID mice by targeting endothelial cells of tumor vasculature with antihuman endoglin immunotoxin. Clin Cancer Res *3*, 1031–1044.

Sessa, C., Guibal, A., Del Conte, G., and Ruegg, C. (2008). Biomarkers of angiogenesis for the development of antiangiogenic therapies in oncology: tools or decorations? Nat Clin Pract Oncol *5*, 378–391.

Shaked, Y., Bertolini, F., Man, S., Rogers, M. S., Cervi, D., Foutz, T., Rawn, K., Voskas, D., Dumont, D. J., Ben-David, Y., *et al.* (2005). Genetic heterogeneity of the vasculogenic phenotype parallels angiogenesis; Implications for cellular surrogate marker analysis of antiangiogenesis. Cancer Cell *7*, 101–111.

Sipkins, D. A., Cheresh, D. A., Kazemi, M. R., Nevin, L. M., Bednarski, M. D., and Li, K. C. (1998). Detection of tumor angiogenesis in vivo by alphaVbeta3-targeted magnetic resonance imaging. Nat Med *4*, 623–626.

Soares, M. M., King, S. W., and Thorpe, P. E. (2008). Targeting inside-out phosphatidylserine as a therapeutic strategy for viral diseases. Nat Med *14*, 1357–1362.

St Croix, B., Rago, C., Velculescu, V., Traverso, G., Romans, K. E., Montgomery, E., Lal, A., Riggins, G. J., Lengauer, C., Vogelstein, B., and Kinzler, K. W. (2000). Genes expressed in human tumor endothelium. Science *289*, 1197–1202.

Thorpe, P. E., and Burrows, F. J. (1995). Antibody-directed targeting of the vasculature of solid tumors. Breast Cancer ResTreat *36*, 237–251.

Tofts, P. S., Brix, G., Buckley, D. L., Evelhoch, J. L., Henderson, E., Knopp, M. V., Larsson, H. B., Lee, T. Y., Mayr, N. A., Parker, G. J., *et al.* (1999). Estimating kinetic parameters from dynamic contrast-enhanced T(1)-weighted MRI of a diffusable tracer: standardized quantities and symbols. J Magn Reson Imaging *10*, 223–232.

Tomillero, A., and Moral, M. A. (2008). Gateways to clinical trials. Methods Find Exp Clin Pharmacol *30*, 643–672.

Tong, R. T., Boucher, Y., Kozin, S. V., Winkler, F., Hicklin, D. J., and Jain, R. K. (2004). Vascular normalization by vascular endothelial growth factor receptor 2 blockade induces a pressure gradient across the vasculature and improves drug penetration in tumors. Cancer Res *64*, 3731–3736.

Tsushima, Y., Funabasama, S., Aoki, J., Sanada, S., and Endo, K. (2004). Quantitative perfusion map of malignant liver tumors, created from dynamic computed tomography data. Acad Radiol *11*, 215–223.

Villanueva, F. S., and Wagner, W. R. (2008). Ultrasound molecular imaging of cardiovascular disease. Nat Clin Pract Cardiovasc Med *5 Suppl 2*, S26–32.

Villanueva, F. S., Jankowski, R. J., Manaugh, C., and Wagner, W. R. (1997). Albumin microbubble adherence to human coronary endothelium: implications for assessment of endothelial function using myocardial contrast echocardiography. J Am Coll Cardiol *30*, 689–693.

Villanueva, F. S., Jankowski, R. J., Klibanov, S., Pina, M. L., Alber, S. M., Watkins, S. C., Brandenburger, G. H., and Wagner, W. R. (1998). Microbubbles targeted to intercellular adhesion molecule-1 bind to activated coronary artery endothelial cells. Circulation *98*, 1–5.

Wang, J. M., Kumar, S., Pye, D., Vanagthoven, A. J., Krupinski, J., and Hunter, R. D. (1993). A monoclonal antibody detects heterogeneity in vascular endothelium of tumours and normal tissues. Int J Cancer *54*, 363–370.

Wang, J. M., Kumar, S., van Agthoven, A., Kumar, P., Pye, D., and Hunter, R. D. (1995). Irradiation induces up-regulation of E9 protein (CD105) in human vascular endothelial cells. Int J Cancer *62*, 791–796.

Weller, G. E., Villanueva, F. S., Tom, E. M., and Wagner, W. R. (2005). Targeted ultrasound contrast agents: in vitro assessment of endothelial dysfunction and multi-targeting to ICAM-1 and sialyl Lewisx. Biotechnol Bioeng *92*, 780–788.

Westphal, J. R., Willems, H. W., Schalkwijk, C. J., Ruiter, D. J., and deWaal, R. M. (1993). A new 180-kDa dermal endothelial cell activation antigen: in vitro and in situ characteristics. J Invest Dermatol *100*, 27–34.

Willett, C. G., Boucher, Y., di Tomaso, E., Duda, D. G., Munn, L. L., Tong, R. T., Chung, D. C., Sahani, D. V., Kalva, S. P., Kozin, S. V., *et al.* (2004). Direct evidence that the VEGF-specific antibody bevacizumab has antivascular effects in human rectal cancer. Nat Med *10*, 145–147.

Willmann, J. K., Lutz, A. M., Paulmurugan, R., Patel, M. R., Chu, P., Rosenberg, J., and Gambhir, S. S. (2008). Dual-targeted contrast agent for US assessment of tumor angiogenesis in vivo. Radiology *248*, 936–944.

Winter, P. M., Caruthers, S. D., Kassner, A., Harris, T. D., Chinen, L. K., Allen, J. S., Lacy, E. K., Zhang, H., Robertson, J. D., Wickline, S. A., and Lanza, G. M. (2003). Molecular imaging of angiogenesis in nascent Vx-2 rabbit tumors using a novel alpha(nu)beta3-targeted nanoparticle and 1.5 tesla magnetic resonance imaging. Cancer Res *63*, 5838–5843.

Xu, J., Rodriguez, D., Kim, J. J., and Brooks, P. C. (2000). Generation of monoclonal antibodies to cryptic collagen sites by using subtractive immunization. Hybridoma *19*, 375–385.

Xu, J., Rodriguez, D., Petitclerc, E., Kim, J. J., Hangai, M., Moon, Y. S., Davis, G. E., Brooks, P. C., and Yuen, S. M. (2001). Proteolytic exposure of a cryptic site within collagen type IV is required for angiogenesis and tumor growth in vivo. J Cell Biol *154*, 1069–1079.

Yankeelov, T. E., Niermann, K. J., Huamani, J., Kim, D. W., Quarles, C. C., Fleischer, A. C., Hallahan, D. E., Price, R. R., and Gore, J. C. (2006). Correlation between estimates of tumor perfusion from microbubble contrast-enhanced sonography and dynamic contrast-enhanced magnetic resonance imaging. J Ultrasound Med *25*, 487–497.

Zhu, A. X., Holalkere, N. S., Muzikansky, A., Horgan, K., and Sahani, D. V. (2008). Early anti-angiogenic activity of bevacizumab evaluated by computed tomography perfusion scan in patients with advanced hepatocellular carcinoma. Oncologist *13*, 120–125.

Part III
Clinical Development

The Clinical Development of Tubulin Binding Vascular Disrupting Agents

Martin Zweifel and Gordon Rustin

Abstract Tubulin binding vascular disrupting agents (VDAs) cause a rapid change in tumour endothelial cell shape, resulting in micro-vessel blockage, loss of blood flow, and eventually tumour cell death. Spindle poisons, such as colchicine and vinblastine, disrupt tumor vasculature only at doses close to their maximum tolerated dose, which has prevented their use as VDAs. Newer agents have since been developed, which have a much wider therapeutic window, such as dolastatins and combretastatins. In this chapter, tubulin binding VDAs currently in clinical development will be discussed, with an emphasis on combretastatin A4 phosphate, which has been the first compound of this class to be discovered and to enter clinical trials.

1 Introduction

Two types of vascular disrupting agents (VDAs) are recognised: the ligand-directed VDAs that use antibodies, peptides, and growth factors to deliver toxins, procoagulants, and proapoptotic effectors to tumor endothelium, and the small molecule VDAs that do not specifically localize to tumor endothelium but exploit pathophysiological differences between tumor and normal tissue endothelia to induce acute vascular shutdown in tumors. Spindle poisons, such as colchicine and vinblastine, disrupt tumor vasculature only at doses close to their maximum tolerated dose (MTD), which has prevented their use as VDAs. Newer agents have since been developed, which have a much wider therapeutic window, such as dolastatins and combretastatins (Chaplin et al. 1996). These agents work by acting near the colchicine binding site of the b subunit of endothelial cell tubulin, resulting in depolymerisation of microtubules and disorganisation of actin and tubulin. Endothelial cells are particularly reliant on the cellular cytoskeleton to maintain their shape.

G. Rustin (✉)
Mount Vernon Cancer Centre, Department of Medical Oncology,
HA6 2RN, Northwood, Middlesex, UK
email: grustin@nhs.net

T. Meyer (ed.), *Vascular Disruptive Agents for the Treatment of Cancer*,
DOI 10.1007/978-1-4419-6609-4_9,

A rapid change in endothelial cell shape (Galbraith et al. 2001) causes micro-vessel blockage and loss of flow; it also disrupts the endothelial cell layer, exposing the basement membrane and increasing tumour vascular permeability. This leads to high interstitial pressures, vessel congestion and further loss of flow. Exposure of the basement membrane may also lead to induction of the coagulation cascade and local thrombus formation. Newly formed endothelial cells in tumour vessels are more sensitive to anti-tubulin drugs because mature cells have a highly developed actin cytoskeleton, which maintains cell shape despite depolymerisation of the tubulin cytoskeleton (Chaplin and Dougherty 1999).

In this chapter, tubulin binding vascular disrupting agents currently in clinical development will be discussed, with an emphasis on combretastatin A4 phosphate (CA4P), which has been the first compound of this class to be discovered and to enter clinical trials.

2 Combretastatin A4

2.1 *Preclinical Development*

2.1.1 Structure and Mechanism of Action

Combretastatin A4 phosphate (CA4P, cis-1-(3,4,5,-trimethoxyphenyl)-2-(4'-methoxyphenyl) ethane-3'-O-phosphate, disodium salt; Fig. 1) is a more water soluble prodrug of combretastatin A4 (CA4) (Pettit et al. 1995). CA4P is activated when it is dephosphorylated into CA4 by non-specific endogenous phosphatases present in plasma and on endothelial cells. It has a structure similar to that of colchicine. CA4P does not bind to tubulin, but CA4 binds at or near the colchicine binding site of β-tubulin (Lin et al. 1988; Woods et al. 1995), causing depolymerization of microtubules. The binding of CA4P is rapid, in contrast to colchicine, which binds in a relatively slow and temperature-dependent manner. However, CA4P dissociates from tubulin over 100 times faster than colchicine, with a half life of 3.6 relative to 405 min at 37°C (Lin et al. 1989). Microtubules are involved in motility, intracellular transport, maintenance of shape, and division of cells. Interference with microtubule assembly, either by inhibition of tubulin polymerisation, or blocking

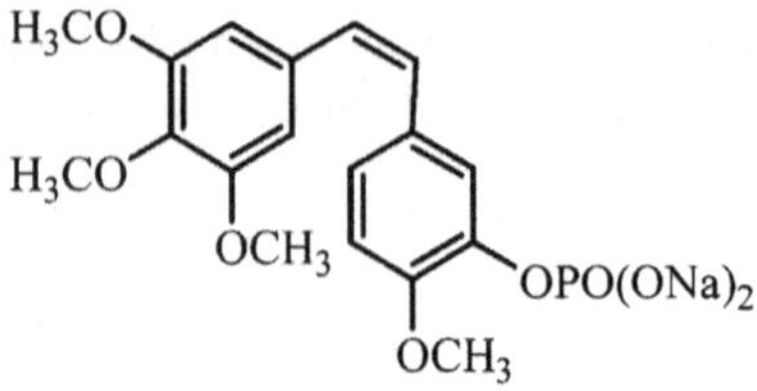

Fig. 1 Molecular structure of combretastatin A4 phosphate (CA4P) (Oxigene 2008)

microtubule disassembly leads to metaphase arrest of the dividing cell (Lin et al. 1989). The trimethoxy unit on ring A was proposed to be essential for interaction with tubulin (Gaukroger et al. 2003). CA4 is active only in its cis configuration (Aprile et al. 2007), which is required to maintain a molecular geometry and a correct orientation of both phenyl groups. Light promotes isomerisation to the less active trans-CA4 form of the drug, so it is stored and administered protected from light. Recently, a two-step stereoselective synthesis of CA4 has been developed by Gaukroger et al., replacing the previous non-stereoselective synthesis (Gaukroger et al. 2001).

2.1.2 In Vivo Antitumor Efficacy

CA4P Single-Agent Activity

The effect of CA4P as a single agent has been examined in rodent and human tumor xenograft models. CA4P was demonstrated to have an effect on the growth of NSCLC tumors grown as xenografts or implanted orthotopically (Boehle et al. 2001). When xenografts of squamous cell carcinoma (KNS-62) or adenocarcinoma cells (Colo-699) implanted into SCID mice were treated with IP CA4P (50 mg/kg daily for 3 weeks), the tumors were approximately threefold smaller in the KNS-62 group and 20-fold smaller in the Colo-699 group as compared to the untreated controls. When mice were injected orthotopically with these same tumors and treated with CA4P, survival was increased by 29% and 35%, respectively, in Colo-699 and KNS-62 implanted animals.

The activity of CA4P (150 mg/kg, once daily over 5 days per week, for a total of 2 weeks) against four anaplastic thyroid cancer (ATC) xenografts was investigated (Dziba et al. 2002). There was a significant decrease in tumor weights of CA4P-treated nude mice with xenografted ARO or DRO tumors, as well as a trend for decreased tumor weights in mice with BHT and KAT-4 xenografts. CA4P treatment did result in toxicity in some animals; especially those injected with the BHT tumors, where four of the six treated animals died. However, when mice with BHT xenografts received treatment with the same dose of CA4P on an every other day schedule for 20 days, toxicity was reduced and there was a statistically significant difference in tumor volume between treated and control animals at the end of the treatment period.

In C3H mouse mammary carcinoma cells grown in the rear foot of female CDF1 mice, CA4P decreased bioenergetic status and pH more rapidly than other VDAs (DMXAA and ZD6126), as assessed by 31P-MR spectroscopy and MRI, and a dose dependent increase in tumour oedema was observed (Breidahl et al. 2006).

In addition to the above studies, CA4P was active as a single agent in a rat rhabdosarcoma model. A single 25 mg/kg (150 mg/m^2) intraperitoneal (IP) dose of CA4P administered to rats bearing large (>7 cm^3) tumors induced tumor regression and growth inhibition (Landuyt et al. 2000; Prise et al. 2002). Interestingly, identical treatment of smaller tumors (3 cm^3) elicited only slight growth delays.

CA4P Combination Activity

Tumors harvested from rodents treated with CA4P characteristically revealed extensive central necrosis, but little effect on tumor size or growth delay was observed. This result is expected however, because CA4P is unable to affect the tumor periphery due to its proximity to the normal vasculature as opposed to the center of the tumor that is fed solely by the tumor vasculature (Dark et al. 1997). Therefore, CA4P has been evaluated in combination studies and has been shown to enhance or act synergistically with the chemotherapeutic agents 5-fluorouracil, paclitaxel, and carboplatin, the antiangiogenic biological therapeutic bevacizumab, biologically active compounds such as cytokines and inhibitors of nitric oxide synthase, and radiotherapy.

CA4P was studied in combination with cisplatin in the treatment of rodents bearing advanced (300 mg) subcutaneous M5076DDP tumours derived from a cisplatin resistant cell line (el Zayat et al. 1993). At the MTD of 7.5 mg/kg administered every 4 days × 3, single agent cisplatin delayed tumour growth equivalent to a 0.8 log cell kill (LCK). Single agent CA4P, administered optimally (250 mg/kg IV daily × 10) produced 1.3 LCK. In comparison, the combination of CA4P (250 mg/kg/inj) + cisplatin (5 mg/kg/inj), administered simultaneously, achieved a 2.0 LCK, which is consistent with a synergistic effect between CA4P and cisplatin. Of note, the combination produced tumour regression, whereas single agent cisplatin and CA4P did not have this effect.

Grosios et al. studied CA4P and 5-fluorouracil in an experimental murine colon adenocarcinoma model (Grosios et al. 2000). Tumor growth delay in MAC-29 colon adenocarcinoma cells implanted subcutaneously (SC) was superior by greater than threefold in the combination treatment group. In tumor bearing C3H/HeJ mice, Li and colleagues noted that the addition of CA4P to radiation increased tumor cell kill rate over that of radiation alone (Li et al. 1998). In another study, the addition of CA4P to radiation also resulted in tumor regression and stabilization for 65 days as well as a 50% cure rate (Chaplin et al. 1999a, b).

In a M5076 model, carboplatin was administered alone at its MTD (90 mg/kg administered IV every 4 days × 3) to yield a 1.4 LCK without causing tumour regression (Landuyt et al. 2000). In comparison, the combination of CA4P and carboplatin, administered simultaneously, resulted in a LCK of 2.0. In contrast, a separate experiment showed that single agent CA4P administered every 4 days × 3 had no activity in this model. As with cisplatin, tumour regression was only observed in the treatment group that received the combination of CA4P and carboplatin. These data are consistent with synergistic anti-tumour activity between CA4P and carboplatin.

The antineoplastic activity of CA4P, paclitaxel, and carboplatin as single agents and in combination was evaluated in nude mice bearing human anaplastic thyroid cancer (ATC) xenografts (Yeung et al. 2007). Following 4 weeks of treatment, the average tumor growth rate was lowest in the triple combination group in both ATC cell lines examined (ARO and KAT-4). In the KAT-4 xenografts, the triple combination group had an average tumor growth rate that was significantly lower than the control and single agent groups. The CA4P and paclitaxel group was the only other group with a significantly lower growth rate than the control group. In the ARO xenografts, only the triple combination group and the carboplatin and paclitaxel group had average tumor growth rates that were significantly lower than the control group. These in vivo results demonstrate that the CA4P, carboplatin and paclitaxel combination exhibits enhanced antitumor activity compared to the single agents alone in mouse tumor models.

Combination of immunotherapeutic procedures is often compromised by the immunosuppressive effects of chemotherapy itself. Combining immunisation with vascular targeting drugs might therefore be an alternative. Concomitant treatment with weekly IL-18/IFNγ-transfected tumour cell immunization and low dose CA4P (2 mg/kg, 5 days a week) enhanced the therapeutic effect as compared with either treatment alone, and resulted in an enhanced antitumour immune activity in a rat model of intrahepatically injected rat colon carcinoma (Badn et al. 2006).

CA4P has been combined with various inhibitors of nitric oxide synthase. This resulted in enhanced tumour necrosis, implying a nitric oxide-related mechanism for this effect (Davis et al. 2002b). Combining the nitric oxide synthase inhibitor N-nitro-l-arginine methyl ester with concomitant weekly IL-18/IFNγ-transfected tumour cell immunization and low dose CA4P (2 mg/kg, 5 days a week) treatment, further retarded tumour growth as compared with either treatment alone (Badn et al. 2006).

Siemann and others examined a combination of antivascular therapy with CA4P and bevacizumab in mice bearing Caki-1 renal cell carcinoma xenografts (Siemann and Shi 2005). This study showed that CA4P or bevacizumab alone had comparable levels of activity, and that the combination was superior to either agent alone, delaying tumor growth nearly twofold longer than that observed with the individual agents. The synergy between CA4P and bevacizumab may be attributable to bevacizumab's ability to prevent reseeding of disrupted vessels with endothelial precursor cells, which repair the damage caused by CA4P (Shaked et al. 2006a, b). Shaked et al. demonstrated, that treatment of tumor-bearing mice with OXi-4503, a vascular disrupting agent closely related to CA4P, led to an acute mobilization of circulating endothelial progenitor cells (CEPs) with a spike at 4 h, which homed to the viable tumor rim that characteristically remains after such therapy. The administration of a monoclonal antibody to vascular endothelial growth factor receptor-2 (VEGFR-2) completely abolished the CEPs spike (Shaked et al. 2006a, b). This finding further supported the administration schedule of concomitant chemotherapy shortly after VDA treatment, because of the ability of chemotherapy to target CEPs. However, paclitaxel has recently been shown to induce proangiogenic CEP mobilization and subsequent tumor homing by systemic induction of SDF-1α, when administered at or near the maximum tolerated dose (Shaked et al. 2008).

2.1.3 Preclinical Administration Schedule: Infusion Frequency and Duration

Several studies in mice have shown that a single administration of CA4 does not significantly affect primary tumour growth (Chaplin et al. 1999a, b; Grosios et al.

1999; Grosios et al. 2000); however, repeated doses can result in substantial growth delays (Griggs et al. 2001).

Hill et al. investigated the effects of multiple daily or twice daily dosing with CA4P on the vascular function, cell survival and growth of syngeneic and spontaneous breast cancers in mice (Hill et al. 2002a). In both transplanted and spontaneous tumors significant growth retardation was observed when CA4P was administrated daily (10 doses × 50 mg/kg), whereas no significant effects were seen if the same total dose was administered as a single bolus injection. This effect was attributed at least in part, to anti-proliferative effects on the tumor and endothelial cells, which retard the revascularization and repopulation of the tumor core that is initially necrosed by the drug treatment. The administration of CA4P in two equal doses separated between 2 and 6 h daily (25 mg/kg twice a day) further enhanced antivascular effects and resulted in enhanced growth retardation. Interestingly, this effect was not observed in the spontaneous T138 tumor model.

Toxicity, as measured by weight loss, was demonstrated to be greater for the twice-daily treatments in both the subcutaneous and the spontaneous tumor model (7% and 6% weight loss, respectively), when compared to the daily dosing group (3% weight loss in both models, and 3% weight gain in untreated animals) (Hill et al. 2002a).

2.1.4 Animal Toxicity

These animal studies demonstrated that at or above MTD, CA4P principally affected tissues with rapid cell division including the gastrointestinal (GI) tract, hematopoietic and lymphoid tissues, and testes (rats only). In rats, 360 mg/m^2 caused severe toxicity or death in 10% of the animals (STD10). Other transient effects included bradycardia, ventricular parasystole, extrasystole, arrhythmia, or ectopic beats in dogs. In vitro safety pharmacology studies were also conducted to assess potential interactions of CA4P and CA4 against a variety of receptors as well as assess effects on I_{Kr} potassium (HERG) and L-type calcium channels and on rabbit Purkinje fibre action potential duration (APD). These studies demonstrated that CA4P and CA4 did not significantly interact with the receptors evaluated in the screen and that CA4P and CA4 were weak blockers of both HERG and L-type calcium channels. Although CA4P did not affect the APD in Purkinje fibers, a concentration-dependent decrease in the duration of the action potential was evident with CA4. The shortening of the APD by CA4 was likely mediated by a relatively greater blockade of L-type calcium channels than of I_{Kr} (HERG) potassium channels. The net effect of these channel-blocking actions in man is difficult to predict. In an in vivo safety pharmacology study, escalating doses of CA4P up to 1,280 mg/m^2 produced minimal to moderate cardiovascular and pulmonary effects in anesthetized dogs, with premature ventricular complexes seen only at the highest dose level. No changes to echocardiograms were observed in any of the animals.

2.2 *Clinical Development*

Fifteen phase I and II trials have been performed or are ongoing, and some of them have been published as paper or abstract by the end of 2008 (Tables 1 and 2). A selection of tubulin binding VDAs currently in clinical development is given in Table 3.

2.2.1 Phase I Trials

The first three trials investigated three different schedules, weekly, 3 weekly, and daily × 5. The weekly trial of CA4P was performed in the United Kingdom at Mount Vernon Cancer Centre under the auspices of the Cancer Research Campaign (CRC) Phase I/II Committee (Rustin et al. 2003). Thirty-four patients with advanced solid tumors were enrolled in this dose-escalation study, receiving weekly doses of a 10 min infusion of 5, 10, 20, 40, 52, 68, 88 or 114 mg/m^2 CA4P for 3 weeks followed by a week gap. Intra-patient dose escalation was allowed in those not experiencing grade 2 or higher drug-related toxicity. All 34 patients experienced at least one adverse event (AE). The most frequently reported drug related AEs were sinus tachycardia (50%), tumor pain and hypertension (35% each), abdominal pain/cramping, sinus bradycardia, headache and fatigue (24% each), dyspepsia/heartburn, nausea, vomiting, hypotension and sweating (21% each). Most of the AEs were grade 1 or 2. The grade 3 AEs, which were deemed related to CA4P, were vasovagal episode, hypotension, fatigue, dehydration, neuropathy, double vision, abdominal pain/cramping, tumor pain (one patient [3%] each). Up to 40 mg/m^2, the only toxicity possibly related to CA4P seen was tumour pain, occurring in 35% of patients a median of 40 min after the start of drug administration. Three dose-limiting toxicities were experienced: reversible ataxia at 114 mg/m^2, vasovagal syncope and motor neuropathy at 88 mg/m^2, and one death associated with CA4P (5 days after the second dose) due to fatal ischemia in small bowel at 52 mg/m^2. The patient had been treated previously with radiation in the area of ischemia, and tumor progression may have contributed to further ischemia. This has led to later trials excluding patients who have had radical RT or have obvious bowel tissue damage following RT. The rationale is that if normal vessels have been damaged by RT, further vascular disruption by a VDA that would normally have no major consequences could result in major normal tissue ischemia.

Twenty-one (61.7%) of the patients were evaluable for response. Four (11.8%) patients were classified as stable disease (SD), 9 (26.5%) patients had early progression (EP) (after 1 cycle) and eight (23.5%) patients had progressive disease (PD) (>28 days). Two of the four patients who had stable disease maintained this response through nine and 12 infusions of treatment.

One patient with adrenocortical carcinoma treated at 68 mg/m^2 was classified as early progression according to the criteria used in this study, as one lesion had increased ≥25% at the end of Cycle 1. The patient continued on CA4P and some

Table 1 Published CA4P phase I trials

	Number of patients	CA4P dose/schedule	Combined with	Results	References
1	34	5–114 mg/m^2 weekly × 3, every 28 days, over 10 min	–	Number of doses of CA4P given: 167 MTD: 68 mg/m^2 DLT: Ataxia; motor neuropathy; syncope; diplopia; tumor pain; dyspnea RP2D: 52–68 mg/m^2	Rustin et al. (2003) Galbraith et al. (2003) Anderson et al. (2003a, b)
2	25	18–90 mg/m^2 every 21 days over 10 min, 60 min in seven patients at 54 mg/m^2	–	Number of doses of CA4P given: 104 MTD: 60 mg/m^2 DLT: Cardiac ischemia; dyspnea RP2D: ≤60 mg/m^2	Dowlati et al. (2002), cardiac safety data in Cooney et al. (2004)
3	37	6–75 mg/m^2/day over 5 days, 3-weekly	–	Number of doses of CA4P given: 700 MTD: 75 mg/m^2 DLT: Tumor pain; sensorimotor neuropathy; syncope; dyspnea RP2D: 52 mg/m^2	Stevenson et al. (2003)
4	18	30–70 mg/m^2 initially a single dose every 21 days, then changed to weekly × 3 every 28 days, over 10 min	–	MTD: 70 mg/m^2 DLT: Tumor pain; cardiac ischemia Decreased tumor blood flow by up to 78% in all five patients assessed	BMS CA 178-002, reviewed in Gaya and Rustin (2005)
5	4	Regionally advanced anaplastic thyroid cancer	Doxorubicin (60 mg/m^2) and cisplatin (100 mg/m^2) day 1, followed by radiotherapy and CA4P	CA4P dose: 45 mg/m^2 weekly during RT Study terminated because of possible cardiotoxicity with this combination of therapies	ClinicalTrials.gov, NCT00077103

6	46	27–54 mg/m² every 21 days over 10 min	Either with paclitaxel 135 or 175 mg/m², and/or carboplatin AUC 4 or 5	MTD: 63 mg/m² DLT: Ataxia; hypertension RP2D: 63 mg/m²	Rustin et al. (2005) (ASCO 2005 Abstract)
7	16	27 or 36 mg/m² every 21 days over 30 min	Carboplatin AUC 4 or 5	Number of doses of CA4P given: 40 MTD 36 mg/m² CA4P, carboplatin AUC 4 DLT: Thrombocytopenia; neutropenia	Bilenker et al. (2005)
8	18	50 mg/m² single dose after two fractions RT versus weekly after 2, 4 and 6 fractions versus twice weekly after every fraction RT; in patients with NSCLC	Radiotherapy, 27 Gy in six fractions over 3 weeks	Perfusion CT demonstrated decrease in whole tumor blood volume 4 h after CA4P in the first and second cohort, not seen in the third cohort	Ng et al. (2007), Mandeville et al. (2008) (ASCO 2008 Abstract)
9	15	Dose levels 45, 54 or 63 mg/m² on day 1, 8 and then every 14 days	Bevacizumab 10 mg/m² stating on day 8 and then every 14 days	DLT: atrial fibrillation; hemorrhage RP2D: 63 mg/m² CA4P + 10 mg/m² bevacizumab every 14 days DCE-MRI showed statistically significant reductions in tumor perfusion	athan et al. (2008) (ASCO 2008 Abstract)

CA4P combretastatin A4 phosphate, *MTD* maximum tolerated dose, *DLT* dose limiting toxicity, *RP2D* recommended phase 2 dose, *RT* radiotherapy

Table 2 Published and ongoing CA4P phase Ib and II trials

	Number of patients	Tumor study design	Combined with	Results	References
10	18	Advanced anaplastic thyroid cancer (ATC)	–	Number of doses of CA4P given: 167 CA4P dose: 45 mg/m^2 weekly×3, every 28 day, over 10 min SD in six patients; PD in 12 patients PFS 7.4 weeks; 28% of patients progression free >3 months Median survival 20 weeks SE: tumor pain; nausea; vomiting; headache	Cooney et al. (2006) (ASCO 2006 Abstract)
11	13	Advanced, by DCE-MRI imageable malignancies; randomized phase II	Paclitaxel 200 mg/m^2; carboplatin AUC 6, on day 2, every 21 day	Number of doses of CA4P given: 234 CA4P dose: 45 or 63 mg/m^2×3, on day 1, every 21 day PR in three patients and SD in six patients after six cycles DCE-MRI demonstrated reduction in blood flow in both dose groups (–46 and –19%, respectively) SE: fatigue; neuropathy; neutropenia; myalgia; nausea; anemia	Akerley et al. (2007) (ASCO 2007 Abstract)
12	12	Advanced gastrointestinal carcinoma; phase Ib/II	Radioimmunotherapy with ^{131}I labeled A5B7 anti-CEA antibody 1,800–1,600 MBq/m^2	Number of doses of CA4P given: CA4P dose: 45–54 mg/m^2 day1+ 2, then weekly up to 7 weeks DLT: Neutropenia (at 66% of the single agent antibody MTD) SD in 1 patient; PD in 9 patients	Meyer et al. (2009)
13	44	Platinum resistant ovarian cancer; phase II extension of the Ib trial	Paclitaxel 175 mg/m^2; carboplatin AUC 5, every 21 day	Number of doses of CA4P given: CA4P dose: 63 mg/m^2 every 21 day Response (GCIG) in 11/34 patients (32%) SE: hypertension, fatigue, nausea/vomiting, pain, alopecia, ataxia, diarrhea, neuropathy, neutropenia, thrombocytopenia	Rustin et al. (2008)

14	60 estimated	Chemotherapy naïve NSCLC	Carboplatin, paclitaxel and bevacizumab ± CA4P	Study started recruiting patients in March 2008	ClinicalTrials.gov, NCT00653939
15	180 estimated	Anaplastic thyroid cancer; randomized phase II	Carboplatin, and paclitaxel ± CA4P (2:1 randomization)	Study started recruiting patients in July 2007 Pivotal registration study design	ClinicalTrials.gov, NCT00507429

CA4P combretastatin A4 phosphate, *CR* complete response, *PR* partial remission, *SD* stable disease, *PD* progressive disease, *PFS* progression free survival, *SE* side effects, *NSCLC* non-small cell lung cancer

Table 3 Selection of tubulin binding VDAs in clinical development

Compound	Company	Trial phase
AVE8062	Sanofi Aventis	II/III
ABT-751	Abbott	II
CA4P	OXiGEN	II
Tasidotin (ILX651)	Genzyme	II
TZT-1027	Daichi Pharmaceuticals	II
Cemadotin (LU103793, NSC D-669356)	BASF	II
Dolastatin-10 (NSC-376128)	NCI	II
ZD6126 (ANG453)	Astra Zeneca/Angiogene	II
NPI-2358	Nereus	I/II
BNC105P	Bionomics	I
CYT997	Cytopia	I
EPC-2407 (MX116407)	EpiCept	I
LP-261	Locus Pharmaceuticals	I
MN-029	MediciNova	I
OXi4503	OXiGEN	I
STA-9584	Synta Pharmaceuticals	Preclinical
Diazonamide A	Joyant Pharmaceuticals	Preclinical

response was seen when comparing lesions to baseline. The sum of the product of four marker lesions compared to baseline had decreased by 51% after three cycles, by 54% after four, 45% after five and by 27% after seven cycles. The improvement was associated with a decrease in both androgen and corticosteroid hormone production. The patient came off study after eight cycles (24 infusions) because of PD.

The once-every-three-weeks phase I trial including 25 patients with advanced solid tumours was carried out in the US (Dowlati et al. 2002). CA4P was administered in escalating doses from 18 to 90 mg/m^2 intravenously over 10 min, or 60 mg/m^2 over 60 min, once every 3 weeks. Data from a total of 107 cycles were valuable. Dose limiting toxicities (DLT) included two episodes of acute coronary syndrome, in the 60 mg/m^2 (10 min), and 90 mg/m^2 group, respectively. Maximum tolerated dose was considered to be 60 mg/m^2 in the 10 min infusion regime. Tumour pain occurred in 10% of cycles, including two grade 4 episodes. Other toxicities observed were short-term and resolved within 24 h, including flush, hot flashes, pruritus, nausea, vomiting, headache, and abdominal cramps. Several ECG changes were noted, mostly QTc prolongations. No significant myelotoxicity, stomatitis or alopecia was noted. A patient with anaplastic thyroid cancer had a complete response and was still alive 30 months after treatment. This report stimulated further research of CA4P activity in anaplastic thyroid cancer (Dziba et al. 2002). However, another patient with anaplastic thyroid cancer died 11 days after treatment due to progressive disease. Another two patients had prolonged progression free survival. A patient with metastatic colon carcinoma received 24 cycles over 19 months and a patient with metastatic medullary thyroid carcinoma received 15 cycles and was progression free for 12 months. A patient with metastatic renal cancer had stabilized disease for 6 months. A patient with non-small cell lung cancer had a 34% disease reduction after two cycles of therapy.

In the daily × 5 trial dose-escalating study of CA4P administered intravenously (IV) at doses of 6–75 mg/m^2/day, 37 patients with advanced cancer received weekly IV administration of CA4P repeated daily × 5 for 1 week every 21 days (Stevenson et al. 2003). The MTD was determined to be 65 mg/m^2/day. The most frequently reported treatment related AEs were fatigue (43%), nausea (41%), headache (38%), paresthesia (35%), vomiting (30%), increased sweating and tumor pain (22%), dyspnea (32%), diarrhea, QTc prolongation, hypoesthesia, somnolence (14% each), chest pain and conjunctivitis (11% each). Most of the AEs were grade 1 or 2. The most frequently reported grade 3 AEs were hypoxia and dyspnea (two patients), and syncope and chest pain (one patient each). Only two types of grade 4 AEs occurred, anorexia (3%) and dyspnea (8%). DLTs included tumor pain (three patients) hypoxia and dyspnea (two patients), and syncope and chest pain (one patient each).

BMS Bristol Myers Squibb, who for a short period owned the rights to CA4P also conducted a small unpublished phase I study, initially with single doses of CA4P 30–70 mg/m^2 every 21 days, in 18 patients. The primary purpose of this study was to evaluate myocardial blood flow and tumour blood flow changes with positron emission tomography. One patient experienced grade 4 tumour pain and subsequently died as a result of progressive disease. Another patient experienced grade 3 hypertension and a non-fatal myocardial infarction; however, this patient had uncontrolled hypertension before the study and did not disclose a history of ischaemic heart disease.

2.2.2 Trials of CA4P in Combination with Cytotoxic Agents

The first clinical trial (Bilenker et al. 2005) of combining CA4P with a cytotoxic drug was in retrospect bound to run into major haematological toxicity due to the scheduling. Preclinical data and PET data from the CRUK phase I trial showed that CA4P reduces renal blood flow, which is therefore likely to reduce renal clearance of carboplatin (Anderson et al. 2003a, b). In the phase I single arm dose escalation trial by Bilenker et al., patients with advanced/metastatic non-hematologic malignancies received on day 1 of each 21-day cycle, a 30 min infusion of carboplatin followed by a 10 min infusion of CA4P at dose levels of 27 or 36 mg/m^2 (Bilenker et al. 2005). The most common treatment-related AEs were fatigue (50%), nausea (44%), thrombocytopenia (38%) vomiting (32%), anemia (25%), and paresthesia (19%). Two patients treated with CA4P 36 mg/m^2 + carboplatin AUC 5 mg/ml-min experienced severe thrombocytopenia. As a result, the protocol was amended to reduce the third dose level to CA4P 36 mg/m^2 + carboplatin AUC 4. After four patients completed treatment at the third dose level, the study was terminated early. Fifty percentage of patients experienced at least one SAE. The most common SAEs were thrombocytopenia (19%) and dyspnea (13%). Six (37.5%) patients showed stable disease with four of the six patients (two with breast cancer, one with head and neck cancer and one with mesothelioma) on study for four cycles. One patient with ovarian cancer remained on study for five cycles. A patient with cancer of the renal pelvis showed stable disease for ten cycles, and subsequently received an additional three cycles with slight dose modification. Pharmacokinetic studies suggested that CA4P reduced renal clearance of carboplatin. The mean ratio of observed to predicted carboplatin AUCs was 1.16, indicating a general mild increase in carboplatin exposure (Bilenker et al. 2005). This study demonstrated the importance of timing the administration of CA4P so that it would not alter the pharmacokinetics of other drugs.

A Phase Ib/II study of CA4P in combination with carboplatin and paclitaxel in patients with advanced cancer and advanced ovarian cancer closed in December 2008, with a total of 46 patients who completed treatment in the Phase Ib portion of the trial and 44 patients in the Phase II portion of the study. This was a multi-center, open-label Investigator sponsored study run from Mount Vernon Cancer Centre, Middlesex, UK. Learning from the experience of Bilenker et al. (Bilenker et al. 2005), patients received CA4P on day 1 and 18–20 h later paclitaxel or carboplatin or both in a 21 day cycle. Patients in the Phase Ib part of the study (Rustin et al. 2005) received treatment with one of the following doublets: CA4P 36 mg/m^2, 45 mg/m^2 or 54 mg/m^2 followed by carboplatin AUC 4 or 5; CA4P 27 mg/m^2, 36 mg/m^2, 45 mg/m^2 or 54 mg/m^2 followed by paclitaxel 135 mg/m^2 or 175 mg/m^2; or triplets CA4P 54 mg/m^2, 63 mg/m^2 or 72 mg/m^2 followed by paclitaxel 175 mg/m^2 then carboplatin 5 AUC. Dose limiting toxicity occurred at the 72 mg/m^2 dose, specifically grade 3 ataxia and grade 3 hypertension. The MTD of the Phase I trial was determined to be 63 mg/m^2 CA4P followed by paclitaxel 175 mg/m^2 then carboplatin 5 AUC, which was the recommended dose in the Phase II trial.

The Phase II trial (Rustin et al. 2008) was a single arm study of up to six cycles of trial therapy in patients with platinum resistant ovarian cancer that required the relapse therapy start within 6 months of the last platinum chemotherapy. It had an interim requirement of >2 responses (RECIST and/or CA125 according to GCIG criteria) in the first 18 patients to proceed to complete enrollment of 43 patients. Seven of first 18 patients achieved a response. At the time this book chapter is published, accrual was completed with 44 patients recruited to the study, and with response data available on 34, and full toxicity data available for 30 patients. Weekly blood counts have demonstrated grade 3/4 neutropenia in 18 and thrombocytopenia in only one patient. Other grade >2 toxicities seen in >1 patient included fatigue, pain, and allergic reactions. Tumour pain, sinus tachycardia, nausea, and hypertension are the commonest CA4P related toxicities. Hypertension never exceeded AECTC grade 1, and was easily controlled by nitroglycerin followed by prophylactic amlodipine. Unlike the Bilenker study, haematological toxicity appeared no worse than what would be expected with carboplatin and paclitaxel alone and remarkably only 15 of 159 cycles of therapy were delayed. Recist and/or CA125 responses have been seen in 10/34 (29%) patients with one unconfirmed PR in an additional patient (no >28 day confirmatory CT scan). This response rate is considerably higher than what would be expected from carboplatin and paclitaxel in a truly platinum resistant population. This has prompted the design of a randomised trial to confirm whether the apparent improvement in response rate is due to the addition of CA4P.

In a randomized phase II study of CA4P in combination with paclitaxel and carboplatin, 13 patients with advanced imageable malignancies were included. Patients were randomized to one of two dose levels of CA4P (45 or 63 mg/m^2) administered weekly on days 1, 8 and 15 with paclitaxel (200 mg/m^2) and carboplatin (AUC 6) administered on day 2. Seventy-eight cycles were administered, with one patient continuing active therapy on cycle 19 at the time the study was presented; the median number of cycles administered was 6. The most frequent AEs were fatigue (69%), neutropenia (62%), myalgia (54%), nausea (46%), anemia (46%), and neuropathy, (39%). More patients dosed with 45 mg/m^2 CA4P experienced AEs that were considered at least possibly related to treatment, however, grade 3–4 AEs were similar between the two dose groups. Tumor responses were observed and were similar between both dose groups. Best overall response through cycle 6 was 3 PR, and 6 SD. Two patients with thyroid cancer were randomized to the low dose group and completed cycle 6. The first had SD and progressed after cycle 6. The second achieved PR and progressed after eight cycles (Akerley et al. 2007).

A phase II, single center study of CA4P in advanced anaplastic carcinoma of the thyroid has been performed under the direction of Dr. Scot Remick at the Ireland Cancer Center, University Hospitals of Cleveland. The study was designed to establish the safety and survival benefit of CA4P in patients with regionally advanced or metastatic anaplastic carcinoma of the thyroid. Patients received CA4P monotherapy at a dose of 45 mg/m^2 as a 10 min infusion every week for 3 weeks followed by 1-week rest. In an interim report presented at the 2006 ASCO annual meeting, a total of 21 patients were enrolled and received at least one dose of study treatment. Most frequent AEs reported were mild to moderate nausea, vomiting and headache. Three patients experienced grade 3 tumor pain. Six of the 18 patients had SD, with overall survival and median survival of 4.4 months (Cooney et al. 2006).

Based on encouraging phase I data on the efficacy of CA4P in patients with anaplastic thyroid carcinoma, a multicenter, open-label, global randomized phase II/III study of approximately 180 patients started recruiting patients in July 2007 randomising patients 2:1 in favour of the experimental arm. Since no effective therapies exist for this rather rare tumor entity, the study has a pivotal registration design, based on a special protocol assessment agreed with the FDA. One arm will receive intravenous 60 mg/m^2 CA4P on days 1, 8, and 15 of each 3-week cycle, followed by paclitaxel and carboplatin on day 2 of each 21-day cycle for up to six cycles. This triplet chemotherapy will be followed by a maintenance dose of CA4P on days 1 and 8, every 21 days until disease progression. The other arm will be treated with paclitaxel and carboplatin on day 1 of each 21-day cycle for up to six cycles.

A randomised phase II study started recruiting patients in March 2008 with stage IIIB or IV NSCLC not previously treated with chemotherapy or other biological agents (ClinicalTrials.gov identifier: NCT00653939). Safety and efficacy of the combination of carboplatin, paclitaxel, and bevacizumab ± CA4P followed by bevacizumab ± CA4P will be assessed. Patients with squamous cell histology are not eligible.

2.2.3 CA4P in Combination with Radiotherapy or Antibodies

A combination study was performed in patients with advanced non-small-cell lung cancer receiving palliative radiotherapy, also receiving CA4P after the second fraction of radiotherapy (Ng et al. 2007; Mandeville et al. 2008). This study is discussed in more detail in a different chapter of this book.

A phase I study assessing combination treatment of CA4P with bevacizumab has terminated recruitment. An abstract has been presented at ASCO 2008 (Nathan et al. 2008). This study is discussed in more detail in a different chapter of this book.

A phase Ib trial of CA4P in combination with radioimmunotherapy with the ^{131}iodine labelled A5B7 anti-CEA antibody in patients with advanced gastrointestinal carcinoma has been performed (Meyer et al. 2009). In pre-clinical models the combination of radioimmunotherapy (RIT) with ^{131}I-A5B7 and vascular disrupting agent (VDA), CA4P proved to be more effective than either agent alone, curing mice with CEA-positive colon carcinoma xenografts (Pedley et al. 2001). A single dose of CA4P was given 1 week before the combination to determine if there was a decrease in DCE-MRI parameters. The starting dose was 1,800 MBq/m^2 of ^{131}I-A5B7 given on day 1 and 45 mg/m^2 CA4P given 48 and 72 h post ^{131}I-A5B7, and then weekly for up to 7 weeks. Twelve patients were treated 11 colorectal, one pancreatic adenocarcinoma, mean age 63 years (32–77), WHO PS 0 (6) and 1 (6). Two out of six patients at the first dose level had DLTs (grade 4 neutropenia) attributed to ^{131}I-A5B7. The dose was reduced to 1,600 MBq/m^2 and CA4P escalated to 54 mg/m^2. Again, 2/6 patients had DLTs (neutropenia). Of ten assessable patients 2 had SD with and nine had PD, confirmed by FDG-PET in four. CA4P and ^{131}I-A5B7 pharmacokinetics were similar to previous studies. SPECT confirmed tumour antibody uptake in all 10 patients studied. DCE-MRI confirmed falls in kinetic parameters (K^{trans}/IAUGC$_{60}$) in nine out of 12 patients. This first trial reporting the combination of radio-immunotherapy and a VDA demonstrated that each component had some effect but that myelosuppression was dose limiting (T. Meyer, March 2009, personal communication). It is not clear whether this was due to the an inherent problem of the radiolabelled antibody or due to an unexpected effect of the CA4P.

2.2.4 Toxicity

In summary of all CA4P single agent trials, adverse events of CA4P were dose related and consisted of nausea, headache, tumor pain, fatigue, vomiting, sinus tachycardia, paresthesia, diarrhea, sweating, and hypertension. As a single agent, CA4P did not appear to have any hematological, hepatic or renal toxicity. The most common drug related adverse events were tumor pain (14%), dyspnea (10%), and hypoxia (8%). There were several adverse events attributable to the nervous system, specifically ataxia, dizziness, paresthesia, weakness, diplopia, and visual disturbances. It is unclear, if direct neurotoxicity of CA4P is involved, particularly since CA4P only binds reversibly to tubulin, and no histological abnormalities were reported in animal toxicity studies. The most common serious adverse events were respiratory distress (9%), tumor pain (6%), and asymptomatic QTc prolongation (6%).

With the exception of the Bilenker et al. trial (Bilenker et al. 2005), where CA4P was administered immediately after carboplatin, the toxicity profile of CA4P appeared similar to that of CA4P single agent studies. Thrombocytopenia, neutropenia, and anemia in the Bilenker et. al. study were observed at rates higher than anticipated for the respective single agent treatments alone, and were attributed to an interaction between the two drugs, resulting in an increased exposure to carboplatin (Bilenker et al. 2005). In subsequent studies, the sequence of administration was changed to CA4P on day 1, followed by carboplatin or/and paclitaxel on day 2.

The frequency of cardiac ischemia appears to be of the order of 1–2%, and seems to be related to hypertension resulting from an increase in peripheral vascular resistance caused by mild stimulation of vascular smooth muscle contraction by CA4P. This effect on vascular contraction is not related to or required for the collapse of tumor vasculature (Anderson et al. 2003a, b). The recognition of hypertension (Fig. 2) and subsequent cardiac ischemia as potentially deleterious side effects of CA4P led to the formulation of a guidance for investigators, starting with excluding patients with uncontrolled hypertension or history of cardiac ischaemia. Sublingual nitroglycerin has been used when systolic blood pressure rose to above 180 mmHg but the dermal patch is now preferred as having less toxicity. Prophylactic use of calcium channel blockers has also been recommended. Consequently, the frequency of myocardial infarction has declined over time from 4% in the first clinical trial to 0.6% in the most recent and ongoing studies.

CA4P at higher doses (>50 mg/m^2) has also been associated with prolongation of the QTc interval on ECG at 3–4 h after infusion, although no arrhythmias have been observed (Dowlati et al. 2002). These electrophysiological changes are consistent with an agent that blocks potassium ion channels. Combretastatin B1 is known to block potassium channels, and prolongs the action potential duration in excitable tissues (Guatteo et al. 1996). CA4P is also a weak inhibitor of L-type calcium channels in vitro.

In initial monotherapy studies, three different regimens were assessed: (1) CA4P IV daily for 5 consecutive days repeated every 3 weeks, (2) CA4P weekly × 3 repeated every 4 weeks, (3) CA4P IV once every 3 weeks. All of these regimens yielded a similar MTD in the range of 60–68 mg/m^2. This suggests that the majority of adverse effects occur in the time period immediately surrounding dosing, and particularly during the first administration. There appeared to be little cumulative toxicity.

2.2.5 Pharmacokinetics

Pharmacokinetic data were obtained from three phase I trials (Dowlati et al. 2002; Rustin et al. 2003; Stevenson et al. 2003). In summary, data from these trials show the following: CA4P is rapidly and extensively metabolised to CA4P, and further glucuronidated to CA4G. Mean plasma terminal $t_{1/2}$ values for CA4P, CA4, and

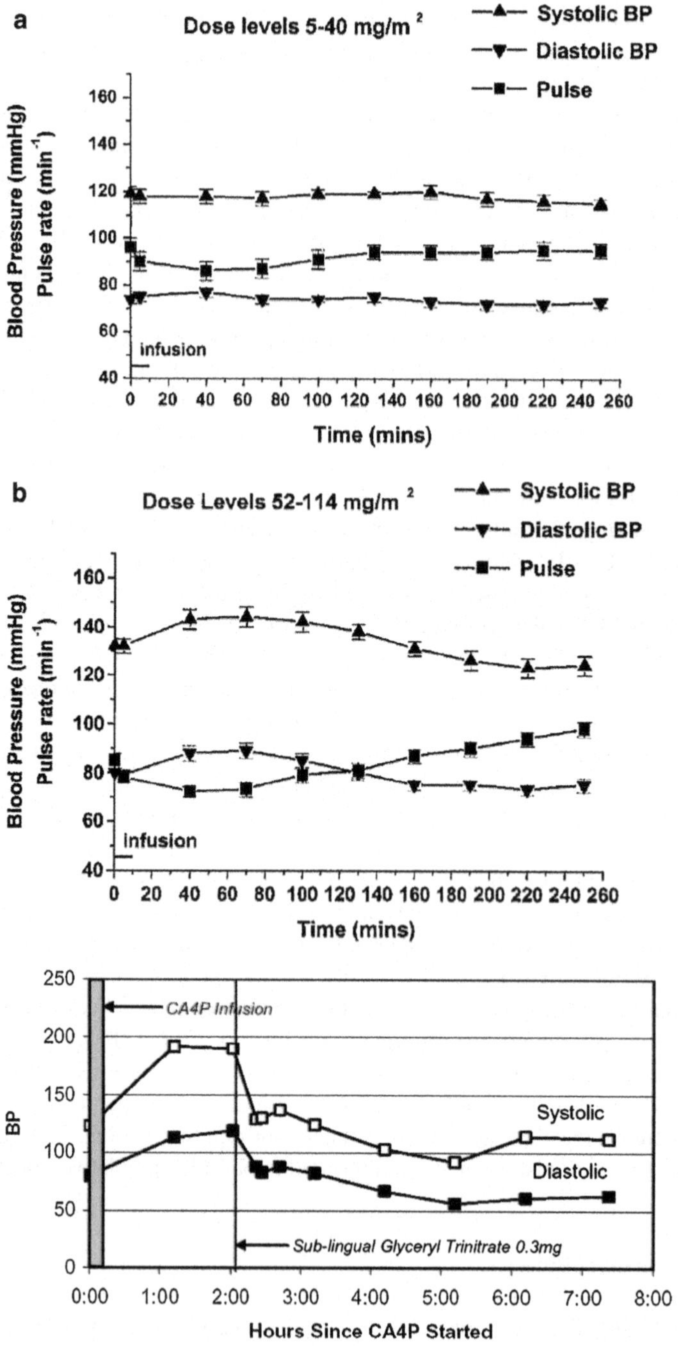

Fig. 2 Mean change in pulse and blood pressure in eight patients treated at 5–40 mg/m² (**a**) and in 22 patients treated at 52–114 mg/m² (**b**) (Rustin et al. 2003). Example of use of nitroglycerine for CA4P induced hypertension (Rustin et al. 2005)

CA4G are 0.4, 3.8, and 4.5 h, respectively. O-Demethylation and aromatic hydroxylation are the major phase I biotransformation pathways, with microsomal oxidation leading to the formation of a number of metabolites of which eight have been identified so far. Isomerization is also observed, contributing to the complexity of the metabolite pattern. Further oxidation gives rise to para-quinones whose role in pharmacodynamic activity is unknown (Aprile et al. 2007).

On average, 58–67% of CA4P dose is excreted as CA4G in the first 24 h of urine collection. The plasma AUC and Cmax of CA4P and CA4 appear to be relatively dose proportional with a moderate level of intersubject variability within dose cohorts. Both CA4 and CA4G display more prolonged disposition profiles, than the parent compound CA4P (Fig. 3).

2.2.6 Pharmacodynamics: Imaging the Effects of Vasculature-Targeting Agents

The clinical development of cytotoxic drugs in oncology traditionally involves the assessment of dose-limiting toxicity (DLT) and maximum tolerated dose (MTD) in phase I trials by dose escalation, based on the paradigm that the highest applicable dose will result in the greatest anti-tumoral effect. MTD is taken forward into single-arm phase II trials with response rate as primary endpoint, assessed by conventional radiologic imaging according to modified guidelines based on modified criteria initially introduced by the International Union Against Cancer and the World Health Organization (Therasse et al. 2000). However, most VDAs are active

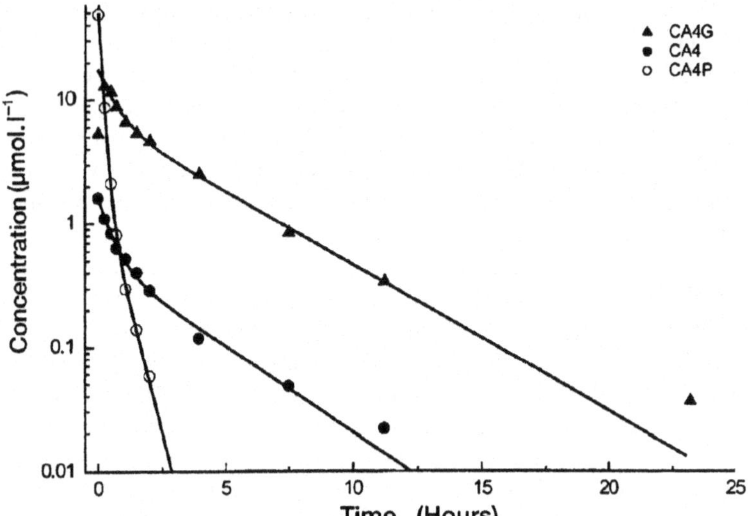

Fig. 3 Typical plasma profile after 68 mg/m^2 CA4P. CA4, combretastatin 4A; CA4G, combretastatin 4° glucuronide (Dowlati et al. 2002; Rustin et al. 2003; Stevenson et al. 2003)

at doses below the MTD in experimental tumors. Furthermore their vascular disrupting activity as single agents might not readily translate into reduced tumor size. As the anti-vascular effects of VDAs nowadays can be measured non-invasively by different imaging approaches, changes in tumor perfusion can directly be visualized and quantified, in particular by dynamic contrast enhanced magnetic resonance imaging (DCE-MRI), positron emission tomography (PET), and perfusion computed tomography (CT) (Collins 2003).

Changes in tumor blood flow following CA4P have been assessed in nine Phase I and II oncology clinical studies. There was considerable variation in dose levels, which ranged from 27 mg/m^2 to 114 mg/m^2. There was considerable technical variability across the studies, which used either perfusion CT, DCE-MRI or PET. A broad spectrum of tumor types was imagined at various stages of disease progression with heterogeneity in size, age, type and/or level of vascularity. The numbers of subjects imagined in each study was small, limiting the power of the analyses. The interval between CA4P infusion and the imaging study was variable. Nonetheless, in all of these studies, decrements were observed in tumor perfusion following CA4P administration, and in most studies these achieved statistical significance.

2.3 Conclusion

In summary, the studies support the interpretation that CA4P causes local disruption of blood flow within the tumor, rather than a more global decrease in blood flow. These include the parameters of heterogeneity of blood flow decrements within the tumor, decreased leakage space, increased non-enhancing pixels, and occasional patterns supportive of macroscopic segmental devascularisation. PET imaging demonstrated approximately a 10% decrease in cardiac output, secondary to an increase in peripheral resistance. There were small changes in perfusion of organs such as the kidneys consistent with the decline in cardiac output, but these changes were smaller and briefer than the changes in tumor blood flow (Anderson et al. 2003a, b). The imaging studies support the specificity of vascular disruption for tumor neovasculature compared to normal tissues.

Dose response relationships in these studies were variable, probably in part due to the small numbers of patients. The relationship may also have been confounded by tumor heterogeneity, since there was a strong correlation in baseline blood flow and decrement post-CA4P, with larger changes observed in more vascular tumors (Stevenson et al. 2003). In two studies (Rustin et al. 2003; Bilenker et al. 2005), there was a correlation between CA4P and/or CA4 exposure; however in the Dowlati et al. study (Dowlati et al. 2002), change in blood flow correlated with Cmax rather than AUC. In the Rustin et al. study (Rustin et al. 2003), significant changes were only seen in the patients who received $\geq$52 mg/m^2. In the Dowlati et al. and the Akerley et al. studies (Dowlati et al. 2002; Akerley et al. 2007) greater effects were observed at the intermediate rather than the higher dose levels. Despite some differences in details, all of these studies indicated that CA4P significantly reduces tumor perfusion, and that the minimal efficacious dose is in the range of 36–52 mg/m^2.

3 Other Tubulin Binding VDAs

3.1 ZD6126 (ANG453)

ZD6126 (ANG453), a water-soluble phosphate prodrug, is rapidly converted by serum phosphatases to N-acetylcolchinol (NAC), a tubulin-binding agent that inhibits tubulin polymerisation and causes microtubule destabilisation. ZD6126 disrupts endothelial cell morphology in a similar manner to CA4P. ZD6126 has significant anti-tumour activity against a broad range of human xenografts in rodent models. The vascular targeting activity of ZD6126 was seen at doses 1/8–1/16 of the MTD, and was selective for tumour blood vessels (Blakey et al. 2002a, b; Davis et al. 2002a). ZD6126 induced a significant dose and time-dependent decrease in tumour perfusion in a C3H mouse mammary carcinoma, reaching a maximal 70% reduction 3 h after injecting 150–300 mg/kg. However, full recovery of perfusion was seen within 6 h (Davis et al. 2002a). A small, but statistically significant 1.4 days inhibition of tumour growth was seen. Muscle and spleen showed transient decreases in blood flow. ZD6126 also enhanced the tumour response to radiation, giving a 1.3-fold increase in the slope of the radiation dose–response curve. The direct effects of ZD6126 on endothelial cells in tumour vessels in vivo have been visualised using electron microscopy. Three ZD6126 phase-I clinical trials have been published as abstracts (DelProposto et al. 2002; Gadgeel et al. 2002; Radema et al. 2002), and one as a paper (LoRusso et al. 2008). These studies demonstrated significant reductions in tumour blood flow by DCE-MRI. Stable disease, lasting four or more cycles, was seen in three patients, and one patient had a minor response lasting 19 cycles. Radema et al. (Radema et al. 2002) reported vascular damage in four out of five patients 4–6 h after infusion of ZD6126, indicated by a doubling of circulating endothelial cells, which were viewed as a surrogate marker for vascular damage. Dose-limiting toxicities were anorexia, constipation, dyspnea, fatigue, headache, (abdominal) pain, nausea, hypokalemia, increased intracranial pressure with brain metastases, and reduced LVEF. In the LoRusso et al. study (LoRusso et al. 2008), 10 min, single-dose escalating intravenous infusions of ZD6126 every 14 (5–112 mg/m^2) or 21 days (40–80 mg/m^2) were compared. ZD6126 was associated with cardiac events approximately 11% (five out of 44) of patients, categorized as dose limiting toxicities. Of the 34 patients on the 21-day schedule who were evaluated for objective tumor response, two had a best overall response of stable disease, the remainder demonstrating disease progression. In the 14-day dosing schedule, 22.2% of patients had an overall response of stable disease and the remaining 77.8% of patients experienced disease progression. During the

Phase I program, pharmacokinetic data of ZD6126 were analyzed from 71 patients. ZD6126 was rapidly hydrolyzed to the active metabolite, ZD6126 phenol, and there was evidence for the presence of circulating metabolites. The dose was eliminated in the urine and faeces, with the majority in the faeces, showing the importance of biliary excretion (Scurr et al. 2004). No clear correlation between BSA and clearance (CL=[Dose/AUC]) of ZD6126 phenol was seen, and a unit dosing strategy has therefore been adopted for the Phase II clinical program (Oliver et al. 2004). In 2003, a phase II study to assess the biological activity of ZD6126 in subjects with newly diagnosed stage IV metastatic renal cell carcinoma was started (NCT000655729), but was closed later on due to toxicity problems (cardiac events), and all rights of the drug were returned to Angiogene Pharmaceuticals Ltd. in 2006 [reviewed in (Lippert 2007)].

3.2 *AVE8062*

AVE8062 is a synthetic water-soluble combretastatin analogue, which has more potent effects on tumour blood flow stasis and anti-tumour effects compared with CA4P (Hori and Saito 2003). AVE8062 suppresses tumour proliferation and prolongs survival in rats (Hori et al. 1999). The drug induced necrosis in 35–40 tumour models within 24 h of treatment (Lejeune et al. 2002). It has been proposed that contractile response of arterioles, rather than a direct effect of this drug on tumour vessels is responsible for its VDA activity (Hori and Saito 2003). Synergism has been seen in animal models when the drug is given in combination with conventional cytotoxic agents (Vrignaud 2004). AVE8062 has undergone a single-agent phase-I trial in humans given as a 30 min IV infusion once weekly for 3 weeks every 28 days (Tolcher et al. 2003). Nine patients with advanced malignancies received 48 weekly infusions at doses between 4.5 and 30 mg/m^2. Asymptomatic systolic hypotension was noted as a side effect. AVE8062 was rapidly eliminated with a t1/2 of 15 min and a clearance of 50 L/h/m^2, leading to an active metabolite, RPR258063, with a t1/2 of 7 h. The Cmax values for AVE8062A and RPR258063 were 2.1 and 0.3 μ/mL at 22 mg/m^2, respectively, levels that portend antitumor and antivascular activity in xenograft models. Decreased vascular flow by DCE-MRI has been observed 4 h post treatment at the 15.5 mg/m^2 dose level. Two clinical trials are currently being performed. A phase Ib trial (ClinicalTrials.gov identifier: NCT00719524) started recruiting up to 28 patients in July 2008 in Italy, France, and Switzerland. Based on dose limiting toxicities, the trial aims to determine the recommended dose of the combination of AVE8062 with cisplatin administered on day 1 followed by docetaxel on day 2, every 3 weeks, in patients with advanced solid tumors for which cisplatin-docetaxel doublet constitutes mainstay of care (i.e., non small cell lung cancer, epithelial ovary cancer, gastric cancer, head and neck cancer). A phase II/III trial (ClinicalTrials.gov identifier: NCT00699517) of AVE8062 in advanced-stage soft tissue sarcoma after failure of anthracycline and ifosfamide chemotherapies, started recruitment in June 2008 in the US, Belgium, France, Hungary, Spain, and Italy. The primary objective of the study is to compare the progression-free survival (PFS) in the two treatment arms. The secondary objectives of the study are to compare the overall survival and the objective response rate in the two treatment arms, and to assess the safety profile of AVE8062 in combination with cisplatin therapy. In addition, the pharmacokinetics of AVE8062 and its main metabolite, RPR258063, are assessed, using a population approach, in all patients enrolled in selected centers. Three-hundred patients are estimated to be enrolled.

3.3 OXi4503

OXi4503 (CA1P; Oxigene Inc, Boston, MA) is the diphosphate prodrug of combretastatin A1 (CA1). OXi4503 shows comparable effects to CA4 in vitro. However, head-to-head comparisons indicate that OXi4503 is at least 10 times more potent in vivo when tumour vascular shutdown is used as the end point (Hill et al. 2002b). Over 50% of the tumour blood vessels are no longer perfused 24 h after a dose as small as 1 mg/kg of OXi4503. Single-dose studies indicate that the MTD in mice is similar to CA4P; therefore, OXi4503 may have a larger therapeutic window (Hill et al. 2002b; Hua et al. 2003). Pre-clinical studies have demonstrated prolonged tumour growth retardation, regressions and even prolonged complete responses in some tumour models (Hill et al. 2002b). Additional activity may be due to the rate of dephosphorylation, or the production of a quinone metabolite with enhanced cytotoxic activity (Thorpe et al. 2003).

A phase I trial is ongoing in the UK at Mount Vernon Hospital, Middlesex, and Christie Hospital, Manchester. Patients with advanced or metastatic solid tumours and WHO performance score 0 or 1 are administered OXi4503 by 10 min iv infusions in an accelerated dose escalation scheme from 0.06 to 15.4 mg/m^2 on days 1, 8 and 15, repeated every 4 weeks. Patient recruitment started in July 2005, and the participating centres later on expanded to the Churchill Hosptial, Oxford (Patterson et al. 2008). By the time this article is published, 36 patients have been treated. Common AEs were pyrexia, fatigue, myelosuppression, nausea and tumour pain. Hypertension is one of the most often recorded drug-related AEs, for which during the course of the trial a protocol amendment has been made, allowing pre-treatment of every patient with prophylactic amlodipine. Drug-related DLTs were seen in patients at 15.4 mg/m^2, one with atrial fibrillation secondary to hypertension, and another patient with tumour lysis syndrome and subsequent bowel fistula formation. PKs showed a dose-dependent linear increase in peak plasma concentrations and AUC of both OXi4503 and it's active metabolite. Five of the last 10 patients who were evaluable by DCE-MRI treated at dose levels above 8 mg/m^2 showed evidence of vascular shutdown.

3.4 *Dolastatin-10 (NSC-376128)*

Dolastatin-10 was first isolated from the mollusc Dolabella auricularia. Dolestatin is thought to be produced by cyanobacteriae, which are ingested by the marine snail. Dolastatin-10 is also a tubulin-binding agent, and binds to distinct sites from vinca alkaloids. In three phase I trials, DLT was granulocytopenia (Pitot et al. 1999; Madden et al. 2000; de Jonge et al. 2005). Stabilization of tumor growth (Madden et al. 2000), and one partial response lasting >54 weeks was observed in an extensively pretreated patient with metastatic liposarcoma (de Jonge et al. 2005). However, there was no objective response of single agent dolastatin-10 in phase II trials including patients with metastatic soft tissue sarcomas (von Mehren et al. 2004), advanced hepatopancreatic and biliary cancers (Kindler et al. 2005), and metastatic melanoma (Margolin et al. 2001), and only minimal activity seen in patients with metastatic breast cancer (Perez et al. 2005), recurrent platinum-sensitive ovarian carcinoma (Hoffman et al. 2003), and advanced colorectal cancer (Saad et al. 2002).

3.5 *Cemadotin (LU103793, NSC D-669356)*

LU-103793 is a water-soluble dolastatin-15 analog (Jordan et al. 1998). In three phase I trials, neutropenia, peripheral edema, liver function test abnormalities, and hypertension, sometimes associated with signs of cardiac ischemia, were dose-limiting. Cardiovascular toxicity appeared to be associated with the magnitude of the peak blood levels of the parent drug or its metabolites. Other significant toxic effects were asthenia and tumor pain. Neither partial nor complete responses were observed although minor tumor regressions were seen in a patient with carcinoma of unknown primary (CUP) and in another patient with liver metastases from a colon cancer (Mross et al. 1998; Villalona-Calero et al. 1998; Supko et al. 2000). In two phase II studies of LU 103793 in patients with advanced non-small-cell lung cancer (SCLC), and metastatic breast cancer, no objective responses were seen. However, in a phase II study including 80 chemotherapy-naïve patients with metastatic melanoma, one complete and three partial responses of median duration 6 months have been observed (Smyth et al. 2001; Kerbrat et al. 2003; Marks et al. 2003).

3.6 *TZT-1027*

TZT-1027 is a synthetic derivative of the cytotoxic pentapeptide dolastatin-10 and has been developed in Japan. The agent interacts with tubulin in the vinca alkaloid binding domain (Kobayashi et al. 1997). Similar to dolastatin-10, it seems to have a unique antitumoral vascular activity resulting in the collapse of the tumor vasculature after exposure to the drug that might potentiate the direct antitumor effect due to the antimicrotubule activity of the drug (Hashiguchi et al. 2004; de Jonge et al. 2005). In four phase I trials, DLTs essentially were neutropenia (Schoffski et al. 2004; Greystoke et al. 2006; Yamamoto et al. 2008), myalgia and neuropathic pain (Horti et al. 2008), fatigue and reversible peripheral neurotoxic syndrome (Schoffski et al. 2004), and paralytic ileus when TZT-1027 was combined with carboplatin (Greystoke et al. 2006). One complete response and three partial responses were observed in a phase I trial including stage III/b or IV NSCLC refractory to conventional therapy or for which no standard therapy was available (Horti et al. 2008). One patient with metastatic esophageal cancer achieved partial response, and each of two patients with non-small cell lung cancer had a minor response (Horti et al. 2008). One patient (pancreatic adenocarcinoma) achieved a partial response lasting 181 days (Greystoke et al. 2006). In a phase II trial in patients with locally advanced or metastatic STS and who had received one prior treatment regimen with an anthracycline-based chemotherapy for metastatic disease, no confirmed objective response was observed (Patel et al. 2006). Similarly, in patients with stage IV or recurrent NSCLC who had received one prior platinum-based chemotherapy regimen, no objective response was observed after TZT-1027 single agent therapy (Riely et al. 2007). Teikoku Hormone Manufacturing Company, which holds the rights to TZT-1027, ended their agreement with Daiichi Pharmaceuticals in 2005, and merged later on to form ASKA Pharmaceutical Company [reviewed in Lippert (2007)].

3.7 ILX651

ILX651 is a novel, third generation, synthetic, water-soluble, dolastatin pentapeptide analog of dolastatin-15, where the carboxyl-terminal ester group of dolastatin-15 has been replaced by a carboxy-terminal tert-butyl amide (Bai et al. 2009). ILX651 is metabolically stable and orally bioavailable. ILX651 has a unique mechanism of action that appears to differ from other microtubule stabilizers such as taxanes and epothilones and tubulin inhibitors such as Vinca alkaloids. Mechanistically, ILX651 is believed to inhibit cell proliferation by suppressing spindle microtubule dynamics through a reduction of the shortening rate, reduction of the switching frequency from growth to shortening and reduction of the time microtubules grow (Ray et al. 2007). Three Phase I dose-escalation studies have been conducted to evaluate ILX651 in adult patients with metastatic or inoperable solid tumors (Cunningham et al. 2005; Ebbinghaus et al. 2005; Mita et al. 2006). Phase II studies have been conducted in the following populations to further evaluate the efficacy of ILX651 administered intravenously (IV): melanoma, non-small cell lung cancer, and hormone-refractory prostate cancer (Genzyme; McDermott et al. 2005). Overall, intravenous ILX651 was well tolerated, but did not show sufficient efficacy to warrant further single agent development using this route of administration. According to Genzyme Oncology, ILX651 will be investigated as an orally administered antineoplastic agent (as the hydrochloride salt) for patients with advanced, refractory neoplasms based on new preclinical data (Genzyme).

3.8 NPI-2358

The diketopiperazine NPI-2358 is a synthetic analog of NPI-2350, a natural product isolated from Aspergillus sp., which depolymerizes microtubules. Although structurally different from the colchicine-binding site agents reported to date, NPI-2358 binds to the colchicine-binding site of tubulin. It has potent in vitro anti-tumor activity. The vascular disrupting activity is comparable with that of CA4P (Nicholson et al. 2006). A Phase 1 study of NPI-2358 was performed in patients with solid tumors and lymphomas. Toxicities included nausea, vomiting, fatigue, fever, tumor pain and transient elevations in blood pressure. DCE-MRI demonstrated decreases in Ktrans of 16–54%. Five patients with pancreatic adenocarcinoma, colorectal carcinoma, anal squamous cell carcinoma, adrenocortical carcinoma and melanoma had stable disease for two or more cycles (Mita et al. 2008). A Phase I/II study of NPI-2358 in combination with docetaxel in patients with advanced non-small cell lung cancer (NCT00630110) started recruiting patients in the US, Australia, and Chile in February 2008. A total of 174 patients are estimated to be enrolled.

3.9 MN-029

MN-029 binds reversibly to the colchicine binding site and has shown activity in cell lines and xenografts (McCreedy et al. 2004). Two phase I clinical trials of MN-029 for the treatment of solid tumors have been completed. In a phase I trial with 34 patients, MN-029 was administered as an intravenous infusion once every 3 weeks. DLT at 180 mg/m^2 in one patient consisted of a reversible episode of acute coronary ischemia. Tumor blood flow reduction assessed by DCE-MRI was recorded at 120 and 180 mg/m^2, but not at 80 mg/m^2. Nine of 34 patients with advanced solid tumors for whom no standard therapy was available had stable disease after three cycles of treatment. Six patients had prolonged (greater than 6 months) stable disease (Medicinova; Ricart et al. 2006). In another Phase I clinical trial, MN-029 was administered as an intravenous infusion every 7 days (Days 1, 8, 15) followed by a 13-day recovery period (one cycle). The maximum dose was limited to 180 mg/m^2 per dose based on the results of the other Phase I trial. The most common side effects of MN-029 in this clinical trial included nausea, vomiting, arthralgia and headache. Eleven of 20 patients with advanced solid tumors for whom no standard therapy was available had stable disease after two cycles of treatment. Four patients continued on extended cycles of MN-029 treatment. Based on RECIST criteria, one patient with metastatic pancreatic cancer had an overall partial response with duration of 74 days. Seven patients had stable disease with a median duration of 83 days (Medicinova).

3.10 ABT-751

ABT-751 is a novel oral sulfonamide antimitotic agent that binds to the colchicine site on beta-tubulin, thus inhibiting polymerization of microtubules. It is considered a cytotoxic agent, but based on its capacity of eliciting selective reduction in tumor blood flow, vascular disrupting properties have been suggested (Segreti et al. 2004). The metronomic daily dose scheduling might confer additional anti-angiogenic properties (Hanahan et al. 2000). Eight phase I and II trials of ABT-751 have been conducted, and it is currently being tested in phase II trials recruiting patients with relapsed pediatric ALL (NCT00439296) and children with neuroblastoma that has relapsed or not responded to previous treatment (NCT00436852).

3.11 BNC-105P

BNC-105P is a VDA that was demonstrated to display selectivity for tumor endothelium. It exhibits strong efficacy in breast and colon tumor models, and was shown to disrupt vasculature in subcutaneous lung, prostate and brain xenograft tumors grown in mice, leading to corresponding increases in tumor necrosis. It is suggested to exhibit a dual mode of action, "locking itself" inside the tumor where it exerts anti-proliferative pressure on the cancer cells. Treatment of tumors with BNC-105P in combination with bevacizumab was shown to prevented tumor re-vascularisation and prolonged vascular shutdown (Bionomics; Kremmidiotis et al. 2008). A phase I two-stage, open-label, dose-escalation trial in patients with advanced solid tumors for whom no standard therapy is available is being conducted in Australia under a US FDA Investigational New Drug application. Patients will be treated with BNC-105P (the pro-drug form of BNC-105) as monotherapy in two 21-day cycles, each cycle consisting of two doses administered 1 week apart (i.e., on days 1 and 8). The safety, tolerance, and the pharmacokinetics of BNC-105 in these patients will be determined. DCE-MRI will be used to assess the vascular disrupting activity (Bionomics).

3.12 EPC-2407

EPC-2407 (MX116407) is a small molecule VDA and apoptosis inducer, binding at or close to the colchicine binding site of tubulin. Vascular disruptive activity was demonstrated at concentrations well below its cytotoxic dose (Kasibhatla et al. 2004). Vascular disruption and tumor necrosis in vivo, and tumor regression in human lung tumor xenografts was demonstrated. Antitumor activity of cisplatin was enhanced (Gourdeau et al. 2004). Pre-clinical studies suggest that the antitumor effects of EPC2407 may be the result of a dual mechanism, a direct effect on disruption of tumor vascular endothelial cells leading to hypoxia and central tumor necrosis, as observed withVDAs, and a second effect on tumor apoptosis (EpiCept). A first in man phase I trial of EPC-2407 in patients with advanced cancer is recruiting patients in the US at the time this article is published (NCT00423410).

3.13 LP-261

LP-261 is another VDA, binding reversibly to tubulin near the colchicine binding site. It has been demonstrated to be a very potent inhibitor of angiogenesis, preventing microvessel outgrowth in the rat aortic ring assay and HUVEC cell proliferation at nanomolar concentrations. Combination treatment of low dose LP-261 with bevacizumab lead to improved tumor inhibition (Gardner et al. 2007). Interim results of a phase I study in patients with advanced malignancies have been reported. Twenty patients had been treated, and MTD had not been reached yet. Only one patient experienced a drug-related (Grade 2) adverse event (diarrhea). Eight of 17 (47%) of patients had stable disease. LP-261 was shown to be rapidly absorbed (1.5–2 h), and eliminated (1.8 h). The reproducible C_{max} and short $t_{1/2}$ may enhance its therapeutic index (Burris et al. 2008).

3.14 CYT-997

CYT-997 is a novel synthetic tubulin binding molecule which demonstrated selective targeting of tumor vasculature and efficacy in preclinical cancer models (Malcontenti-Wilson et al. 2005). In a phase I study, CYT997 was administered by continuous infusion over 24 h every 3 weeks to patients with advanced cancer. No dose-limiting toxicity was observed. Toxicities included injection site reactions, renal toxicity in a patient with abnormal baseline kidney function, grade-1 QT_c prolongation in one patient. No myelosuppression, gastrointestinal toxicity or clinically-significant cardiac toxicity were observed. Seven of 31 patients achieved stable disease for a period of 4–5 months. Two patients with symptomatic progressive disease were stabilized for 5–6 months (Cytopia; Lickliter et al. 2008). CYT997 can be administered both intravenously and orally. Enrolment in a second Phase I study, where CYT997 is administered as a capsule dose, is ongoing. Early data from this study indicates that CYT997 is well absorbed in cancer patients following presentation as a capsule dose (Cytopia). A phase I/II study of intravenous CYT-997 in combination with carboplatin and etoposide in relapsed glioblastoma multiforme (NCT00650949), and a phase I study of intravenous CYT-997 in relapsed and refractory multiple myeloma (NCT00664378) are recruiting patients at the time this article is published.

3.15 Other Tubulin Binding VDAs in Development

STA-9584 is a new VDA that has been demonstrated to block blood flow of tumors in mouse models by specifically disrupting tumor microvasculature, not only in the center, but also at the periphery (Foley et al. 2008). STA-9584 is in preclinical development.

Diazonamide A is another tubulin binding agent, equivalent in activity to dolastatin-10. Observations suggest, that it either has a unique binding site on tubulin differing from the vinca alkaloid and dolastatin-10 binding sites, or that diazonamide A binds weakly to unpolymerized tubulin but strongly to microtubule ends. Diazonamide A and its oxygen analog could have uniquely potent inhibitory effects on the dynamic properties of microtubules (Cruz-Monserrate et al. 2003).

Symplostatin and *Malevamide* are marine compounds structurally related to the dolastatins (Harrigan et al. 1998; Horgen et al. 2002).

References

Akerley, W. L., M. Schabel, et al. (2007). "A randomized phase 2 trial of combretatstatin A4 phosphate (CA4P) in combination with paclitaxel and carboplatin to evaluate safety and efficacy in subjects with advanced imageable malignancies." *J Clin Oncol, ASCO Annual Meeting Proceedings Part I* **25**(18S): 14060.

Anderson, H., J. T. Yap, et al. (2003). "Measurement of renal tumour and normal tissue perfusion using positron emission tomography in a phase II clinical trial of razoxane." *Br J Cancer* **89**(2): 262–7.

Anderson, H. L., J. T. Yap, et al. (2003). "Assessment of pharmacodynamic vascular response in a phase I trial of combretastatin A4 phosphate." *J Clin Oncol* **21**(15): 2823–30.

Aprile, S., E. Del Grosso, et al. (2007). "In vitro metabolism study of combretastatin A-4 in rat and human liver microsomes." *Drug Metab Dispos* **35**(12): 2252–61.

Badn, W., S. Kalliomaki, et al. (2006). "Low-dose combretastatin A4 phosphate enhances the immune response of tumor hosts to experimental colon carcinoma." *Clin Cancer Res* **12**(15): 4714–19.

Bai, R., M. C. Edler, et al. (2009). "Intracellular activation and deactivation of tasidotin, an analog of dolastatin 15: correlation with cytotoxicity." *Mol Pharmacol* **75**(1): 218–26.

Bilenker, J. H., K. T. Flaherty, et al. (2005). "Phase I trial of combretastatin a-4 phosphate with carboplatin." *Clin Cancer Res* **11**(4): 1527–33.

Bionomics http://www.bionomics.com.au/page.php?section=129 (accessed March 2009).

Blakey, D. C., S. E. Ashton, et al. (2002). "ZD6126: a novel small molecule vascular targeting agent." *Int J Radiat Oncol Biol Phys* **54**(5): 1497–502.

Blakey, D. C., F. R. Westwood, et al. (2002). "Antitumor activity of the novel vascular targeting agent ZD6126 in a panel of tumor models." *Clin Cancer Res* **8**(6): 1974–83.

Boehle, A. S., B. Sipos, et al. (2001). "Combretastatin A-4 prodrug inhibits growth of human non-small cell lung cancer in a murine xenotransplant model." *Ann Thorac Surg* **71**(5): 1657–65.

Breidahl, T., F. U. Nielsen, et al. (2006). "The effects of the vascular disrupting agents combretastatin A-4 disodium phosphate, 5,6-dimethylxanthenone-4-acetic acid and ZD6126 in a murine tumour: a comparative assessment using MRI and MRS." *Acta Oncol* **45**(3): 306–16.

Burris, H., S. Freedman, et al. (2008). "A phase 1 study of LP-261 in patients with advanced solid malignancies." *AACR Meeting Abstracts* **2008**(1 Annual Meeting): 1421.

Chaplin, D. and G. Dougherty (1999). "Tumour vasculature as a target for cancer therapy." *Br J Cancer* **80**(Suppl 1): 57–64.

Chaplin, D. J., G. R. Pettit, et al. (1996). "Antivascular approaches to solid tumour therapy: evaluation of tubulin binding agents." *Br J Cancer* **74**(Suppl 27): S86–S88.

Chaplin, D. J., G. R. Petit, et al. (1999). "Anti-vascular approaches to solid tumour therapy: evaluation of combretastatin A4-phosphate." *Anticancer Res* **19**: 189–196.

Chaplin, D. J., G. R. Pettit, et al. (1999). "Anti-vascular approaches to solid tumour therapy: evaluation of combretastatin A4 phosphate." *Anticancer Res* **19**(1A): 189–95.

Collins, J. M. (2003). "Functional imaging in phase I studies: decorations or decision making?" *J Clin Oncol* **21**(15): 2807–9.

Cooney, M. M., T. Radivoyevitch, et al. (2004). "Cardiovascular safety profile of combretastatin a4 phosphate in a single-dose phase I study in patients with advanced cancer." *Clin Cancer Res* **10**(1 Pt 1): 96–100.

Cooney, M. M., P. Savvides, et al. (2006). "Phase II study of combretastatin A4 phosphate (CA4P) in patients with advanced anaplastic thyroid carcinoma (ATC)." *J Clin Oncol, ASCO Annual Meeting Proceedings Part I*(18S): 5580.

Cruz-Monserrate, Z., H. C. Vervoort, et al. (2003). "Diazonamide A and a synthetic structural analog: disruptive effects on mitosis and cellular microtubules and analysis of their interactions with tubulin." *Mol Pharmacol* **63**(6): 1273–80.

Cunningham, C., L. J. Appleman, et al. (2005). "Phase I and pharmacokinetic study of the dolastatin-15 analogue tasidotin (ILX651) administered intravenously on days 1, 3, and 5 every 3 weeks in patients with advanced solid tumors." *Clin Cancer Res* **11**(21): 7825–33.

Cytopia http://www.cytopia.com.au/glance.html#pcvprogram (accessed March 2009).

Dark, G. G., S. A. Hill, et al. (1997). "Combretastatin A-4, an agent that displays potent and selective toxicity toward tumor vasculature." *Cancer Res* **57**(10): 1829–34.

Davis, P. D., G. J. Dougherty, et al. (2002). "ZD6126: a novel vascular-targeting agent that causes selective destruction of tumor vasculature." *Cancer Res* **62**(24): 7247–53.

Davis, P. D., G. M. Tozer, et al. (2002). "Enhancement of vascular targeting by inhibitors of nitric oxide synthase." *Int J Radiat Oncol Biol Phys* **54**(5): 1532–6.

de Jonge, M. J., A. van der Gaast, et al. (2005). "Phase I and pharmacokinetic study of the dolastatin 10 analogue TZT-1027, given on days 1 and 8 of a 3-week cycle in patients with advanced solid tumors." *Clin Cancer Res* **11**(10): 3806–13.

DelProposto, Z., P. LoRusso, et al. (2002). "MRI evaluation of the effects of the vascular-targeting agent ZD6126 on tumor vasculature." *Proc Am Soc Clin Oncol* **21**: abstract 440.

Dowlati, A., K. Robertson, et al. (2002). "A phase I pharmacokinetic and translational study of the novel vascular targeting agent combretastatin A-4 phosphate on a single-dose intravenous schedule in patients with advanced cancer." *Cancer Res* **62**(June 15): 3408–16.

Dziba, J. M., R. Marcinek, et al. (2002). "Combretastatin A4 phosphate has primary antineoplastic activity against human anaplastic thyroid carcinoma cell lines and xenograft tumors." *Thyroid* **12**(12): 1063–70.

Ebbinghaus, S., E. Rubin, et al. (2005). "A phase I study of the dolastatin-15 analogue tasidotin (ILX651) administered intravenously daily for 5 consecutive days every 3 weeks in patients with advanced solid tumors." *Clin Cancer Res* **11**(21): 7807–16.

el Zayat, A. A., D. Degen, et al. (1993). "In vitro evaluation of the antineoplastic activity of combretastatin A-4, a natural product from *Combretum caffrum* (arid shrub)." *Anticancer Drugs.* **4**(1): 19–25.

EpiCept http://www.epicept.com/Product_Pipeline/Cancer/EPC2407/(accessed March 2009).

Foley, K., C. Borella, et al. (2008). "Vascular disrupting agent STA-9584 selectively targets microvasculature at both the center and periphery of tumors." *AACR Meeting Abstracts* **2008**(1 Annual Meeting): 1444.

Gadgeel, S. M., P. M. LoRusso, et al. (2002). "A dose-escalation study of the novel vascular-targeting agent, ZD6126, in patients with solid tumors." *Proc Am Soc Clin Oncol* **21**: abstract 438.

Galbraith, S. M., Chaplin, D. J. et al. (2001). "Effects of combretastatin A4 phosphate on endothelial cell morphology in vitro and relationship to tumour vascular targeting activity in vivo." *Anticancer Res* **21**(1A): 93–102.

Galbraith, S. M., R. J. Maxwell, et al. (2003). "Combretastatin A4 phosphate has tumor antivascular activity in rat and man as demonstrated by dynamic magnetic resonance imaging." *J Clin Oncol* **21**(15): 2831–42.

Gardner, E., E. Springman, et al. (2007). "Antiangiogenic and antitumor activity of LP-261, a novel oral tubulin binding agent, alone and in combination with bevacizumab." *AACR Meeting Abstracts* **2007**(1 Annual Meeting): 1423.

Gaukroger, K., J. A. Hadfield, et al. (2001). "Novel syntheses of cis and trans isomers of combretastatin A-4." *J Org Chem* **66**(24): 8135–8.

Gaukroger, K., J. A. Hadfield, et al. (2003). "Structural requirements for the interaction of combretastatins with tubulin: how important is the trimethoxy unit?" *Org Biomol Chem* **1**(17): 3033–7.

Gaya, A. M. and G. J. Rustin (2005). "Vascular disrupting agents: a new class of drug in cancer therapy." *Clin Oncol (R Coll Radiol)* **17**(4): 277–90.

Genzyme http://www.genzymeoncology.com/onc/research/onc_p_research.asp (accessed March 2009).

Gourdeau, H., L. Leblond, et al. (2004). "Antivascular and antitumor evaluation of 2-amino-4-(3-bromo-4,5-dimethoxy-phenyl)-3-cyano-4H-chromenes, a novel series of anticancer agents." *Mol Cancer Ther* **3**(11): 1375–84.

Greystoke, A., S. Blagden, et al. (2006). "A phase I study of intravenous TZT-1027 administered on day 1 and day 8 of a three-weekly cycle in combination with carboplatin given on day 1 alone in patients with advanced solid tumours." *Ann Oncol* **17**(8): 1313–9.

Griggs, J., J. C. Metcalfe, et al. (2001). "Targeting tumour vasculature: the development of combretastatin A4." *Lancet Oncol* **2**(2): 82–7.

Grosios, K., S. E. Holwell, et al. (1999). "In vivo and in vitro evaluation of combretastatin A-4 and its sodium phosphate prodrug." *Br J Cancer* **81**(8): 1318–27.

Grosios, K., P. M. Loadman, et al. (2000). "Combination chemotherapy with combretastatin A-4 phosphate and 5-fluorouracil in an experimental murine colon adenocarcinoma." *Anticancer Res* **20**(1A): 229–33.

Guatteo, E., L. Bianchi, et al. (1996). A novel K+channel blocker isolated from "hiccup nut" toxin. *Neuroreport* **7**(15–17): 2575–9.

Hanahan, D., G. Bergers, et al. (2000). "Less is more, regularly: metronomic dosing of cytotoxic drugs can target tumor angiogenesis in mice." *J Clin Invest* **105**(8): 1045–7.

Harrigan, G. G., H. Luesch, et al. (1998). "Symplostatin 1: A dolastatin 10 analogue from the marine cyanobacterium *Symploca hydnoides*." *J Nat Prod* **61**(9): 1075–7.

Hashiguchi, N., T. Kubota, et al. (2004). "TZT-1027 elucidates antitumor activity through direct cytotoxicity and selective blockade of blood supply." *Anticancer Res* **24**(4): 2201–8.

Hill, S. A., D. J. Chaplin, et al. (2002). "Schedule dependence of combretastatin A4 phosphate in transplanted and spontaneous tumour models." *Int J Cancer* **102**(1): 70–4.

Hill, S. A., G. M. Tozer, et al. (2002). "Preclinical evaluation of the antitumour activity of the novel vascular targeting agent Oxi 4503." *Anticancer Res.* **22**(3): 1453–58.

Hoffman, M. A., J. A. Blessing, et al. (2003). "A phase II trial of dolastatin-10 in recurrent platinum-sensitive ovarian carcinoma: a Gynecologic Oncology Group study." *Gynecol Oncol* **89**(1): 95–8.

Horgen, F. D., E. B. Kazmierski, et al. (2002). "Malevamide D: isolation and structure determination of an isodolastatin H analogue from the marine cyanobacterium *Symploca hydnoides*." *J Nat Prod* **65**(4): 487–91.

Hori, K. and S. Saito (2003). "Microvascular mechanisms by which the combretastatin A-4 derivative AC7700 (AVE8062) induces tumour blood flow stasis." *Br J Cancer* **89**(7): 1334–44.

Hori, K., S. Saito, et al. (1999). "Antitumor effects due to irreversible stoppage of tumor tissue blood flow: evaluation of a novel combretastatin A-4 derivative, AC7700." *Jpn J Cancer Res* **90**(9): 1026–38.

Horti, J., E. Juhasz, et al. (2008). "Phase I study of TZT-1027, a novel synthetic dolastatin 10 derivative, for the treatment of patients with non-small cell lung cancer." *Cancer Chemother Pharmacol* **62**(1): 173–80.

Hua, J., Y. Sheng, et al. (2003). "Oxi4503, a novel vascular targeting agent: effects on blood flow and antitumor activity in comparison to combretastatin A-4 phosphate." *Anticancer Res.* **23**(2B): 1433–40.

Jordan, M. A., D. Walker, et al. (1998). "Suppression of microtubule dynamics by binding of cemadotin to tubulin: possible mechanism for its antitumor action." *Biochemistry* **37**(50): 17571–8.

Kasibhatla, S., H. Gourdeau, et al. (2004). "Discovery and mechanism of action of a novel series of apoptosis inducers with potential vascular targeting activity." *Mol Cancer Ther* **3**(11): 1365–74.

Kerbrat, P., V. Dieras, et al. (2003). "Phase II study of LU 103793 (dolastatin analogue) in patients with metastatic breast cancer." *Eur J Cancer* **39**(3): 317–20.

Kindler, H. L., P. K. Tothy, et al. (2005). "Phase II trials of dolastatin-10 in advanced pancreaticobiliary cancers." *Invest New Drugs* **23**(5): 489–93.
Kobayashi, M., T. Natsume, et al. (1997). "Antitumor activity of TZT-1027, a novel dolastatin 10 derivative." *Jpn J Cancer Res* **88**(3): 316–27.
Kremmidiotis, G., T. Lavranos, et al. (2008). "BNC105P is a vascular disruption agent that exhibits dual mode of action in a number of cancer indications and works additively in combination with bevacizumab." *AACR Meeting Abstracts* **2008**(1 Annual Meeting): 1445.
Landuyt, W., O. Verdoes, et al. (2000). "Vascular targeting of solid tumours: a major "inverse" volume-response relationship following combretastatin A-4 phosphate treatment of rat rhabdomyosarcomas." *Eur J Cancer* **36**(14): 1833–43.
Lejeune P, H. T., Vrignaud P et al (2002). In vivo antitumour activity and tumor necrosis induced by AVE8062A, a tumour vascular targeting agent. *Proc AACR* **43**(156): Abstr 781.
Li, L., A. Rojiani, et al. (1998). "Targeting the tumor vasculature with combretastatin A-4 disodium phosphate: effects on radiation therapy." *Int J Radiat Oncol Biol Phys* **42**(4): 899–903.
Lickliter, J., A. Francesconi, et al. (2008). "Phase I evaluation of CYT997, a novel cytotoxic and vascular-disrupting agent, in patients with advanced cancer." *J Clin Oncol* **26**(May 20 suppl): abstr 3504.
Lin, C. M., S. B. Singh, et al. (1988). "Interactions of tubulin with potent natural and synthetic analogs of the antimitotic agent combretastatin: a structure-activity study." *Mol Pharmacol* **34**(2): 200–8.
Lin, C. M., H. H. Ho, et al. (1989). "Antimitotic natural products combretastatin A-4 and combretastatin A-2: studies on the mechanism of their inhibition of the binding of colchicine to tubulin." *Biochemistry* **28**(17): 6984–91.
Lippert, J. W., 3rd (2007). "Vascular disrupting agents." *Bioorg Med Chem* **15**(2): 605–15.
LoRusso, P. M., S. M. Gadgeel, et al. (2008). "Phase I clinical evaluation of ZD6126, a novel vascular-targeting agent, in patients with solid tumors." *Invest New Drugs* **26**(2): 159–67.
Madden, T., H. T. Tran, et al. (2000). "Novel marine-derived anticancer agents: a phase I clinical, pharmacological, and pharmacodynamic study of dolastatin 10 (NSC 376128) in patients with advanced solid tumors." *Clin Cancer Res* **6**(4): 1293–301.
Malcontenti-Wilson, C., I. D. Phillips, et al. (2005). "Selective targeting of tumor vasculature by the novel synthetic molecule CYT997 and its efficacy in preclinical cancer models." *AACR Meeting Abstracts* **2005**(1): 808.
Mandeville, H. C., V. Goh, et al. (2008). "Volumetric perfusion CT assessment of concurrent combretastatin-A4-phosphate (CA4P) and radiotherapy (RT) in non-small cell lung cancer." *J Clin Oncol* **26**(May 20 suppl): abstr 14517.
Margolin, K., J. Longmate, et al. (2001). "Dolastatin-10 in metastatic melanoma: a phase II and pharmokinetic trial of the California Cancer Consortium." *Invest New Drugs* **19**(4): 335–40.
Marks, R. S., D. L. Graham, et al. (2003). "A phase II study of the dolastatin 15 analogue LU 103793 in the treatment of advanced non-small-cell lung cancer." *Am J Clin Oncol* **26**(4): 336–7.
McCreedy, B. K., T Locke, KW (2004). "The novel vascular disrupting agent, MN-029, shows potent and selective anti-tumour activity in preclinical animal models." *Proc 2nd International Conference On Vascular Targeting, Miami, Florida*: Abstract 23.
McDermott, D. F., E. Hersh, et al. (2005). "ILX651 administered daily for five days every 3 weeks (qdx5dq3w) in patients (pts) with inoperable locally advanced or metastatic melanoma:phase II experience." *ASCO Annual Meeting Proceedings* **23**(16S, Part I of II (June 1 Supplement)): 7556.
Medicinova http://www.medicinova.com/html/research_cancer.html (accessed March 2009).
Meyer, T., A. M. Gaya, et al. (2009). "A phase I trial of radioimmunotherapy with 131I-A5B7 anti-CEA antibody in combination with combretastatin-A4-phosphate in advanced gastrointestinal carcinomas." *Clin Cancer Res* **15**(13): 4484–92.
Mita, A. C., L. A. Hammond, et al. (2006). "Phase I and pharmacokinetic study of tasidotin hydrochloride (ILX651), a third-generation dolastatin-15 analogue, administered weekly for 3 weeks every 28 days in patients with advanced solid tumors." *Clin Cancer Res* **12**(17): 5207–15.
Mita, A. C., L. K. Yee, et al. (2008). "Phase I study of NPI-2358 (a novel vascular disrupting agent) in patients with solid tumors and lymphomas." *J Clin Oncol* **26**(May 20 suppl): abstr 3525.

Mross, K., W. E. Berdel, et al. (1998). "Clinical and pharmacologic phase I study of Cemadotin-HCl (LU103793), a novel antimitotic peptide, given as 24-hour infusion in patients with advanced cancer. A study of the Arbeitsgemeinschaft Internistische Onkologie (AIO) Phase I Group and Arbeitsgruppe Pharmakologie in der Onkologie und Haematologie (APOH) Group of the German Cancer Society." *Ann Oncol* **9**(12): 1323–30.

Nathan, P., I. Judson, et al. (2008). "A phase I study of combretastatin A4 phosphate (CA4P) and bevacizumab in subjects with advanced solid tumors." *J Clin Oncol* **26**(May 20 suppl): 3550.

Ng, Q. S., V. Goh, et al. (2007). "Tumor antivascular effects of radiotherapy combined with combretastatin a4 phosphate in human non-small-cell lung cancer." *Int J Radiat Oncol Biol Phys.* **67**(5): 1375–80.

Nicholson, B., G. K. Lloyd, et al. (2006). "NPI-2358 is a tubulin-depolymerizing agent: in-vitro evidence for activity as a tumor vascular-disrupting agent." *Anticancer Drugs.* **17**(1): 25–31.

Oliver, R., C. Wheeler, et al. (2004). "Evaluation of the role of body-surface-area dose adjustment of ZD6126, a novel vascular-targeting agent." *ASCO Annual Meeting Proceedings* **22**(14S): 3065.

Oxigene (2008). Investigator's brochure CA4P (Edition 15).

Patel, S., M. L. Keohan, et al. (2006). "Phase II study of intravenous TZT-1027 in patients with advanced or metastatic soft-tissue sarcomas with prior exposure to anthracycline-based chemotherapy." *Cancer* **107**(12): 2881–7.

Patterson, D. M., N. Charnley, et al. (2008). "Phase I evaluation of vascular disrupting agent OXi4503." *J Clin Oncol* **26**(May 20 suppl): abstract 3551.

Pedley, R. B., S. A. Hill, et al. (2001). "Eradication of colorectal xenografts by combined radioimmunotherapy and combretastatin a-4 3-O-phosphate." *Cancer Res.* **61**(12): 4716–22.

Perez, E. A., D. W. Hillman, et al. (2005). "Phase II trial of dolastatin-10 in patients with advanced breast cancer." *Invest New Drugs* **23**(3): 257–61.

Pettit, G. R., C. Temple, Jr., et al. (1995). "Antineoplastic agents 322. synthesis of combretastatin A-4 prodrugs." *Anticancer Drug Des* **10**: 299–309.

Pitot, H. C., E. A. McElroy, Jr., et al. (1999). "Phase I trial of dolastatin-10 (NSC 376128) in patients with advanced solid tumors." *Clin Cancer Res* **5**(3): 525–31.

Prise, V. E., D. J. Honess, et al. (2002). "The vascular response of tumor and normal tissues in the rat to the vascular targeting agent, combretastatin A-4-phosphate, at clinically relevant doses." *Int J Oncol* **21**(4): 717–26.

Radema, S. A., L. V. Beerepoot, et al. (2002). "Clinical evaluation of the novel vascular-targeting agent, ZD6126: assessment of toxicity and surrogate markers of vascular damage." *Proc Am Soc Clin Oncol* **21**: abstract 439.

Ray, A., T. Okouneva, et al. (2007). "Mechanism of action of the microtubule-targeted antimitotic depsipeptide tasidotin (formerly ILX651) and its major metabolite tasidotin C-carboxylate." *Cancer Res* **67**(8): 3767–76.

Ricart, A. D., M. Cooney, et al. (2006). "A phase I pharmacokinetic (PK) and pharmacodynamic (PD) study of MN-029, a novel vascular disrupting agent (VDA), in patients (pts) with advanced solid tumors." *J Clin Oncol, ASCO Annual Meeting Proceedings Part I* **24**(18S (June 20 Supplement)): 3096.

Riely, G. J., S. Gadgeel, et al. (2007). "A phase 2 study of TZT-1027, administered weekly to patients with advanced non-small cell lung cancer following treatment with platinum-based chemotherapy." *Lung Cancer* **55**(2): 181–5.

Rustin, G. J., S. M. Galbraith, et al. (2003). "Phase I clinical trial of weekly combretastatin A4 phosphate: clinical and pharmacokinetic results." *J Clin Oncol* **21**(15): 2815–22.

Rustin, G. J., P. D. Nathan, et al. (2005). "A Phase Ib Trial Of Combretastatin A4 Phosphate (CA4P) In Combination With Carboplatin Or Paclitaxel Chemotherapy In Patients With Advanced Cancer." *Proc ASCO* **23**: Abstract 3103: 217s.

Rustin, G., G. Jayson, et al. (2008). *Fosbretabulin combretastatin A-4 phosphate [CA4P] carboplatin and paclitaxel is active in patients with platinum resistant ovarian cancer.* IGCS 2008, 12th Biennial Meeting, International Gynecologic Cancer Society, Bangkok, Thailand.

Saad, E. D., E. H. Kraut, et al. (2002). "Phase II study of dolastatin-10 as first-line treatment for advanced colorectal cancer." *Am J Clin Oncol* **25**(5): 451–3.

Schoffski, P., B. Thate, et al. (2004). "Phase I and pharmacokinetic study of TZT-1027, a novel synthetic dolastatin 10 derivative, administered as a 1-hour intravenous infusion every 3 weeks in patients with advanced refractory cancer." *Ann Oncol* **15**(4): 671–9.

Scurr, M., I. Judson, et al. (2004). "Assessment of metabolism, excretion and pharmacokinetics of a single dose of [14C]-ZD6126 in patients with solid malignant tumors." *ASCO Annual Meeting Proceedings* **22**(14S): 3083.

Segreti, J. A., J. S. Polakowski, et al. (2004). "Tumor selective antivascular effects of the novel antimitotic compound ABT-751: an in vivo rat regional hemodynamic study." *Cancer Chemother Pharmacol* **54**(3): 273–81.

Shaked, Y., A. Ciarrocchi, et al. (2006). "Impact of circulating endothelial progenitor cells on the growth of viable tumor rim after treatment with a vascular disrupting agent." *AACR Meeting Abstracts* **2006**(1): 1343.

Shaked, Y., A. Ciarrocchi, et al. (2006). "Therapy-induced acute recruitment of circulating endothelial progenitor cells to tumors." *Science* **313**(5794): 1785–87.

Shaked, Y., E. Henke, et al. (2008). "Rapid chemotherapy-induced acute endothelial progenitor cell mobilization: implications for antiangiogenic drugs as chemosensitizing agents." *Cancer Cell* **14**(3): 263–73.

Siemann, D. and W. Shi (2005). *Dual agent targeting of the tumor vasculature: combining avastin with CA4P or OXi4503.* AACR-NCI-EORTC International Conference on Molecular Targets and Cancer Therapeutics.

Smyth, J., M. E. Boneterre, et al. (2001). "Activity of the dolastatin analogue, LU103793, in malignant melanoma." *Ann Oncol* **12**(4): 509–11.

Stevenson, J. P., M. Rosen, et al. (2003). "Phase I trial of the antivascular agent combretastatin A4 phosphate on a 5-day schedule to patients with cancer: magnetic resonance imaging evidence for altered tumor blood flow." *J Clin Oncol* **21**(23): 4428–38.

Supko, J. G., T. J. Lynch, et al. (2000). "A phase I clinical and pharmacokinetic study of the dolastatin analogue cemadotin administered as a 5-day continuous intravenous infusion." *Cancer Chemother Pharmacol* **46**(4): 319–28.

Therasse, P., S. G. Arbuck, et al. (2000). "New guidelines to evaluate the response to treatment in solid tumors. European Organization for Research and Treatment of Cancer, National Cancer Institute of the United States, National Cancer Institute of Canada." *J Natl Cancer Inst* **92**(3): 205–16.

Thorpe, P. E., D. J. Chaplin, et al. (2003). "The first international conference on vascular targeting: meeting overview." *Cancer Res* **63**(5): 1144–7.

Tolcher, A. W., L. Forero, P. Celio, L. A. Hammond, A. Patnaik, M. Hill, C. Verat-Follet, M. Haacke, M. Besenval, E. K. Rowinsky (2003). "Phase I, pharmacokinetic, and DCE-MRI correlative study of AVE8062A, an antivascular combretastatin analogue, administered weekly for 3 weeks every 28 days." *Proc Am Soc Clin Oncol* **22**: Abstract 834.

Villalona-Calero, M. A., S. D. Baker, et al. (1998). "Phase I and pharmacokinetic study of the water-soluble dolastatin 15 analog LU103793 in patients with advanced solid malignancies." *J Clin Oncol* **16**(8): 2770–9.

von Mehren, M., S. P. Balcerzak, et al. (2004). "Phase II trial of dolastatin-10, a novel anti-tubulin agent, in metastatic soft tissue sarcomas." *Sarcoma* **8**(4): 107–11.

Vrignaud, P. (2004). "In vivo synergy between cytotoxic agents and AVE8062A, a tumour vascular targeting agent." *Proc 2nd International Conference On Vascular Targeting, Miami, Florida*: Abstract 8.

Woods, J. A., J. A. Hadfield, et al. (1995). "The interaction with tubulin of a series of stilbenes based on combretastatin A-4." *Br J Cancer* **71**: 705–11.

Yamamoto, N., M. Andoh, et al. (2008). "Phase I study of TZT-1027, a novel synthetic dolastatin 10 derivative and inhibitor of tubulin polymerization, given weekly to advanced solid tumor patients for 3 weeks." *Cancer Sci* Dec 8 [Epub ahead of print].

Yeung, S. C., M. She, et al. (2007). "Combination chemotherapy including combretastatin A4 phosphate and paclitaxel is effective against anaplastic thyroid cancer in a nude mouse xenograft model." *J Clin Endocrinol Metab* **92**(8): 2902–9.

ASA404 (DMXAA): New Concepts in Tumour Vascular Targeting Therapy

Bruce C. Baguley

Abstract ASA404 (DMXAA; 5,6-dimethylxanthenone-4-acetic acid) was detected as a potential Tumour-Vascular Disrupting Agent (Tumour-VDA) by its ability to induce necrosis of experimental tumours. This was found to correlate with the cessation of tumour blood flow and in some cases to a dramatic curative effect. Studies on possible mechanisms demonstrated that ASA404 induced apoptosis in tumour endothelial cells, as well as elevating the tumour tissue concentration of cytokines, particularly of tumour necrosis factor (TNF). Cytokines were found to be important for both the action and the toxicity of the drug. Thus, ASA404 is likely to act both directly on tumour vasculature and indirectly through effects on other host cells, particularly macrophages. Phase II clinical trials established that at doses associated with acceptable toxicity, ASA404 in combination with cytotoxic drugs was effective against non-small cell lung cancer.

1 Introduction

The tumour vasculature, which contributes not only oxygen and nutrients to tumour cells but responds to multiple signals from the surrounding microenvironment, is an integral part of this complex, ever-changing tissue. The design of successful tumour therapy requires an understanding of the unique properties and dynamic nature of this microenvironment, and unexpected observations of the effects of a new chemotherapeutic drug can sometimes help us to advance this understanding. The Tumour-Vascular Disrupting Agent (Tumour-VDA) ASA404 (DMXAA) is a good example of how this can occur and while further studies aimed at elucidating the biochemical target of action are still ongoing, it is clear that its action cannot be understood by considering tumour vascular endothelial cells alone. A stream of

B.C. Baguley (✉)
Auckland Cancer Society Research Centre,
The University of Auckland, Auckland, New Zealand
e-mail: b.baguley@auckland.ac.nz

T. Meyer (ed.), *Vascular Disruptive Agents for the Treatment of Cancer*,
DOI 10.1007/978-1-4419-6609-4_10,

unexpected results was a feature of preclinical investigations, among which was the observation that combination of ASA404 with a variety of chemotherapeutic agents led to enhanced experimental antitumour activity. A further feature emerging from recent research is the extent to which the action of ASA404 in humans differs from that in mice. It is clear from current clinical studies that the potential utility of ASA404 lies in combination therapy and it is therefore essential that the principles involved in such combinations can be appreciated. This review commences with a brief summary of the preclinical development of this fascinating drug and follows with a discussion on its cellular action and clinical development.

2 Preclinical Development

ASA404 was originally synthesised at the Auckland Cancer Society Research Centre in a programme to develop more active analogues of the drug flavone acetic acid (FAA) (Fig. 1). FAA was produced in a programme aimed at developing anti-inflammatory agents, but showed unexpectedly high activity against murine Colon 38 tumours during testing at the US National Cancer Institute (Plowman et al. 1986). Experiments in this laboratory demonstrated that FAA did not cause histological changes typical of a cytotoxic drug but rather induced tumour necrosis in a manner that resembled the action of tumour necrosis factor (TNF) (Finlay et al. 1988; Smith et al. 1987). Since no cell-based or biochemical assays were available to characterise this activity, the in vivo assay (induction of tumour necrosis 24 h after drug administration, with histological assessment) was used to screen for other agents with similar activity. Several drugs, including fostriecin (a phosphorus-containing antibiotic), homoharringtonine, colchicine, podophyllotoxin, vincristine and vinblastine were identified using this assay (Baguley et al. 1989, 1991).

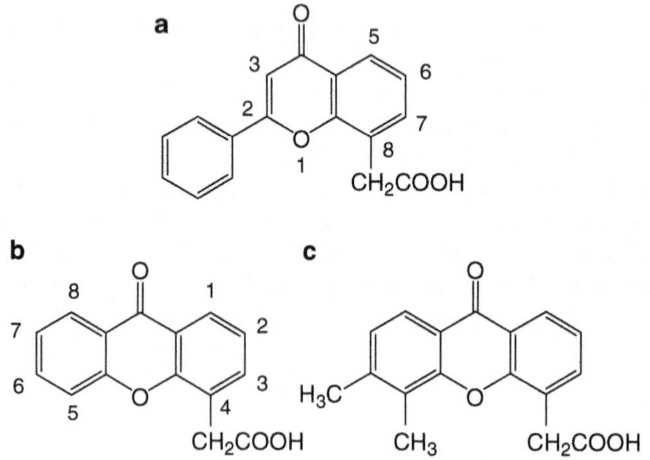

Fig. 1 Structures of flavone acetic acid (**a**) and xanthenone-4-acetic acid (**b**) and ASA404 (**c**)

Xanthenone acetic acid (XAA) (Fig. 1), which, like FAA, had earlier been synthesised as an anti-inflammatory drug (Nakanishi et al. 1976) was also found to have activity with this assay, and a programme was initiated to identify active derivatives of XAA (Atwell et al. 1990), as well as other more distantly related compounds (Rewcastle et al. 1991b). The 5-methyl derivative of XAA was identified as the most potent of the derivatives tested, and further work revealed the 5,6-dimethyl derivative (DMXAA; ASA404) to be over tenfold more dose-potent and more active than either FAA or XAA. A single intraperitoneal dose (30 mg/kg) cured 80% of mice with 5–10 mm diameter subcutaneous tumours (Rewcastle et al. 1991a). The in vivo assay in tumour-bearing mice, using 24 h histological assay as an endpoint, therefore, proved to be effective for the identification of Tumour-VDAs.

2.1 *Tumour Vasculature as a Target*

Studies on the modes of action of FAA and ASA404 elucidated two seemingly distinct mechanisms – the induction of cytokines and the disruption of tumour blood flow (Baguley 2003). Effects on tumour vasculature were investigated by labelling with two fluorescent dyes, one administered before and the other after treatment with either FAA or ASA404. Rapid (within 60 min) cessation of tumour blood flow was demonstrated, accompanied by rupture of blood vessels and the subsequent onset of tumour necrosis (Zwi et al. 1989, 1994a, b). The disruption of tumour blood flow was correlated with the induction of vascular endothelial cell apoptosis, as measured by DNA breaks (TUNEL assays) (Ching et al. 2002, 2004) and to an increase in tumour vascular permeability (Chung et al. 2008; Zhao et al. 2005). A further consequence of tumour blood flow inhibition was the induction of tumour hypoxia, measured scintigraphically in response to ASA404 or to the tubulin-binding vascular disrupting agent combretastatin A4, using a Technetium-labelled hypoxia-specific probe 2,2'-(1,4-diaminobutane)bis(2-methyl-3-butanone) dioxime (99mTc-labeled HL-91; Prognox (Siim et al. 2000)).

Induction of immunoreactivity to von Willebrand factor in tumour vasculature was observed in response to ASA404 (Siim and Baguley 2006), suggesting activation of platelets. A consequence of such activation is the release of serotonin (5-hydroxytryptamine), which was detected in plasma following treatment with either FAA or ASA404 (Baguley et al. 1997). Serotonin is converted by the liver to 5-hydroxyindole-3-acetic acid (5-HIAA), and extended 5-HIAA responses to ASA404 were observed in tumour bearing versus non-tumour bearing mice (Zhao et al. 2005). 5-HIAA responses were also observed for the mitotic poisons colchicine, vinblastine (Baguley et al. 1997) and combretastatin A4 (Q Ding and BC Baguley, unpublished) indicating that this is likely to be a general response to administration of vascular disrupting agents.

The mechanism underlying the response of endothelial cells to ASA404 is likely to involve the enzyme p38 MAP kinase. Some tumour cell lines form endothelial cell-like networks when cultured on Matrigel (vasculogenic mimicry). Addition of ASA404 inhibited network formation by a process that was sensitive to an inhibitor of p38 MAP kinase (Zhao et al. 2007). ASA404 similarly affected network formation by a cultured human vascular endothelial cell line, and this was also reversed by inhibitors of p38 kinase (X Zhan, GJ Finlay and BC Baguley, unpublished). The combretastatin A4 has a similar p38 kinase dependent effect on network formation (Tozer et al. 2005).

2.2 Cytokine Induction as a Target for ASA404

Local production of TNF was identified in response to both FAA (Evelhoch et al. 1988; Wiltrout et al. 1988) and ASA404 (Philpott et al. 1995) but has not been observed for other tumour VDAs. The time course of plasma and tissue TNF response to FAA and ASA404, which peaks at around 3 h after treatment, implies that TNF is not mediating the early changes in tumour blood flow. The importance of TNF in the action of ASA404 was established by showing that mice lacking the gene for either TNF (Ching et al. 1999) or the TNFR1 receptor (Zhao et al. 2002) did not respond to ASA404 at the efficacious dose (27.5 mg/kg). However, these knockout mice did respond to higher doses of ASA404, suggesting that alternative factors could substitute for TNF. Tumours in mice lacking the gene for interferon-β (IFN-β) (Roberts et al. 2008) or interferon-γ (IFN-γ) (Pang et al. 1998) did not respond to a standard dose of ASA404, suggesting that other cytokines could be involved. Since vascular endothelial cells have receptors for TNF, IFN-β and IFN-γ, it can be conjectured that treatment of mice with ASA404 can induce vascular endothelial cell disruption by a variety of interconnected, cytokine-dependent pathways. TNF can bind to TNFR1/2 receptors on vascular endothelial cells to induce apoptosis (Lucas et al. 1998), suggesting that TNF forms part of an indirect action of ASA404. TNF, IFN-β and IFN-γ, together with other cytokines as well as chemokines such as IP-10 (Cao et al. 2001), are induced simultaneously in mice treated with ASA404, and all potentially have effects on tumour endothelial function.

In addition to cytokines and chemokines, FAA and ASA404 induce nitric oxide both in vivo (Thomsen et al. 1991) and, with activated peritoneal macrophages, in vitro (Thomsen et al. 1990). Consequent reaction of nitric oxide with water leads to formation of nitrite and nitrate, which are potential biomarkers in plasma. The high plasma concentration of nitrite suggests that the nitric oxide is produced by iNOS (inducible nitric oxide synthase), which is thought to be induced maximally by ASA404 after approximately 6 h (Veszelovsky et al. 1995). Nitric oxide, at the low concentrations secreted by eNOS (endothelial nitric oxide synthase), binds to G-protein coupled receptors (GPCRs) on endothelial cells and associated smooth muscle cells, activating the enzyme soluble guanylyl cyclase, which has a number of functions, including maintenance of a low degree of vascular permeability. Higher concentrations of nitric oxide, as formed by iNOS in activated macrophages, leads to S-nitrosation of multiple proteins in vascular endothelial cells, including soluble guanylyl cyclase (Mayer et al. 2009) and a consequent increased vascular permeability.

Endotoxin (bacterial lipopolysaccharide) is a well known inducer of TNF, other cytokines and nitric oxide, raising the question of whether ASA404 acts through a pathway similar to that of endotoxin. Such a relationship appears to be supported by the observation that endotoxin and ASA404 also induce cross tolerance to each other (Roberts et al. 2007). However, endotoxin, unlike ASA404, causes little growth delay of murine Colon 38 tumours despite decreasing tumour blood flow and increasing 5-HIAA, nitric oxide and tumour haemorrhagic necrosis (Ching et al. 1994). Endotoxin induces a spectrum of cytokines different from that induced by ASA404 (Perera et al. 1994). The activation of TLR4 receptors by endotoxin leads to the formation of complexes containing a number of proteins including Myd88 and TRIF. This initiates the activation of several signalling cascades including NFκB and p38 kinase, leading to the production of cytokines (Rakoff-Nahoum and Medzhitov 2009). However, evidence from knockout mice indicates that neither the MyD88 nor the TRIF pathway is directly activated by ASA404 (Roberts et al. 2007).

The synergy between endotoxin and ASA404 (10 μg/ml) in the induction of TNF by cultured splenic macrophages (Wang et al. 2004) as well as between endotoxin and higher concentrations of ASA404 (800 μg/ml) in cultured human peripheral blood mononuclear cells (Philpott et al. 2001) suggests an indirect involvement of the TLR4 pathway. One possible mechanism for such involvement is through the facilitation of assembly of receptor complexes that include TLR4, MD2 (myeloid differentiation factor-2) and CD14. Assembly occurs on lipid rafts and requires ceramides (Cuschieri et al. 2007). Treatment of tumour-bearing mice with ASA404 causes increased concentrations of ceramides in spleen (Q Ding, P Kestell, S Alix, BC Baguley, unpublished), as well as increased plasma concentrations of the ceramide metabolite sphingosine (Baguley et al. 2008). This is consistent with the hypothesis that while ASA404 stimulates the formation of TLR4 receptors, it does not directly activate them.

In attempting to delineate which pathways are selectively targeted by ASA404, it is important to keep in mind that TLR4 complexes are involved in processes other than activation of the Myd88/TRIF pathway. One of these involves the translocation of TLR4 receptors to endosomes, where they associate with the bridging adaptor protein TRAM and lead to the activation of IRF-3 (interferon releasing factor-1) and its downstream transcription products (Kenny and O'Neill 2008). There is evidence for both activation of IRF-3 and the induction of interferon-β in murine peritoneal macrophages cultured in the presence of moderately high concentrations (100 μM) of ASA404 (Roberts et al. 2007).

It should be noted that the effects of ASA404 on macrophages might equally apply to tumour endothelial cells, since they also have surface receptors containing TLR4, MD2 and CD14. Receptor activation leads to signalling through the Myd88/TRIF and p38 kinase pathways, as well as to cytokine production, increased vascular permeability and an increased rate of endothelial apoptosis (Dauphinee and Karsan 2006). Although not yet proven, it is possible that ASA404 activates similar signalling pathways in macrophages and endothelial cells and thus stimulates extensive cross-talk between these host cell populations in tumour tissue.

2.3 ASA404 Combination Treatment in Mice

ASA404 is highly active as a single agent against the murine Colon 38 tumour, particularly when administered in an optimal schedule (Zhao et al. 2003). However, in other murine tumours, as well as in human tumour xenografts in immunodeficient mice, responses to ASA404 as a single agent are often only moderate. In these models, it is clear that combination with a variety of cytotoxic drugs, as well as ionising radiation, radioimmunotherapy, photodynamic therapy and hyperthermia, lead to increased antitumour activity that is sometimes more than additive (Baguley and Wilson 2002; Kelland 2005; Seshadri et al. 2005).

In a preclinical study using the mouse mammary MDAH-MCa-4 tumour, ASA404 as a single agent provided an average tumour growth delay of 6.7 days. ASA404 was also evaluated in combination with a number of cytotoxic drugs. In some cases, host toxicity necessitated a reduction in ASA404 dose. With the exception of 5-fluorouracil, which showed no advantage, all drugs tested provided evidence of a productive effect, with the following order of increasing activity: etoposide, carboplatin, cyclophosphamide, doxorubicin, cisplatin < vincristine, docetaxel < paclitaxel (Siim et al. 2003). Co-administration of paclitaxel provided a particularly striking effect, with the median tumour growth delay being extended from 0.3 to 80 days, with three of seven animals cured.

It will be interesting to determine the degree of interaction between ASA404 and targeted therapies. One report has described a positive interaction between ASA404 and bevacizumab, an anti-vascular endothelial growth factor (VEGF) monoclonal antibody in a human tumour xenograft (Djeha et al. 2006). In view of the role of cytokines in the action of ASA404, it is interesting that both thalidomide (Ching et al. 1995) and non-steroidal anti-inflammatory agents (Wang et al. 2008), which are known to suppress inflammatory cytokine production, potentiate the action of ASA404. The mechanisms underlying these results, and their possible clinical implications, are not yet clear.

3 Clinical Development of ASA404

Phase I evaluation of ASA404 employed two dosage schedules (single dose repeated weekly or every 3 weeks) and with a starting dose of 5.9 mg/m^2, calculated as 10% of the expected maximum tolerated dose (MTD) from data with mice. The MTD in humans was 3,700 mg/m^2 and side effects at high doses included confusion, tremor, slurred speech, visual disturbance, anxiety, urinary incontinence toxicity, and increases in the cardiac QT interval (Jameson et al. 2000; Jameson et al. 2003; McKeage et al. 2006; Rustin et al. 2003).

The difference in toxicity in mice and rats is a feature of ASA404; if the Phase I starting dose had been calculated from rat data, it would have been approximately 200 mg/m^2. The MTD in humans was predicted more accurately by rat toxicity than by mouse toxicity and the likely reason is that murine toxicity is dictated by systemic TNF production. Plasma concentrations of TNF were clearly elevated in mice but were not detectable in either rats (Liu et al. 2007) or humans (Jameson et al. 2000); increases in tumour TNF concentrations were detectable in all three species but were much higher in mice than rats or humans. Furthermore, the MTD in mice with targeted knockout of the gene for TNF (Ching et al. 1999) or its receptor TNFR1 (Zhao et al. 2002), was at least fourfold higher than in wild-type mice, suggesting that TNF, with characteristic effects on skin temperature and host vascular permeability (Chung et al. 2008), was responsible for the dose-limiting toxicity in mice. The very steep dose response curve observed in mice, in which the difference between a non-toxic and a toxic dose was very small, was not observed in either rats or humans, presumably for the same reason.

Only two unconfirmed partial responses were seen in the Phase I trials of ASA404. However, the exciting preclinical data on combination therapy (Siim et al. 2003), together with the argument that a Tumour-VDA and a cytotoxic drug may act by complementary mechanisms (Baguley and Wilson 2002), led to the initiation of Phase II trials in non-small cell lung cancer (NSCLC), ovarian and prostate cancer. In these trials, ASA404 was added to the standard cytotoxic drug regimen, which was carboplatin-paclitaxel in NSCLC and ovarian cancer, and docetaxel in prostate cancer. Increased response rates with addition of ASA404 were seen in all three trials, with a large effect in NSCLC (McKeage et al. 2008) and an encouraging effect in prostate cancer (McKeage 2008). Side effects caused by the addition of ASA404 to the treatment arm were minimal.

In the first phase II NSCLC trial, 73 patients not previously treated with chemotherapy, were randomised to receive up to six cycles of standard therapy comprising carboplatin (area under curve of 6 mg/ml.min) and paclitaxel (175 mg/m^2), either together with ASA404 at a dose of 1,200 mg/m^2 (37 patients) or without ASA404 (36 patients). Tumour response rate (31% versus 22%), median time to tumour progression (5.4 versus 4.4 months) and median survival (14.0 versus 8.8 months, hazard ratio: 0.73, 95%; confidence interval: 0.39, 1.38; P=0.33) were all improved in the ASA404 combination group as compared with the standard therapy group. An extension of this trial with ASA404 administered to 64 patients at a higher dose (1,800 mg/m^2) also reported positive efficacy findings, with a median survival of 14.5 months (McKeage et al. 2007; 2009). In a trial of 75 patients with recurrent ovarian cancer receiving carboplatin (area under curve of 6 mg/ml.min) and paclitaxel (175 mg/m^2), either together with ASA404 at 1,200 mg/m^2 (37 patients) or without ASA404 (38 patients), the response rate was 63.9% in the ASA404 and 48.6% in the standard arm (Gabra and Jameson 2007). In a trial of 75 patients with hormone refractory metastatic prostate cancer receiving docetaxel (75 mg/m^2), either together with ASA404 at 1,200 mg/m^2 (33 patients) or without ASA404 (38 patients), the response rate was 23.1% in the ASA404 arm and 9.1% in the standard arm (Pili et al. 2008). Two randomised, double-blind, placebo-controlled, multicentre studies Phase III trials have been initiated in NSCLC. In the first (ATTRACT-1), ASA404 (1800 mg/m^2 of free base) was administered together with carboplatin (AUC = 6 mg/ml.min) and paclitaxel (200 mg/m^2) every 21 days in patients with previously untreated disease.

However, this trial was halted when interim analysis showed no survival benefit (http://www.antisoma.com). In the second (ATTRACT-2), ASA404 (1800 mg/m^2) was administered together with docetaxel (75 mg/m^2) every 21 days in patients as second-line treatment. No safety concerns were apparent and at the time of writing this trial is ongoing.

3.1 Biomarkers

The Phase I and Phase II trials have provided opportunities to develop biomarkers that might allow estimation of the vascular disrupting effects of ASA404 on the tumour vascular endothelium in a clinical situation. The properties of this endothelium can change in several ways in response to both the stress caused either directly by ASA404 (for instance through the p38 MAP kinase pathway) or indirectly through the products of macrophages and other cells (for instance TNF, reactive oxygen species and nitric oxide). These result in changes in cell shape and/or the induction of endothelial apoptosis, both of which cause increased vascular permeability. Permeability changes lead firstly to a loss of plasma from the vasculature, with consequent increased haematocrit and reduced blood flow, and secondly to activation of platelets. Both of these processes have been used to devise biomarkers that have been applied to preclinical studies and to clinical trials.

Increased permeability of the vascular endothelium leads to a release of plasma proteins, particularly albumin, into the surrounding tissue, and this can be detected in several ways. One of the simplest methods, applicable to experimental systems, is to label the albumin with a dye such as Evans Blue, which binds strongly to albumin (Chung et al. 2008; Zhao et al. 2005). As measured by extraction of Evans Blue from tissue extracts, ASA404 selectively increases tumour vascular permeability and the increase correlates with a decrease in tumour blood flow (Zhao et al. 2005). In clinical trials, the same rationale can be used by administering the paramagnetic contrast agent gadopentetate dimeglumine (Gd-DTPA), which binds strongly to albumin, as a rapid intravenous bolus. Diffusion of the protein-bound drug from the blood vessels into the extravascular extracellular space can then be measured by dynamic contrast-enhanced magnetic resonance imaging (DCE-MRI) (Galbraith et al. 2002). This method also allows measurement of the rate of entry of the contrast agent into the tumour, thus providing a measure of tumour blood flow. One of the difficulties of the method is that while increased vascular permeability results in an increase in signal intensity, the associated decrease in blood flow results in a decrease in signal intensity. These opposing effects can be separated by appropriate experimental design and were used to demonstrate a vascular effect of ASA404 in a Phase I clinical trial (Galbraith et al. 2002). A second imaging technique, involving positron emission tomography, can be used in an analogous fashion and preliminary studies have been completed (Thorpe et al. 2003).

A second biomarker involves the serotonin metabolite 5-HIAA, which can be measured in plasma samples by high performance liquid chromatography. Distortion or death of vascular endothelial cells results in the exposure to collagen on the underlying basement membrane, which induces degranulation of platelets. Serotonin, one of the products released from platelets, is highly susceptible to oxidation and is therefore a poor candidate for a biomarker. However, the liver is able to distinguish free serotonin from that contained in platelets, converting the former to its comparatively stable metabolite 5-HIAA (Baguley et al. 1997; Kestell et al. 2001). In mice, increases in plasma 5-HIAA concentration correlated with both tumour increased vascular permeability and decreased blood flow (Zhao et al. 2005). In a Phase I clinical trial, increases in plasma 5-HIAA correlated with administered dose (McKeage et al. 2006) and in a Phase II NSCLC trial, the mean 5-HIAA concentration 2 h after ASA404 treatment point was 137.2±46.6 nM, representing an increase of 80.6±26.0 nM above baseline (McKeage et al. 2007).

4 Perspective

There is increasing recognition that the tumour microenvironment plays a major role both in the growth of tumours and in their response to treatment. Vascular endothelial cells are an important component of the tumour microenvironment and the concept that they might be selectively targeted in cancer has been a highly active area of research. Macrophages constitute 10–15% of most tissues and are especially prominent in tumours (Medzhitov 2008), sharing many features with endothelial cells including the expression of TLR4 receptors; making them also potential targets for cancer therapy. Macrophages can be divided into three overlapping classes, those potentially able to kill tumour cells, those involved in wound healing and those that suppress the action of the first two classes (Mosser and Edwards 2008). The interactions between these classes of macrophages provide a complex biological control network that includes the vascular endothelium. It is within this network that we might search for the action of ASA404.

A suggested scheme for the action of ASA404 is provided in Fig. 2. The vertical arrows represent the "classical" pathway for interaction between a Tumour-VDA and a cytotoxic regimen. The Tumour-VDA is most effective against poorly diffused areas of the tumour, where drug-induced increases in vascular permeability lead to catastrophic failure of blood flow, rupture of blood vessels and the onset of extensive tumour necrosis. In well perfused areas, particularly at the periphery of the tumour (Baguley and Wilson 2002), good vascular access to conventional cytotoxic chemotherapy is more effective, providing a good theoretical basis for the combination.

The other arrows in Fig. 2 indicate likely interactions within the tumour microenvironment that might also contribute to the distinctive properties of ASA404. Stressed or dying tumour cells generated by cytotoxic therapy release factors such as calreticulin and the nuclear protein HMGB1, which interact with TLR4 receptors (Apetoh et al. 2007; Apetoh et al. 2008). These receptors are

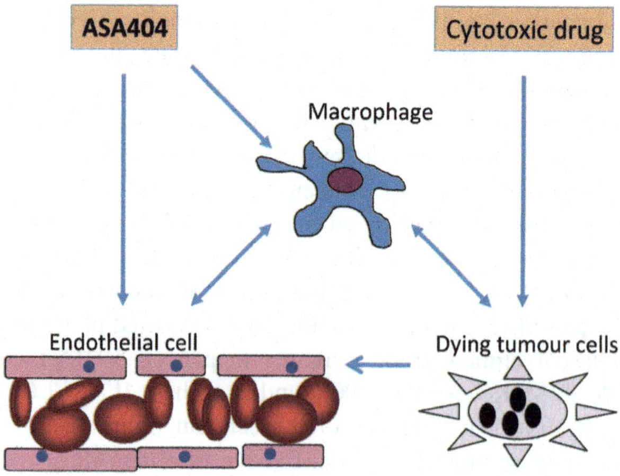

Fig. 2 Simplified scheme for the combined actions of ASA404 and cytotoxic drugs. While targeting separate populations (*vertical arrows*) they also stimulate macrophage involvement (*other arrows*). Products of dying tumour cells are thought to stimulate TLR4 receptors of macrophages and endothelial cells, leading to activation of signalling pathways. ASA404 in some way amplifies these pathways, leading to further effects on both endothelial cells and surviving tumour cells

present on macrophages, dendritic cells and vascular endothelial cells and can activate analogous pathways in the different cell types. While some activated macrophages and dendritic cells are capable of killing tumour cells directly through the production of reactive oxygen species and nitric oxide, activated endothelial cells can cause indirect killing by inducing failure of the vascular system.

The unexpected findings from both preclinical and clinical studies with ASA404 have served to highlight our lack of knowledge of many aspects of human cancer therapy. However, further clinical development of ASA404, together with ongoing research on the tumour microenvironment, may well open up exciting new areas of knowledge of tumour physiology in the future.

References

Apetoh L, Ghiringhelli F, Tesniere A, Obeid M, Ortiz C, Criollo A, Mignot G, Maiuri MC, Ullrich E, Saulnier P, Yang H, Amigorena S, Ryffel B, Barrat FJ, Saftig P, Levi F, Lidereau R, Nogues C, Mira JP, Chompret A, Joulin V, Clavel-Chapelon F, Bourhis J, Andre F, Delaloge S, Tursz T, Kroemer G, Zitvogel L (2007) Toll-like receptor 4-dependent contribution of the immune system to anticancer chemotherapy and radiotherapy. Nat Med 13: 1050–1059

Apetoh L, Tesniere A, Ghiringhelli F, Kroemer G, Zitvogel L (2008) Molecular interactions between dying tumor cells and the innate immune system determine the efficacy of conventional anticancer therapies. Cancer Res 68: 4026–4030

Atwell GJ, Rewcastle GW, Baguley BC, Denny WA (1990) Potential antitumor agents. 60. Relationships between structure and in vivo colon 38 activity for 5-substituted 9-oxoxanthene-4-acetic acids. J Med Chem 33: 1375–1379

Baguley BC (2003) Antivascular therapy of cancer: DMXAA. The Lancet Oncology 4: 141–148
Baguley BC, Wilson WR (2002) Potential of DMXAA combination therapy for solid tumors. Expert Rev Anticancer Ther 2: 593–603
Baguley BC, Calveley SB, Crowe KK, Fray LM, O'Rourke SA, Smith GP (1989) Comparison of the effects of flavone acetic acid, fostriecin, homoharringtonine and tumour necrosis factor alpha on colon 38 tumours in mice. Eur J Cancer Clin Oncol 25: 263–269
Baguley BC, Holdaway KM, Thomsen LL, Zhuang L, Zwi LJ (1991) Inhibition of growth of colon 38 adenocarcinoma by vinblastine and colchicine: evidence for a vascular mechanism. Eur J Cancer 27: 482–487
Baguley BC, Zhuang L, Kestell P (1997) Increased plasma serotonin following treatment with flavone-8-acetic acid, 5,6-dimethylxanthenone-4-acetic acid, vinblastine, and colchicine: relation to vascular effects. Oncol Res 9: 55–60
Baguley BC, Ding Q, Kestell P, Alix S (2008) Potential importance of the ceramide pathway in the action of the tumour vascular disrupting agent ASA404 (DMXAA, 5,6-dimethylxanthenone-4-acetic acid). Eur J Cancer 6: 32
Cao Z, Baguley BC, Ching LM (2001) Interferon-inducible protein 10 induction and inhibition of angiogenesis in vivo by the antitumor agent 5,6-dimethylxanthenone-4-acetic acid (DMXAA). Cancer Res 61: 1517–1521
Ching LM, Joseph WR, Zhuang L, Baguley BC (1994) Interaction between endotoxin and the anti-tumour agent 5,6- dimethylxanthenone-4-acetic acid in the induction of tumour necrosis factor and haemorrhagic necrosis of colon 38 tumours. Cancer Chemother Pharmacol 35: 153–160
Ching LM, Xu ZF, Gummer BH, Palmer BD, Joseph WR, Baguley BC (1995) Effect of thalidomide on tumour necrosis factor production and anti- tumour activity induced by 5,6-dimethylxanthenone-4-acetic acid. Br J Cancer 72: 339–343
Ching LM, Goldsmith D, Joseph WR, Korner H, Sedgwick JD, Baguley BC (1999) Induction of intratumoral tumor necrosis factor (TNF) synthesis and hemorrhagic necrosis by 5,6-dimethylxanthenone-4-acetic acid (DMXAA) in TNF knockout mice. Cancer Res 59: 3304–3307
Ching LM, Cao Z, Kieda C, Zwain S, Jameson MB, Baguley BC (2002) Induction of endothelial cell apoptosis by the antivascular agent 5,6-dimethylxanthenone-4-acetic acid. Br J Cancer 86: 1937–1942
Ching LM, Zwain S, Baguley BC (2004) Relationship between tumour endothelial cell apoptosis and tumour blood flow shutdown following treatment with the antivascular agent DMXAA in mice. Br J Cancer 90: 906–910
Chung F, Liu J, Ching LM, Baguley BC (2008) Consequences of increased vascular permeability induced by treatment of mice with 5,6-dimethylxanthenone-4-acetic acid (DMXAA) and thalidomide. Cancer Chemother Pharmacol 61: 497–502
Cuschieri J, Bulger E, Billgrin J, Garcia I, Maier RV (2007) Acid sphingomyelinase is required for lipid Raft TLR4 complex formation. Surg Infect (Larchmt) 8: 91–106
Dauphinee SM, Karsan A (2006) Lipopolysaccharide signaling in endothelial cells. Lab Invest 86: 9–22
Djeha H, Shah K, McGeever G, Dobinson D, Green C (2006) Combination of the vascular disrupting agent DMXAA (AS1404) with bevacizumab and paclitaxel produces synergistic antitumor activity in lung cancer xenografts. AACR 47: #233
Evelhoch JL, Bissery MC, Chabot GG, Simpson NE, McCoy CL, Heilbrun LK, Corbett TH (1988) Flavone acetic acid (NSC 347512)-induced modulation of murine tumor physiology monitored by in vivo nuclear magnetic resonance spectroscopy. Cancer Res 48: 4749–4755
Finlay GJ, Smith GP, Fray LM, Baguley BC (1988) Effect of flavone acetic acid on Lewis lung carcinoma: evidence for an indirect effect. J Natl Cancer Inst 80: 241–245
Gabra H, Jameson MB (2007) Update of phase II study of DMXAA (AS1404) combined with carboplatin and paclitaxel in recurrent ovarian cancer. EJC Supplements 5 319
Galbraith SM, Rustin GJ, Lodge MA, Taylor NJ, Stirling JJ, Jameson M, Thompson P, Hough D, Gumbrell L, Padhani AR (2002) Effects of 5,6-dimethylxanthenone-4-acetic acid on human tumor microcirculation assessed by dynamic contrast-enhanced magnetic resonance imaging. J Clin Oncol 20: 3826–3840

Jameson MB, Thompson PI, Baguley BC, Evans BD, Harvey VJ, Porter DJ, McCrystal MR, Kestell P (2000) Phase I pharmacokinetic and pharmacodynamic study of 5,6-dimethylxanthenone-4-acetic acid (DMXAA), a novel antivascular agent. Proc Am Soc Clin Oncol 19: 705

Jameson MB, Thompson PI, Baguley BC, Evans BD, Harvey VJ, Porter DJ, McCrystal MR, Small M, Bellenger K, Gumbrell L, Halbert GW, Kestell P (2003) Clinical aspects of a phase I trial of 5,6-dimethylxanthenone-4-acetic acid (DMXAA), a novel antivascular agent. Br J Cancer 88: 1844–1850

Kelland LR (2005) Targeting established tumor vasculature: a novel approach to cancer treatment. Curr Canc Ther Rev 1: 1–9

Kenny EF, O'Neill LA (2008) Signalling adaptors used by Toll-like receptors: an update. Cytokine 43: 342–349

Kestell P, Zhao L, Jameson MB, Stratford MR, Folkes LK, Baguley BC (2001) Measurement of plasma 5-hydroxyindoleacetic acid as a possible clinical surrogate marker for the action of antivascular agents. Clin Chim Acta 314: 159–166

Liu J, Ching LM, Goldthorpe N, Sutherland R, Baguley BC, Kirker J, McKeage MJ (2007) Antitumour action of 5,6-dimethylxanthenone-4-acetic acid (DMXAA) in rats bearing chemically-induced primary mammary tumours. J Clin Oncol 59: 661–669

Lucas R, Garcia I, Donati YR, Hribar M, Mandriota SJ, Giroud C, Buurman WA, Fransen L, Suter PM, Nunez G, Pepper MS, Grau GE (1998) Both TNF receptors are required for direct TNF-mediated cytotoxicity in microvascular endothelial cells. Eur J Immunol 28: 3577–3586

Mayer B, Kleschyov AL, Stessel H, Russwurm M, Munzel T, Koesling D, Schmidt K (2009) Inactivation of soluble guanylate cyclase by stoichiometric S-nitrosation. Mol Pharmacol 75: 886–891

McKeage MJ (2008) The potential of DMXAA (ASA404) in combination with docetaxel in advanced prostate cancer. Expert Opin Investig Drugs 17: 23–29

McKeage MJ, Fong P, Jeffery M, Baguley BC, Kestell P, Ravic M, Jameson MB (2006) 5,6-Dimethylxanthenone-4-acetic acid in the treatment of refractory tumors: a phase I safety study of a vascular disrupting agent. Clin Cancer Res 12: 1776–1784

McKeage MJ, Reck M, Jameson MB, Rosenthal MA, Gibbs D, Mainwaring PN, Freitag L, Sullivan R, von Pawel J (2009) Phase II study of ASA404 (vadimezan, 5,6-dimethylxanthenone-4-acetic acid/DMXAA) 1800mg/m^2 combined with carboplatin and paclitaxel in previously untreated advanced non-small cell lung cancer. Lung Cancer 65: 192–197

McKeage MJ, von Pawel J, AS1404-201 Study Group Investigators (2007) Phase II study of DMXAA (ASA404) 1800 mg/m^2 combined with carboplatin and paclitaxel in non-small cell lung cancer. World Conference on Lung Cancer, Seoul, South Korea. J Thoracic Oncol 2: 728

McKeage MJ, von Pawel J, Reck M, Jameson MB, Rosenthal MA, Sullivan R, Gibbs D, Mainwaring PN, Serke M, Lafitte JJ, Chouaid C, Freitag L, Quoix E (2008) Randomised phase II study of ASA404 combined with carboplatin and paclitaxel in previously untreated advanced non-small cell lung cancer. Br J Cancer 99: 2006–2012

Medzhitov R (2008) Origin and physiological roles of inflammation. Nature 454: 428–435

Mosser DM, Edwards JP (2008) Exploring the full spectrum of macrophage activation. Nat Rev Immunol 8: 958–969

Nakanishi M, Oe T, Tsuruda M, Matsuo H, Sakuragi S, Maruyama Y (1976) Studies on Anti-inflammatory Agents. XXXI. Studies on the synthesis and anti-inflammatory activity of xanthenyl- and benzo-pyranopyridinylacetic acid derivatives. J Pharm Soc Japan 96: 99–109

Pang JH, Cao Z, Joseph WR, Baguley BC, Ching LM (1998) Antitumour activity of the novel immune modulator 5,6- dimethylxanthenone-4-acetic acid (DMXAA) in mice lacking the interferon- gamma receptor. Eur J Cancer 34: 1282–1289

Perera PY, Barber SA, Ching LM, Vogel SN (1994) Activation of LPS-inducible genes by the antitumor agent 5,6- dimethylxanthenone-4-acetic acid in primary murine macrophages. Dissection of signaling pathways leading to gene induction and tyrosine phosphorylation. J Immunol 153: 4684–4693

Philpott M, Baguley BC, Ching LM (1995) Induction of tumour necrosis factor-alpha by single and repeated doses of the antitumour agent 5,6-dimethylxanthenone-4-acetic acid. Cancer Chemother Pharmacol 36: 143–148

Philpott M, Ching L, Baguley BC (2001) The antitumour agent 5,6-dimethylxanthenone-4-acetic acid acts in vitro on human mononuclear cells as a co-stimulator with other inducers of tumour necrosis factor. Eur J Cancer 37: 1930–1937

Pili R, Rosenthal M, AS1404-2-3 Study Group Investigators (2008) Addition of DMXAA (ASA404) to docetaxel in patients with hormone-refractory metastatic prostate cancer (HRMPC): update from a randomized, phase II study. Proc Am Soc Clin Oncol 26 Suppl Abstract 5007

Plowman J, Narayanan VL, Dykes D, Szarvasi E, Briet P, Yoder OC, Paull KD (1986) Flavone acetic acid: a novel agent with preclinical antitumor activity against colon adenocarcinoma 38 in mice. Cancer Treat Rep 70: 631–635

Rakoff-Nahoum S, Medzhitov R (2009) Toll-like receptors and cancer. Nat Rev Cancer 9: 57–63

Rewcastle GW, Atwell GJ, Baguley BC, Boyd M, Thomsen LL, Zhuang L, Denny WA (1991a) Potential antitumor agents. 63. Structure-activity relationships for side-chain analogues of the colon 38 active agent 9-oxo-9H-xanthene-4- acetic acid. J Med Chem 34: 2864–2870

Rewcastle GW, Atwell GJ, Palmer BD, Boyd PD, Baguley BC, Denny WA (1991b) Potential antitumor agents. 62. Structure-activity relationships for tricyclic compounds related to the colon tumor active drug 9-oxo-9H- xanthene-4-acetic acid. J Med Chem 34: 491–496

Roberts ZJ, Goutagny N, Perera PY, Kato H, Kumar H, Kawai T, Akira S, Savan R, van Echo D, Fitzgerald KA, Young HA, Ching LM, Vogel SN (2007) The chemotherapeutic agent DMXAA potently and specifically activates the TBK1-IRF-3 signaling axis. J Exp Med 204: 1559–1569

Roberts ZJ, Ching LM, Vogel SN (2008) IFN-beta-dependent inhibition of tumor growth by the vascular disrupting agent 5,6-dimethylxanthenone-4-acetic acid (DMXAA). J Interferon Cytokine Res 28: 133–139

Rustin GJ, Bradley C, Galbraith S, Stratford M, Loadman P, Waller S, Bellenger K, Gumbrell L, Folkes L, Halbert G (2003) 5,6-dimethylxanthenone-4-acetic acid (DMXAA), a novel antivascular agent: phase I clinical and pharmacokinetic study. Br J Cancer 88: 1160–1167

Seshadri M, Spernyak JA, Mazurchuk R, Camacho SH, Oseroff AR, Cheney RT, Bellnier DA (2005) Tumor vascular response to photodynamic therapy and the antivascular agent 5,6-dimethylxanthenone-4-acetic acid: implications for combination therapy. Clin Cancer Res 11: 4241–4250

Siim BG, Baguley BC (2006) Flavones and xanthenones as vascular disrupting agents. In Vascular-targeted Therapies in Oncology, Sieman DW (ed) pp 159–177. John Wiley & Sons Ltd: London

Siim BG, Laux WT, Rutland MD, Palmer BN, Wilson WR (2000) Scintigraphic imaging of the hypoxia marker (99 m)technetium-labeled 2,2′-(1,4-diaminobutane)bis(2-methyl-3-butanone) dioxime (99mTc-labeled HL-91; prognox): noninvasive detection of tumor response to the antivascular agent 5,6-dimethylxanthenone-4-acetic acid. Cancer Res 60: 4582–4588

Siim BG, Lee AE, Shalal-Zwain S, Pruijn FB, McKeage MJ, Wilson WR (2003) Marked potentiation of the antitumour activity of chemotherapeutic drugs by the antivascular agent 5,6-dimethylxanthenone-4-acetic acid (DMXAA). Cancer Chemother Pharmacol 51: 43–52

Smith GP, Calveley SB, Smith MJ, Baguley BC (1987) Flavone acetic acid (NSC 347512) induces haemorrhagic necrosis of mouse colon 26 and 38 tumours. Eur J Cancer Clin Oncol 23: 1209–1211

Thomsen LL, Ching LM, Baguley BC (1990) Evidence for the production of nitric oxide by activated macrophages treated with the antitumor agents flavone-8-acetic acid and xanthenone- 4-acetic acid. Cancer Res 50: 6966–6970

Thomsen LL, Ching LM, Zhuang L, Gavin JB, Baguley BC (1991) Tumor-dependent increased plasma nitrate concentrations as an indication of the antitumor effect of flavone-8-acetic acid and analogues in mice. Cancer Res 51: 77–81

Thorpe PE, Chaplin DJ, Blakey DC (2003) The first international conference on vascular targeting: meeting overview. Cancer Res 63: 1144–1147

Tozer GM, Kanthou C, Baguley BC (2005) Disrupting tumour blood vessels. Nature Reviews Cancer 5: 423–435

Veszelovsky E, Holford NH, Thomsen LL, Knowles RG, Baguley BC (1995) Plasma nitrate clearance in mice: modeling of the systemic production of nitrate following the induction of nitric oxide synthesis. Cancer Chemother Pharmacol 36: 155–159

Wang LC, Reddy CB, Baguley BC, Kestell P, Sutherland R, Ching LM (2004) Induction of tumour necrosis factor and interferon-gamma in cultured murine splenocytes by the antivascular agent DMXAA and its metabolites. Biochem Pharmacol 67: 937–945

Wang LC, Ching LM, Paxton JW, Kestell P, Sutherland R, Zhuang L, Baguley BC (2008) Enhancement of the action of the antivascular drug 5,6-dimethylxanthenone-4-acetic acid (DMXAA; ASA404) by non-steroidal anti-inflammatory drugs. Invest New Drugs

Wiltrout RH, Boyd MR, Back TC, Salup RR, Arthur JA, Hornung RL (1988) Flavone-8-acetic acid augments systemic natural killer cell activity and synergizes with IL-2 for treatment of murine renal cancer. J Immunol 140: 3261–3265

Zhao L, Ching LM, Kestell P, Baguley BC (2002) The antitumour activity of 5,6-dimethylxanthenone-4-acetic acid (DMXAA) in TNF receptor-1 knockout mice. Br J Cancer 87: 465–470

Zhao L, Ching LM, Kestell P, Baguley BC (2003) Improvement of the antitumor activity of intraperitoneally and orally administered 5,6-dimethylxanthenone-4-acetic acid by optimal scheduling. Clin Cancer Res 9: 6545–6550

Zhao L, Ching LM, Kestell P, Kelland LR, Baguley BC (2005) Mechanisms of tumor vascular shut-down induced by 5,6-dimethylxanthenone-4-acetic acid (DMXAA); increased tumor vascular permeability. Int J Cancer 116: 322–326

Zhao L, Marshall ES, Kelland LR, Baguley BC (2007) Evidence for the involvement of p38 MAP kinase in the action of the vascular disrupting agent 5,6-dimethylxanthenone-4-acetic acid (DMXAA). Invest New Drugs 25: 271–276

Zwi LJ, Baguley BC, Gavin JB, Wilson WR (1989) Blood flow failure as a major determinant in the antitumor action of flavone acetic acid. J Natl Cancer Inst 81: 1005–1013

Zwi LJ, Baguley BC, Gavin JB, Wilson WR (1994a) Correlation between immune and vascular activities of xanthenone acetic acid antitumor agents. Oncol Res 6: 79–85

Zwi LJ, Baguley BC, Gavin JB, Wilson WR (1994b) The morphological effects of the anti-tumor agents flavone acetic acid and 5,6-dimethyl xanthenone acetic acid on the colon 38 mouse tumor. Pathology 26: 161–169

Vascular Disruptive Agents in Combination with Radiotherapy

Henry C. Mandeville and Peter J. Hoskin

Abstract Despite early promise, clinical trials of single agent VDAs have not demonstrated the ability to consistently produce significant tumour shrinkage or durable remissions. Contributing to this effect is the persistence of viable residual tumour rim following treatment with a VDA and this provides a strong rationale for combining them with other anti-cancer strategies, including radiotherapy. With evidence suggesting that the overall anti-tumour effect of radiotherapy is in part related to resultant damage to the tumour vasculature, this provides additional support for combining these two therapeutic modalities. As described in this chapter, the preclinical and early phase clinical trials to date have demonstrated that VDAs can improve the therapeutic index of radiotherapy through improved anti-tumour effect, spatial cooperation and with non-overlapping toxicities. There remains scope to further improve the anti-tumour effects produced by VDAs in combination with radiotherapy. Strategies that have shown promise when combined with VDAs and irradiation include hyperthermia, bioreductive agents and other vascular directed therapies.

1 Introduction

As early as the first half of the nineteenth century, Walshe reported that some solid tumours could be eradicated when their circulation is interrupted (Walsh 1844). The key turning point, leading to the development of current vascular directed treatments, was in 1971 when Folkman proposed tumour growth to be angiogenesis dependent and the inhibition of angiogenesis as a treatment for cancer (Folkman 1971). This paper resulted in intensification of work exploring this concept and other strategies for vascular directed therapies.

P.J. Hoskin (✉)
Marie Curie Research Wing, Mount Vernon Hospital, Northwood, UK
e-mail: peterhoskin@nhs.net

T. Meyer (ed.), *Vascular Disruptive Agents for the Treatment of Cancer*,
DOI 10.1007/978-1-4419-6609-4_11,

The concept of vascular disruptive therapies arose following the discovery that endothelial cells in tumours rapidly proliferate, in contrast to the non-proliferating endothelial cells in normal tissue, a finding that has now been demonstrated in both rodent and human tumour blood vessels (Denekamp and Hobson 1982; Ebhard et al. 2000). It was this finding that led Denekamp to propose the exploitation of the functional and morphological differences between tumour and normal blood vessels through the selective targeting of tumour blood supply (Denekamp 1982). Early work exploring this concept demonstrated tumour regression, growth delay and long term tumour control as a result of compromised tumour blood flow (Denekamp et al. 1983). Over the last 25 years this concept has been extensively studied, resulting in the development of potent new vascular disruptive agents.

Radiotherapy is one of the key components of modern cancer treatment and is second only to surgery in the number of cancers that it cures. In recent years there has been rapid and extensive development in the technology available, which has resulted in an equally rapid revolution in the delivery of radiotherapy treatments. Complex techniques such as intensity modulated radiotherapy and image guided radiotherapy are now becoming readily available. These new techniques hold the promise of more precise radiotherapy and as a result should produce better tolerance, reduction of the associated late effects and ultimately enable escalation of radiotherapy dose with the aim of improving treatment efficacy and cure rate.

Efforts to improve the efficacy of radiotherapy have led to the widespread adoption of combination schedules with cytotoxic chemotherapeutic and hormonal agents in a variety of cancers. As knowledge of molecular and cellular targets increases this has resulted in the instigation of trials to explore the optimal therapeutic deployment of targeted agents and determine whether they can enhance the effects of radiotherapy. It had been assumed that combining vascular directed therapies with radiotherapy would result in increased tumour hypoxia, therefore negatively impacting the anti-tumour effect of ionising radiation (O'Reilly 2006). Contrary to this hypothesis, preclinical studies of antivascular agents, both vascular disruptive and anti-angiogenic, combined with radiation have in fact demonstrated enhanced anti-tumour activity.

2 Vascular Effects of Radiation

The damage to the microvasculature of normal tissues following radiotherapy is well documented. This tumour bed effect has been demonstrated in preclinical models where tumours implanted in a previously irradiated site grow back more slowly than control tumours at an unirradiated site (Leith et al. 1992). Radiotherapy appears to affect the tumour microvasculature through activation of the RhoA/Rho kinase pathway, resulting in rapid and persistent remodelling of the endothelial cytoskeleton and increase in the permeability of the microvasculature (Gabryś et al. 2007). It has been postulated that tumour radiosensitivity may be related to microvascular sensitivity, with more resistant cells lines displaying reduced endothelial cell apoptosis, although this theory has been contested (Garcia-Barros et al. 2003). The normal tissue effects including the gastrointestinal sequelae of radiotherapy may also be contributed to by this effect. Endothelial cell apoptosis has been shown to occur in microvasculature of the gut following a single high dose of radiotherapy, an effect that can be pharmacologically inhibited following the administration of an intravenous infusion of bFGF (Paris et al. 2001). Radiation-induced necrosis, a late normal tissue effect resulting from endothelial cell dysfunction, has been shown to be associated with increased vascular permeability and raised levels of VEGF. Exploratory clinical trials have been undertaken where the monoclonal antibody inhibitor of VEGF-A, bevacizumab, has been used in the treatment of radiation necrosis of the brain (Gonzalez et al. 2007).

Radiotherapy is also thought to have local and systemic effects on angiogenesis and has been shown to induce the expression of VEGF (Gorski et al. 1999). The formation of recurrent tumours after radiotherapy is preceded by angiogenesis, usually occurring within 20 days of completing radiotherapy (Hast et al. 2002). Upregulation and stabilisation of HIF1α occurs as a result of radiotherapy producing increased VEGF expression, which has the effect of increasing endothelial cell survival, angiogenesis and also tumour cell survival and proliferation (Dewhirst et al. 2008). Reduced levels of the endogenous angiogenesis inhibitor angiostatin have also been observed as a result of radiotherapy to the primary tumour, with a subsequent increase in growth of previously dormant metastases (Camphausen et al. 2001). However enhanced inhibition of distal angiogenesis following tumour irradiation has also been described, but no effect on angiogenesis has been demonstrated with irradiation of normal tissues (Hartford et al. 2000). Despite these apparent contradictory findings, the interaction of radiotherapy with tumour vasculature undoubtedly plays an important in the response to treatment and has the potential to be exploited further.

3 Rationale for Combining VDAs and Radiotherapy

Radiotherapy is a highly effective treatment in a large number of malignancies, yet there are still a significant proportion of patients receiving radical treatment that are not cured of their disease. Radiotherapy has been combined with other cancer treatments to improve its efficacy and the use of concurrent cytotoxic chemotherapy is the standard of care for specific tumours, in particular squamous cell carcinomas of the uterine cervix, anus, oesophagus and head and neck region. In assessing the potential benefits of adding a new treatment to radiotherapy, the key features to ascertain are whether it offers improved antitumour effect, spatial cooperation or non-overlapping toxicities (Steel and Peckham 1979) (Table 1).

There are potential exploitable non-interactive mechanisms supporting the concept for combining vascular directed therapies and radiotherapy, with each individual treatment exerting independent effects. Interactive mechanisms may also potentially result from these combinations, where the vascular effects of radiotherapy and

Table 1 Advantages and disadvantages of combining VDAs and radiotherapy

Advantages	Disadvantages
Enhanced tumour control	VDA-induced tumour hypoxia
Spatial cooperation	Cardiovascular effects
Increased endothelial cell apoptosis	Acute blood pressure changes
Non-overlapping toxicities	Reversible neurological sequelae
No enhancements of normal tissue effects of radiotherapy	Loss of beneficial effects with incorrect timing and sequence

these vascular directed therapies enhance the effects of one or even both. An ideal combination therapy enhances tumour cell kill without enhancing damage to critical normal tissues, defined with radiotherapy as the therapeutic index: the tumour response produced for a given level of normal tissue damage (Steel 2002). The critical events that result in radiation-induced cell killing are thought to be DNA damage, in particular double strand breaks. The mechanisms of how vascular directed therapies actually exert their therapeutic effect on tumour vasculature are complex and dependent on the agent employed.

Timing, sequence and schedule are of particular importance when combining vascular directed therapies with radiotherapy. The vascular effects of each component of these combination treatments have to be considered, in addition to any potential interaction between the individual treatments. As vascular disruptive agents produce markedly different effects to the effects seen with antiangiogenic agents, strategies to incorporate them must reflect these differences. These effects on tumour vasculature can produce significant acute and chronic changes in the tumour microenvironment, which in turn can affect the radioresponsiveness of the tumour or even how it responds to the vascular directed therapy. The main concern expressed regarding the concept of combining vascular treatments and radiotherapy has been the potential for increased tumour hypoxia. Tumour oxygenation is an important radiobiological factor in determining the potential response to radiation and therefore is an important consideration in the sequencing of these treatments (Gray et al. 1953).

Since the introduction of VDAs, there has been extensive investigation into strategies to therapeutically exploit their potent effects on tumour vasculature. The effects of VDAs are most marked in the central portion of tumours, where significant necrosis is seen in tumours sensitive to this treatment. Despite this VDAs, when given as single agent, have demonstrated only minimal impact on tumour growth, in both preclinical and clinical studies. The persistence of a viable residual rim of tumour following treatment with VDAs is thought to be a significant contributing factor facilitating tumour regrowth. Combining radiotherapy with VDAs offers a potential means for enhancing the effects of both treatments.

Due to the inadequate nature of tumour vasculature the central regions of tumours are usually chronically hypoxic, which has the effect of rendering the cells in this region relatively resistant to radiotherapy. By comparison, the peripheral and more highly oxygenated regions are more sensitive to the effects of ionising radiation. Combining radiotherapy with VDAs offers potential spatial cooperation, with VDAs more effective in the centre and radiotherapy more effective at the rim. Following treatment with a VDA the remaining cells surviving in the peripheral tumour rim are likely to be well oxygenated; combined treatment with radiotherapy has been demonstrated to reduce the proportion of hypoxic cells compared to radiotherapy alone (Li et al. 1998).

Despite this apparent spatial cooperation the exact mechanism for interaction between these two therapeutic modalities remains unclear. Radiation-induced damage to the tumour vasculature is thought to be an important determinant of tumour cell survival, with the resultant endothelial cell apoptosis contributing to the overall anti-tumour effect (Garcia-Barros et al. 2003). The addition of a VDA could produce an increase in endothelial cell apoptosis and it is possible that the damage to tumour blood vessels from radiotherapy may enhance the sensitivity of endothelial cells to the effects of VDAs.

The fact that radiotherapy and VDAs appear to have non-overlapping toxicities further supports combining these treatments. Radiotherapy produces mainly localised toxicities, with acute effects such as inflammation, swelling, and erythema, and late effects including fibrosis. These treatment-related normal tissue sequelae are very much dependant on the tumour site and the dose, technique and fractionation of radiotherapy used. This is in contrast to VDAs where the main side effects described are acute blood pressure changes, cardiovascular and reversible neurological effects.

4 Tubulin-Binding VDAs and Radiotherapy

Colchicine is the classic example of a tubulin-binding agent. Studies as far back as 1937 have explored its effects on tumour vasculature and demonstrated, in both animal and human tumours, the ability to induce haemorrhage and extensive necrosis (Boyland and Boyland 1937; Seed et al. 1940). Significant vascular effects have also been observed with the cytotoxic and potent tubulin-binding vinca alkaloids, vincristine and vinblastine (Hill et al. 1993). The vascular effects observed with both colchicines and the vinca alkaloids occur only at doses close to the maximum tolerated dose (MTD), with a very narrow therapeutic window, which has limited the therapeutic exploitation of their vascular disruptive effects.

Newer tubulin-binding vascular disrupting agents offering a larger therapeutic window, including the combretastatins, have since been developed. These act at the colchicine-binding site of β-subunit of endothelial cell tubulin (Lin et al. 1988). Typically they produce a rapid reduction in tumour perfusion with maximal tumour vascular shutdown seen 1–6 h post administration, with substantial recovery of tumour blood flow by 24 h (Prise et al. 2002). Activation of the Rho/Rho-kinase pathway causes microtubule depolymerisation and remodelling of the actin cytoskeleton (Kanthou and Tozer 2002). Activation of stress-activated protein 2 (SAPK2) also occurs. These effects produce three-dimensional changes in shape of endothelial cells, more pronounced in newly formed ones as they lack a well-developed actin cytoskeleton and pericytic infiltration. Increased vascular resistance and also increased vascular permeability occurs, as there is disruption of the molecular engagement of the endothelial cell-specific junctional molecules, including vascular endothelial-cadherin (VE-cadherin) (Vincent et al. 2005). Combretastatin-induced vascular collapse, observed with CA4P and AC7700, may be related to arteriolar vasoconstriction reducing intravascular pressure, which results in an increase in the differential between interstitial fluid pressure and the intravascular capillary pressure (Tozer et al. 2001; Hori and Saito 2003). Contrary to previous conjecture as to the mechanism leading to this vascular collapse, direct measurements of tumour interstitial fluid pressures following CA4P in an in vivo tumour model revealed no resultant increase (Ley et al. 2007).

4.1 Combretastatin A4 Phosphate

Combretastatin A4 phosphate (CA4P) is the VDA that has been most extensively studied in combination with radiotherapy. CA4P (fosbretabulin [Zybrestat]) is a synthetic, water soluble, phosphorylated prodrug of the natural product combretastatin A4 (CA4). Originally isolated from the bark of the Cape bushwillow, *Combretum caffrum,* CA4 is a tubulin-binding agent that has potent activity in preventing tubulin polymerization and microtubule assembly (Dark et al. 1997). Studies have been undertaken in a variety of preclinical rodent tumour models using both single fraction radiotherapy and fractionated radiotherapy. Given the known concerns, regarding potential VDA-induced acute hypoxia compromising the effects of radiotherapy, exploration of the optimal timing for the administration of CA4P has been has been a key component to this work.

The majority of studies that have been undertaken have used a single fraction of radiotherapy. Intraperitoneal (i.p.) CA4P at doses of 10 mg/kg to 100 mg/kg administered 30–60 mins after a single fraction of radiotherapy, at a dose per fraction of 5 Gy up to 20 Gy, was investigated using the KHT sarcoma tumour model (Li et al. 1998). In this study the addition of CA4P, 100 mg/kg, to radiotherapy reduced tumour cell survival by 10–500-fold compared to radiotherapy alone. Further work using the KHT sarcoma cell line showed the addition of synchronous CA4P 100 mg/kg i.p. to a single 10 Gy fraction of radiotherapy significantly reduced the surviving fraction irrespective of whether it was administered 1 h prior to, synchronously or 30 min after radiotherapy (Murata et al. 2001a). These findings were in contrast to their findings with the C3H murine mammary tumour when following administration of a single fraction of radiotherapy, at doses of 25 Gy up to 70 Gy, they determined the TCD50 value for radiation alone to be 53.2 Gy. This was reduced significantly to 45.1 Gy by the addition of CA4P 250 mg/kg i.p., given synchronously or 30 min after radiotherapy. No improvement in the TCD50 was seen when the CA4P was administered 1 h prior to radiotherapy.

The effect of tumour size on the outcome with combined vascular disruption and radiation has been explored. Studies using a syngenic rat rhabdomyosarcoma model have reported tumour size to be an important factor in determining which of these tumours will benefit from the addition of CA4P to radiotherapy. In this work a significant tumour growth delay was demonstrated when CA4P 25 mg/kg i.p. was given 24 h after a single 8 Gy fraction of radiotherapy (Landuyt et al. 2001). Interestingly however this effect was only significant in large tumours, deemed to be those measuring between 7 and 14 cm^3. Further work using this rhabdomyosarcoma model has examined whether tumour size continues to be a factor when CA4P was combined with fractionated radiotherapy (Ahmed et al. 2006). Five daily fractions of 3 Gy were delivered on successive days then CA4P 25 mg/kg i.p. was given, 24 h after the final irradiation, with the tumour growth delay in small tumours (2 cm^3) compared to that in large tumours (10 cm^3). Only the group with large tumours showed a small delay in tumour growth with the combination treatment compared to radiotherapy alone, whereas no difference was seen between the treatment groups with small tumours.

Studies using single fractions of radiotherapy are logistically easier to undertake and provide an excellent means for screening for the effects of new targeted therapies when added to radiotherapy. However fractionated radiotherapy remains the mainstay of modern radiotherapy, especially with radical and curative treatments where generally a greater number of fractions and smaller fraction sizes are used.

Fractionated radiotherapy schedules have been looked at in combination with CA4P. Using the murine adenocarcinoma CaNT eight daily fractions of radiotherapy were delivered over 2 weeks, at a dose per fraction of 5 Gy and four fractions per week (Chaplin et al. 1999). CA4P 100 mg/kg i.p. was administered 24 h after the final fraction of radiotherapy each week (i.e. fourth and eighth fractions). In addition to minimise the effects of any resultant hypoxia the radiotherapy was delivered whilst the mice were breathing Carbogen (95% O_2, 5% CO_2). A 63% increase in tumour regression compared to radiotherapy alone, plus complete regression of 50% of the tumours in the combination group with neither radiotherapy nor CA4P alone producing any complete regressions. In another study using the C3H mammary carcinoma model CA4P was administered at a dose of 250 mg/kg i.p. 30 min after the fifth and tenth fractions of radiotherapy, with 10 fractions given over 2 weeks at a dose per fraction of 4–8 Gy (Murata et al. 2000). The addition of CA4P to fractionated radiotherapy reduced the TCD50 value significantly to 65.6 Gy compared to 70.6 Gy for radiotherapy alone.

When combining any new agent with radiotherapy it is critical to determine whether the normal tissue effects of radiotherapy are increased by the combination treatment. The study by Murata et al. (2001a) looked at the acute skin toxicity of CA4P 250 mg i.p. given immediately following single fraction radiotherapy. There was no significant difference in the percentage of animals with moist desquamation between the group receiving the combined treatment and those receiving radiotherapy alone. In addition to assessing the early responding skin effects of CA4P in combination with radiotherapy, the late effects of this combination have also been examined looking at the late responding bladder and lung effects (Horsman et al. 2002). No significant difference in bladder reserve or ventilation rate was observed. This work demonstrated no enhancement of radiation response or damage in either the early or late responding normal tissues studied.

Another strategy to exploit the complimentary effects of VDAs and irradiation that is being investigated is the use of CA4P encapsulated in liposomes. These anti-E-selectin conjugated liposomes have specific peptide sequences on their surface for preferential targeting of irradiated tumour blood vessels via intergrin $\alpha V\beta 3$. Enhanced tumour growth delay has been seen in both B16-F10 melanoma and Mca-4 mammary tumours with a single 5 Gy fraction radiotherapy in combination with immunoliposomes at a CA4P concentration of 15 mg/kg, given 5 min post irradiation via retro-orbital injection (Pattillo et al. 2005, 2009). In these experiments free CA4P at a dose of 81 mg/kg did not significantly improve tumour growth delay in combination with single fraction radiotherapy. However when fractionated radiotherapy (20 Gy in 10# over 10 days) was used in combination with CA4P or immunoliposomes given every other day (at the same dose as in the single fraction studies), both enhanced tumour growth delay and there was no significant difference between the two treatments.

4.2 Other Combretastatins

OXi4503 (CA1P) is a sodium phosphate prodrug of combretastatin A-1 shown to be ten times more potent than CA4P in terms of tumour vascular shutdown, with preclinical studies demonstrating a similar MTD to CA4P (Hill et al. 2002). The vascular disruption is again most pronounced in central regions, although CA1P produces greater vascular disruption at the tumour periphery compared to CA4P. In addition to its effect on the tumour vasculature it also displays a potent antitumour effect with tumour regression seen in preclinical studies at doses greater than 25 mg/kg (Hua et al. 2003). The additional cytotoxicity of CA1P, despite comparatively lower tumour concentrations than are seen with CA4P, may be the result of the generation of the more reactive quinone species, ortho-quinone Q1 (Kirwan et al. 2004; Folkes et al. 2007). OXI4503 has been looked at in combination with single fraction radiotherapy in the C3H mammary carcinoma model. When given i.p. 1 h after radiotherapy, at a dose of 50 mg/kg, it significantly reduced the TCD50 value to 41 Gy compared to a value of 52 Gy for radiotherapy alone (Hokland and Horsman 2007).

AC7700 (AVE8062A) is a water-soluble synthetic analogue of CA4. It is a prodrug cleaved by aminopeptidases to produce the active drug. AC7700 combined with radiotherapy has been investigated in a variant of Yoshida sarcoma, LY80, examining the effects on tumour blood flow and tumour growth (Hori et al. 2008). A single dose of 10 mg/kg i.v. was administered at 2 h, 2 days, 3 days or 4 days following radiotherapy. There were significant increases in tumour blood flow at 48 h with radiotherapy alone, reaching its maximum value at 3–4 days post treatment. A marked reduction in tumour blood flow was produced by the co-administration of AC7700 irrespective of when it was given. A greater than additive tumour growth delay was produced by AC7700 when given post irradiation and additionally it prevented locoregional lymph node metastasis in 50% of the mice receiving the combined treatment. In the groups receiving radiotherapy alone or in combination with AC7700 given 48 h prior to radiotherapy, 100% of the mice developed lymph node metastases.

4.3 ZD6126

N-acetylcolchinol-O-phosphate (ZD6126) a colchicine analogue and phosphate prodrug of N-acetylcolchinol is currently undergoing both preclinical and clinical evaluation. It has been shown to produce similar effects on tumour vasculature to CA4P. ZD6126 has been studied in combination with radiotherapy in a number of preclinical tumour models. Using the U87 glioblastoma model, ZD6126 was given at a dose of 150 mg/kg i.p. either 1 h prior to or 1 h after a single 10 Gy fraction of radiotherapy (Wachsberger et al. 2005). When given 1 h prior to radiotherapy acute hypoxia was detected and this resulted in reduced tumour growth delay compared to radiotherapy alone. The tumour growth delay seen with ZD6126 given 1 h after radiotherapy was comparable but not greater than radiotherapy alone.

The effects of this combined treatment on HUVECs have shown augmented cell killing in clonogenic survival assays, reduced irradiated endothelial cell survival and radiation induced apoptosis (Hoang et al. 2006). In this work, using Matrigel plug assay with lung carcinoma xenograft, the greatest reduction in vascularisation was observed with combined ZD6126 and radiotherapy. Tumour growth delay, using head and neck squamous cell carcinoma xenografts, was also examined. 2.5 Gy was delivered twice weekly for 4–5 weeks with ZD6126, 200 mg/kg i.p. given once per week, 1 h after the second fraction of radiotherapy each week producing only non significant enhancement of tumour growth delay.

The optimal timing for combining these treatments has been explored in work using the KHT sarcoma model (Siemann and Rojiani 2002). With ZD6126 at a dose of 150 mg/kg, tumour cell survival was reduced when given either prior to or after radiotherapy. The greatest cell kill was observed if ZD6126 was given 1–4 h after or 24 h prior to radiotherapy. Fractionated radiotherapy, 25 Gy in 10 fractions over 2 weeks, combined with ZD6126, at a dose of 150 mg/kg i.p. given 1 h after the final fraction of radiotherapy each week, produced a significant delay in tumour regrowth compared to radiotherapy alone. Further work has looked at whether tumour size has an impact on the effect of ZD6126 and radiation (Siemann and Rojiani 2005). A decrease in size of tumour surviving fraction post treatment was observed with increasing tumour size.

5 Flavonoid VDAs and Radiotherapy

The flavonoids work by causing partial dissolution of the actin cytoskeleton, resulting in DNA strand breaks and the induction of endothelial cell apoptosis. Inhibition of endothelial cell migration and tubulogenesis, leads to the formation of imperfect blood vessels and increases the probability of apoptosis. The antitumour effect is mediated through the activation of macrophages causing the release of cytokines, in particular TNF. Antivascular effect is aided by the activation of platelets, which causes the release of serotonin. Both TNF and serotonin act as VDAs in their own right.

5.1 Flavone Acetic Acid

Flavone acetic acid ester, a flavonoid initially screened by the National Cancer Institute, showed sufficient in vivo anti-tumour activity for it to be selected for phase I testing by the Cancer Research Campaign in the United Kingdom (Bibby and Double 1993). It did not proceed to phase II trials as significant hypotension was observed and it was also determined to be a prodrug of flavone acetic acid (FAA). FAA was found to have high anti-tumour action in murine tumour models and noted to induce haemorrhagic necrosis (Plowman et al. 1986; Smith et al. 1987). Mechanistic studies revealed FAA to cause selective shutdown of tumour blood vessels (Hill et al. 1989; Zwi et al. 1989). Both phase I and II clinical testing were subsequently undertaken, examining FAA as a single agent and also in combination with other anti-cancer treatments. These trials of FAA did not demonstrate any significant clinical activity, which has lead to further research focusing on new analogues, in an effort to clinically harness the anti-tumour effect of these compounds and overcome this apparent species-specific effect of FAA.

FAA was one of the first VDAs to be examined in combination with radiotherapy. When given at a dose of 170 mg/kg i.v. it was shown to enhance the tumour response to a single 10 Gy fraction of radiotherapy in Glasgow's murine ^{239}Pu-induced osteogenic sarcoma model (De Neve et al. 1990). This enhancement was only seen when FAA was given immediately prior to radiotherapy and was not seen when administered either 1 h prior or 48 h after. FAA has also been shown to be more effective than TNF in inhibiting the growth of irradiated HUVECs (Lin et al. 1996). The TCD50 in C3H mammary carcinoma, treated with a single fraction, was reduced from 52 Gy with radiotherapy alone to 42 Gy with the addition of FAA administered i.p. 1 h after radiotherapy, at a dose of 150 mg/kg (Horsman et al. 2001).

5.2 5,6-Dimethylxanthenone-4-Acetic Acid

The tricyclic analogue of FAA, xanthenone-4-acetic acid (XAA), is highly amenable to synthesis of derivatives, including 5,6-dimethylxanthenone-4-acetic acid (DMXAA [ASA404]), which is 16-fold more potent than FAA (Baguley 2003). DMXAA induces apoptosis in a significant proportion of both murine and human tumour endothelial cells (Ching et al. 2002).

Simultaneous administration of DMXAA, 20 mg/kg i.p. and a single 15 Gy fraction of radiotherapy increased the mean tumour growth time (time to grow to three times treatment volume), in the C3H mammary carcinoma model, to 18.5 days compared to 15.5 days with radiation alone (Murata et al. 2001b). When the timing of administration was altered to 1–3 h post radiotherapy this produced a further significant improvement in the mean tumour growth time extending it to 21–22 days. However DMXAA given 24 h post radiation was no better than simultaneous administration and if given prior to radiotherapy any beneficial effect was lost with the mean tumour growth time then similar to radiotherapy alone. The survival of KHT sarcoma cells was also studied following a 10 Gy single fraction in combination with DMXAA 17.5 mg/kg. The greatest cell killing was seen when DMXAA was given 1–3 h after radiotherapy, compared to just prior and 6 h after. The final component of this study examined the acute cutaneous toxicity of the combination treatment, with the feet of CDF1 mice irradiated with or without DMXAA, given 1 h after irradiation. The dose at which 50% of the animals developed moist desquamation was not significantly different between the two groups; 33 Gy for the combined treatments and 32 Gy for radiotherapy alone.

Potentiation of the radiation response has been seen in both RIF-1 fibrosarcoma and the MDAH-Mca-4 mammary carcinoma models (Wilson et al. 1998). DMXAA (80 μmol/kg i.p.) was given 5 min after a single 20 Gy fraction of radiotherapy, producing a calculated dose modification factor of 2.3 and 3.9 respectively in the two tumour models. The effect of timing was examined in the MDAH-Mca-4 tumour model. All of the combination schedules with DMXAA and radiotherapy produced a greater tumour growth delay than radiotherapy alone, although the effect was less when DMXAA was given 1–4 h prior to radiotherapy. In this work DMXAA was also looked at in combination with a fractionated radiotherapy schedule of 20 Gy in eight fractions over 4 days. Following the final fraction of radiotherapy DMXAA, 80 μmol/kg i.p., was given immediately and produced a tumour growth delay of 9 days compared to 3.1 days for radiotherapy alone. This fractionation was then used, in both the RIF-1 and MDAH-Mca-4 models, to examine the effect of concurrent daily i.p. DMXAA. This was given 5 min after the second fraction of radiotherapy each day and also at a reduced dose of 56 μmol/kg, due to the associated increased toxicity of the daily treatment. The combined treatment produced the greatest tumour growth delay in both models and was significantly better than radiotherapy alone.

6 Hyperthermia, VDAs and Radiotherapy

Hyperthermia has been extensively investigated as an anticancer treatment. The most promising component of this research has been the beneficial effects of its combination with radiotherapy. It is known to be a potent radiosensitiser of both tumour cells and normal tissue (Horsman and Overgaard 2007). This interaction is dependent on the temperature used, length of administration, sequence and interval between treatments. Sequential treatment, with radiotherapy followed by hyperthermia seems to provide the best combination, with antitumour effects still seen when heating is delivered 4–6 h after irradiation. At an interval of 4 h there is negligible enhancement of normal tissue effects whilst some enhancement of radiation damage in tumours still occurs. This is attributed to the killing of radioresistant hypoxic tumour cells by hyperthermia, with this differential effect due to the fact that significant hypoxia is not seen in normal tissues.

There is evidence that tumour blood flow is important in determining response to heat. The efficacy of hyperthermia can be improved through a reduction in blood flow resulting in both better tumour heating and increased tumour damage (Horsman et al. 1989; Honess et al. 1991). This has led to work looking at combining VDAs with hyperthermia and subsequently with radiotherapy too. The C3H mammary carcinoma model has been used to compare the effects of CA4P, FAA and DMXAA in combination with both radiotherapy and hyperthermia, delivered by tumour immersion in a circulating water bath (Horsman and Murata 2002). There was a marked improvement on the TCD50 for radiotherapy alone (53 Gy) with the addition of CA4P (25 mg/kg), DMXAA (20 mg/kg) or FAA (150 mg/kg). These were administered i.p. 30–60 min after the single fraction of radiotherapy and produced TCD50 values of 48 Gy, 45 Gy and 42 Gy respectively. The addition of hyperthermia, heating tumours to 41.5°C for 1 h starting 4 h after radiotherapy, further improved tumour control lowering TCD50 values to between 28 and 33 Gy. The addition of a VDA to radiotherapy and hyperthermia using either 41.5°C or even 43°C improved tumour control by a greater extent than radiotherapy and hyperthermia alone. OXI4503 has also been studied in combination with thermoradiotherapy using this same model (Hokland and Horsman 2007). The optimal combination was with hyperthermia, again using 41.5°C for 1 h, delivered 3 h after OXI4503, 50 mg/kg i.p. The TCD50 value for radiotherapy alone was 52 Gy; for OXI4503 and radiotherapy it was 41 Gy and the addition of hyperthermia produced a further reduction to 37 Gy.

The effects on tumour control of combining DMXAA with a single fraction of radiotherapy and hyperthermia have been further examined, again in the C3H mammary carcinoma model (Murata and Horsman 2004). One hour after radiotherapy, DMXAA was delivered at a dose of 20 mg/kg i.p., then followed by heating of the tumour to 41.5°C after a further 3 h. Radiotherapy alone produced a TCD50 value of 52 Gy, which was reduced to 47 Gy by the addition of DMXAA. The triple combination of radiotherapy, DMXAA and hyperthermia lowered the TCD50 value even further to 30 Gy, producing an enhancement ratio of 1.75. This beneficial effect was still evident with a reduction in the temperature used; 40.5°C improved tumour control producing an enhancement ratio of 1.29, equivalent to the effect seen with radiotherapy and hyperthermia at a higher temperature of 43°C without DMXAA.

7 Other Novel Agents in Combination with VDAs and Radiotherapy

7.1 *Bioreductive Agents*

With tumour hypoxia providing a major stumbling block to the success of conventional anticancer strategies this has led to the development of bioreductive agents, such as tirapazamine, a hypoxia-activated topoisomerase II poison. Given the increased hypoxia resulting following the administration of VDAs, preclinical studies have explored their combined effects. DMXAA has been shown to enhance the anti-tumour effects, in MDAH-Mca-4 tumours, of the bioreductive drugs tirapazamine, CI-1010 and SN23816 (Lash et al. 1998). Enhanced tumour growth delay has also been reported with the addition of CA4P to both tirapazamine and AQ4N, in experiments using the mouse mammary tumour CaNT (Tozer et al. 2008). With both VDAs and bioreductive agents being demonstrated to potentially enhance the anti-tumour effects of radiotherapy, this provides a rationale for looking at all three treatments together.

Additional preclinical work using the MDAH-Mca-4 tumour model has examined DMXAA in combination with fractionated radiotherapy, 20 Gy in eight fractions over 4 days, and tirapazamine (Wilson et al. 1998). When i.p. tirapazamine was administered 5 min after each fraction of radiotherapy at a dose of 75 μmol/kg, this extended the tumour growth delay to 8 days, compared to 3.1 days for radiotherapy alone. DMXAA, 80 μmol/kg i.p. given immediately after the final fraction of radiotherapy, produced an enhanced tumour growth delay of 9 days, but the combination of treatments displaying the greatest anti-tumour effect was radiotherapy, tirapazamine and DMXAA, with a tumour growth delay of 12 days.

7.2 *Nitric Oxide Synthase Inhibition*

Nitric oxide (NO) has a significant role in the mediation of tumour vascular function and angiogenesis (Fukumura et al. 2001). Tumour cells often express one or multiple isoforms of nitric oxide synthase (NOS), dependent on the tumour type. The functions of NO depend on concentration and localisation of NO produced by these enzymes (Fukumura et al. 2006). Non-selective NOS inhibition with L-NNA can produce a selective increase in tumour vascular resistance and decrease in tumour blood flow (Tozer et al. 1995, 1997). This has lead to it being investigated in the clinical setting where a recent clinical Phase 1 study has reported significant vascular effects even at relatively low doses (Ng et al. 2007b). Combined L-NNA and CA4P produces a tumour specific vascular effect, with enhanced reduction of perfused vascular volume and necrosis (Tozer et al. 1999; Davis et al. 2002).

In a study looking at the combination of ZD6126 and radiotherapy, nitric oxide synthase inhibition was incorporated as the U87 glioblastoma model is known to be relatively resistant to the induction of tumour necrosis by ZD6126 (Wachsberger et al. 2005). The addition of L-NNA (20 mg/kg) to ZD6126 (200 mg/kg), both given i.p., increased the percentage of necrosis produced at 24 h post treatment to 89–95%, compared with 10–38% with ZD6126 alone. However this combination of L-NNA and ZD6126, when given after a single 10 Gy of radiotherapy did not show any additional benefit compared with radiotherapy and ZD6126 alone.

The murine mammary carcinoma model, CaNT, has been used to examine the effects of L-NNA in combination with CA4P and fractionated radiotherapy, 40 Gy in eight fractions over 2 weeks (Mandeville et al. 2008). Tumour growth delay was significantly increased with both schedules of i.p. CA4P studied, weekly 100 mg/kg and 50 mg/kg 5 days a week, when combined with continuous oral L-NNA, 1 mg/ml in the drinking water. CA4P, 100 mg/kg given i.p. 24 h after the final fraction of RT each week, significantly increased tumour growth delay but the addition of L-NNA to radiotherapy and CA4P again did not confer any additional benefit.

Despite the increased tumour vascular effect of combined nitric oxide synthase inhibition and VDAs, neither of these studies has managed to show an increased anti-tumour effect when they are combined with radiotherapy. This may be due to enhanced tumour hypoxia as a result of the combined treatment increasing tumour radioresistance, but further scheduling studies are warranted to examine the interaction in more detail.

7.3 *Other Targeted Therapies*

Novel agents targeting other cellular processes, including proliferation, have been demonstrated to indirectly inhibit angiogensis. The monoclonal antibodies cetuximab (C225), which targets EGFR, and trastuzumab, which targets the erbB2/neu, have both been shown to reduce expression of VEGF (Petit et al. 1997). In further preclinical studies cetuximab has been shown to also reduce the expression of IL-8 and bFGF (Perrotte et al. 1999). Selectively targeting EGFR with the small molecule tyrosine kinase inhibitor, gefitinib (Iressa), also inhibits angiogenesis, decreasing the production of VEGF, bFGF and TGF-α (Ciardiello et al. 2001). With these antiangiogenic effects only contributing partially to the overall antitumour action of these agents it is likely that there is further scope to combine them with vascular directed therapies.

The poorly differentiated squamous cell carcinoma xenograft, FaDu, has been used to look at the combination of radiotherapy, CA4P and cetuximab (Mandeville et al. 2009). Tumours were irradiated in three groups with eight fractions given over 2 weeks, using 2 Gy, 2.5 Gy or 3 Gy per fraction. Cetuximab at a dose of 1 mg i.p. was administered every 3 days for four doses, with the first dose given prior to starting RT. CA4P 100 mg/kg i.p. was given on the fifth day of each week. Compared to radiotherapy alone only the combination of cetuximab, CA4P and radiotherapy (2.5 Gy per fraction) produced a significant delay in tumour regrowth. This suggests CA4P-induced tumour vascular disruption enhances the effect of cetuximab and radiotherapy in FaDu human squamous cell carcinoma. Increasing fraction size produced a greater delay in tumour regrowth, which was non-significant.

Other EGFR inhibitors have also been looked at in combination with VDAs and radiotherapy. Gefitinib has been combined with ZD6126 and fractionated radiotherapy, 16 Gy in four fractions over 2 weeks, in the NSCLC xenograft model, A549 (Raben et al. 2004). ZD6126 was given weekly at a dose of 150 mg/kg i.p. after the completion of radiotherapy each week and gefitinib was given at a dose of 100 mg/kg daily for 2 weeks. This triple combination of radiotherapy, gefitininib and ZD6126 significantly increased tumour growth delay compared to radiotherapy and either gefitinib or ZD6126 alone.

8 Clinical Trials of Combined VDAs and Radiotherapy

A phase Ib study of CA4P in combination with radiotherapy in patients with advanced lung, head and neck or prostate cancers has recently finished recruitment. CA4P was given, at a dose of either 50 mg/m^2 or 63 mg/m^2 i.v., 2 h after radiotherapy and, in the majority of treatment groups, after the final fraction of radiotherapy for the week. Preliminary results confirm that CA4P alone and radiotherapy have different side effects, with no significant overlap or enhancement of the normal tissue effects of radiotherapy.

Functional imaging has been used to assess the resultant intratumoural changes of the combined treatment. Perfusion CT has been used to assess the tumour vascular changes in the cohorts with advanced NSCLC, receiving 27 Gy in six fractions over 3 weeks (Ng et al. 2007a). Of eight patients treated six showed an increase in permeability surface area product after the second fraction of radiotherapy and also a reduction in blood volume at 4 h after the first dose of CA4P, 50 mg/m^2. This reduction in blood volume was sustained at 72 h post CA4P. From this initial analysis radiotherapy seems to enhance the vascular effects of CA4P and result in sustained vascular shutdown in NSCLC.

9 Conclusions

The preclinical and early phase clinical trials to date have demonstrated that VDAs can improve the therapeutic index of radiotherapy through improved anti-tumour effect, spatial cooperation and with non-overlapping toxicities. The timing and sequencing of administration of VDA is critical to successfully combining them with radiotherapy. Administering a VDA prior to radiotherapy results in loss of the beneficial effects of the combination, which is likely to be the result of induction of acute tumour hypoxia. Phase I/II clinical trials of VDAs and radiotherapy have been undertaken, with preliminary functional imaging data demonstrating enhancement of the tumour vascular effects. There remains scope to further improve the anti-tumour effects produced with VDAs in combination with radiotherapy through the addition of other therapeutic strategies such as hyperthermia, bioreductive agents and other vascular directed therapies. In order to determine whether the beneficial effects seen in preclinical studies can be translated into clinical practice further clinical studies, especially phase II and phase III studies, are required.

References

Ahmed B, Landuyt W, Griffioen AW, Van Oosterom A, Van den Bogaert W, Lambin P (2006). In vivo antitumour effect of combretastatin A-4 phosphate added to fractionated irradiation. Anticancer Res 26(1A):307–10.

Baguley BC (2003). Antivascular therapy of cancer: DMXAA. Lancet Oncol 4(3):141–8.

Bibby MC, Double JA (1993). Flavone acetic acid – From laboratory to clinic and back. Anticancer Drugs 4(1):3–17.

Boyland E, Boyland ME (1937). Studies in tissue metabolism: the action of colchicines and B. typhus extract. Biochem J 31(3):454–60.

Camphausen K, Moses MA, Beecken W D, Khan MK, Folkman J, O'Reilly MS (2001). Radiation therapy to a primary tumor accelerates metastatic growth in mice Cancer Res 61(5):2207–11.

Chaplin DJ, Pettit GR, Hill SA (1999). Anti-vascular approaches to solid tumour therapy: evaluation of combretastatin A4 phosphate. Anticancer Res 19(1A):189–95.

Ching LM, Cao Z, Kieda C, Zwain S, Jameson MB, Baguley BC (2002). Induction of endothelial cell apoptosis by the antivascular agent 5,6-Dimethylxanthenone-4-acetic acid. Br J Cancer 86:1937–42.

Ciardiello F, Caputo R, Bianco R, Damiano V, Fontanini G, Cuccato S, De Placido S, Bianco AR, Tortora G (2001). Inhibition of growth factor production and angiogenesis in human cancer cells by ZD1839 (Iressa), a selective epidermal growth factor receptor tyrosine kinase inhibitor. Clin Cancer Res 7(5):1459–65.

Dark GG, Hill SA, Prise VE, Tozer GM, Pettit GR, Chaplin DJ (1997). Combretastatin A-4, an agent that displays potent and selective toxicity toward tumor vasculature. Cancer Res 57(10):1829–34.

Davis PD, Tozer GM, Naylor MA, Thomson P, Lewis G, Hill SA (2002). Enhancement of vascular targeting by inhibitors of nitric oxide synthase. Int J Radiat Oncol Biol Phys 54(5):1532–6.

De Neve W, Evelhoch J, Everett C, Simpson N, Bissery MC, Corbett T, Valeriote F (1990). Interaction between flavone acetic acid (LM-975, NSC 349512) and radiation in Glasgow's osteogenic sarcoma in vivo. Int J Radiat Oncol Biol Phys 18(6):1359–65.

Denekamp J (1982). Endothelial cell proliferation as a novel approach to targeting tumour therapy. Br J Cancer 46: 711–20.

Denekamp J, Hobson B (1982). Endothelial cell proliferation in experimental tumours. Br J Cancer 46:711–20.

Denekamp J, Hill SA, Hobson B (1983). Vascular occlusion and tumour cell death. Eur J Cancer Clin Oncol 19:271–5.

Dewhirst MW, Cao Y, Moeller B (2008). Cycling hypoxia and free radicals regulate angiogenesis and radiotherapy response. Nat Rev Cancer 8(6):425–37.

Ebhard A, Kahlert S, Goede V, Hemmerlein B, Plate KH, Augustin HG (2000). Heterogeneity of angiogenesis and blood vessel maturation in human tumors: implications for antiangiogenic tumor therapies. Cancer Res 60:1388–93.

Folkes LK, Christlieb M, Madej E, Stratford MR, Wardman P (2007). Oxidative metabolism of combretastatin A-1 produces quinone intermediates with the potential to bind to nucleophiles and to enhance oxidative stress via free radicals. Chem Res Toxicol 20(12):1885–94.

Folkman J (1971). Tumor angiogenesis: therapeutic implications. N Engl J Med 285:1182–6.

Fukumura D, Gohongi T, Kadambi A, Izumi Y, Ang J, Yun CO, Buerk DG, Huang PL, Jain RK (2001). Predominant role of endothelial nitric oxide synthase in vascular endothelial growth factor-induced angiogenesis and vascular permeability. Proc Natl Acad Sci U S A 98(5):2604–9.

Fukumura D, Kashiwagi S, Jain RK (2006). The role of nitric oxide in tumour progression. Nat Rev Cancer 6(7):521–34.

Gabry D, Greco O, Patel G, Prise KM, Tozer GM, Kanthou C (2007). Radiation effects on the cytoskeleton of endothelial cells and endothelial monolayer permeability. Int J Radiat Oncol Biol Phys 69(5):1553–62.

Garcia-Barros M, Paris F, Cordon-Cardo C, Lyden D, Rafii S, Haimovitz-Friedman A, Fuks Z, Kolesnick R (2003). Tumor response to radiotherapy regulated by endothelial cell apoptosis. Science 300(5622):1155–9.

Gonzalez J, Kumar AJ, Conrad CA, Levin VA (2007). Effect of bevacizumab on radiation necrosis of the brain. Int J Radiat Oncol Biol Phys 67(2):323–6.

Gorski DH, Beckett MA, Jaskowiak NT, Calvin DP, Mauceri HJ, Salloum RM, Seetharam S, Koons A, Hari DM, Kufe DW, Weichselbaum RR (1999). Blockage of the vascular endothelial growth factor stress response increases the antitumor effects of ionizing radiation. Cancer Res 59(14):3374–8.

Gray LH, Conger AD, Ebert M, Hornsey S, Scott OC (1953). The concentration of oxygen dissolved in tissues at the time of irradiation as a factor in radiotherapy. Br J Radiol 26(312):638–48.

Hartford AC, Gohongi T, Fukumura D, Jain RK (2000). Irradiation of a primary tumor, unlike surgical removal, enhances angiogenesis suppression at a distal site: potential role of host-tumor interaction. Cancer Res 60(8):2128–31.

Hast J, Schiffer IB, Neugebauer B, Teichman E, Schreiber W, Brieger J, Kim DW, Gebhard S, Born CJ, Strugala M, Sagemüller J, Brenner W, Mann WJ, Oesch F, Thelen M, Hengstler JG (2002). Angiogenesis and fibroblast proliferation precede formation of recurrent tumors after radiation therapy in nude mice. Anticancer Res 22(2A):677–88.

Hill SA, Williams KB, Denekamp J (1989). Vascular collapse after flavone acetic acid: a possible mechanism of its anti-tumour action. Eur J Cancer Clin Oncol 25:1419–24.

Hill SA, Lonergan SJ, Denekamp J, Chaplin DJ (1993). Vinca alkaloids: anti-vascular effects in a murine tumour. Eur J Cancer 9:1320–4.

Hill SA, Tozer GM, Pettit GR, Chaplin DJ (2002). Preclinical evaluation of the antitumour activity of the novel vascular targeting agent Oxi 4503. Anticancer Res 22:1453–8.

Hoang T, Huang S, Armstrong E, Eickhoff J C, Harari P M (2006). Augmentation of radiation response with the vascular targeting agent ZD6126. Int J Radiat Oncol Biol Phys 64(5):1458–65.

Hokland SL, Horsman MR (2007). The new vascular disrupting agent combretastatin-A1-disodium-phosphate (OXi4503) enhances tumour response to mild hyperthermia and thermoradiosensitization. Int J Hyperthermia 23(7):599–606.

Honess DJ, Hu DE, Bleehen NM (1991). A study of the mechanism of hydralazine enhancement of thermal damage in the KHT tumour. Int J Hyperthermia 7(4):667–79.

Hori K, Saito S (2003). Microvascular mechanisms by which the combretastatin A-4 derivative AC7700 (AVE8062) induces tumour blood flow stasis. Br J Cancer 89(7):1334–44.

Hori K, Furumoto S, Kubota K (2008). Tumor blood flow interruption after radiotherapy strongly inhibits tumor regrowth. Cancer Sci 99(7):1485–91.

Horsman MR, Murata R (2002). Combination of vascular targeting agents with thermal or radiation therapy. Int J Radiat Oncol Biol Phys 54(5):1518–23.

Horsman MR, Overgaard J (2007). Hyperthermia: a potent enhancer of radiotherapy. Clin Oncol (R Coll Radiol) 19(6):418–26.

Horsman MR, Christensen KL, Overgaard J (1989). Hydralazine-induced enhancement of hyperthermic damage in a C3H mammary carcinoma in vivo. Int J Hyperthermia 5(2): 123–36.

Horsman MR, Murata R, Overgaard J (2001). Improving local tumour control by combing vascular targeting drugs, mild hyperthermia, and radiation. Acta Oncol 40(4):497–503.

Horsman MR, Murata R, Overgaard J (2002). Combination studies with combretastatin radiation: effects in early and late responding tissues. Radiother Oncol 64:S50.

Hua J, Sheng Y, Pinney KG, Garner CM, Kane RR, Prezioso JA, Pettit GR, Chaplin DJ, Edvardsen K (2003). Oxi4503, a novel vascular targeting agent: effects on blood flow and antitumour activity in comparison to combretastatin A-4 phosphate. Anticancer Res 23(2B):1433–40.

Kanthou C, Tozer G M (2002). The tumor vascular targeting agent combretastatin A-4-phosphate induces reorganization of the actin cytoskeleton and early membrane blebbing in human endothelial cells. Blood 99(6):2060–9.

Kirwan IG, Loadman PM, Swaine DJ, Anthoney DA, Pettit GR, Lippert JW 3rd, Shnyder SD, Cooper PA, Bibby MC (2004). Comparative preclinical pharmacokinetic and metabolic studies of the combretastatin prodrugs combretastatin A4v phosphate and A1 phosphate. Clin Cancer Res 10:1446–53.

Landuyt W, Ahmed B, Nuyts S, Theys J, Op de Beeck M, Rijnders A, Anné J, van Oosterom A, van den Bogaert W, Lambin P (2001). In vivo antitumor effect of vascular targeting combined with either ionizing radiation or anti-angiogenesis treatment. Int J Radiat Oncol Biol Phys 49(2):443–50.

Lash C J, Li A E, Rutland M, Bagueley B C, Zwi L J, Wilson W R (1998). Enhancement of the anti-tumour effects of the antivascular agent 5,6-dimethylxanthenone-4-acetic acid (DMXAA) by combining with 5-hydroxytryptamine and bioreductive drugs. Br J Cancer 78(4):439–45.

Leith JT, Padfield G, Quaranto L, Michelson S (1992). Effect of preirradiation of transplantation site on growth characteristics and hypoxic fractions in human colon tumor xenografts. Cancer Res 52(8):2162–6.

Ley CD, Horsman MR, Kristjansen PE (2007). Early effects of combretastatin-A4 disodium phosphate on tumor perfusion and interstitial fluid pressure. Neoplasia 9(2):108–12.

Li L, Rojiani A, Siemann DW (1998). Targeting the tumor vasculature with combretastatin A-4 disodium phosphate: effects on radiation therapy. Int J Radiat Oncol Biol Phys 42(4):899–903.

Lin CM, Singh SB, Chu PS, Dempcy RO, Schmidt JM, Pettit GR, Hamel E (1988). Interactions of tubulin with potent natural and synthetic analogs of the antimitotic agent combretastatin: a structure-activity study. Mol Pharmacol 34(2):200–8.

Lin PS, Ho KC, Tsai S (1996). Tumor necrosis factor-alpha suppresses the regrowth of fractionated irradiated endothelial cells in vitro. Cancer Biother Radiopharm 11(4):251–7.

Mandeville HC, Hoskin PJ, Lewis G, Prise VE, Saunders MI, Tozer GM, Hill SA (2008). Nitric oxide synthase inhibition and the effects combination with combretastatin-A4-phosphate and radiotherapy. Radiother Oncol 88(Suppl.2):S156.

Mandeville HC, Hill SA, Goh VJ, Milner J, Lewis G, Saunders MI, Tozer GM, Hoskin PJ. (2009) Preclinical and clinical investigation of combretastatin-A4-phosphate induced vascular disruption in combination with the EGFR inhibitor cetuximab and fractionated radiotherapy in HNSCC. Radiother Oncol 90(Suppl.3):S54.

Murata R, Horsman MR (2004). Tumour-specific enhancement of thermoradiotherapy at mild temperatures by the vascular targeting agent 5,6-dimethylxanthenone-4-acetic acid. Int J Hyperthermia 20(4):393–404.

Murata R, Overgaard J, Horsman MR (2000). Combining combretastatin A-4 disodium phosphate and radiation in a fractionated schedule to improve local control in mice. Radiother Oncol 56:S98.

Murata R, Siemann DW, Overgaard J, Horsman MR (2001a). Interaction between combretastatin A-4 disodium phosphate and radiation in murine tumors. Radiother Oncol 60(2):155–61.

Murata R, Siemann DW, Overgaard J, Horsman MR (2001b). Improved tumor response by combining radiation and the vascular-damaging drug 5,6-dimethylxanthenone-4-acetic acid. Radiat Res 156(5 Pt 1):503–9.

Ng QS, Goh V, Milner J, Stratford MR, Folkes LK, Tozer GM, Saunders MI, Hoskin, PJ (2007a). Effect of nitric-oxide synthesis on tumour blood volume and vascular activity: a phase I study. Lancet Oncol 8(2):111–8.

Ng QS, Goh V, Carnell D, Meer K, Padhani AR, Saunders MI, Hoskin PJ (2007b). Tumor antivascular effects of radiotherapy combined with combretastatin a4 phosphate in human non-small-cell lung cancer. Int J Radiat Oncol Biol Phys 67(5):1375–80.

O'Reilly MS (2006). Radiation combined with antiangiogenic and antivascular agents. Semin Radiat Oncol 16(1):45–50.

Paris F, Fuks Z, Kang A, Capodieci P, Juan G, Ehleiter D, Haimovitz-Friedman A, Cordon-Cardo C, Kolesnick R (2001). Endothelial apoptosis as the primary lesion initiating intestinal radiation damage in mice. Science 293(5528):293–7.

Pattillo CB, Sari-Sarraf F, Nallamothu R, Moore BM, Wood GC, Kiani MF (2005).Targeting of the antivascular drug combretastatin to irradiated tumors results in tumor growth delay. Pharm Res 22(7):1117–20.

Pattillo CB, Venegas B, Donelson FJ, Del Valle L, Knight LC, Chong PL, Kiani MF (2009). Radiation-guided targeting of combretastatin encapsulated immunoliposomes to mammary tumors. Pharm Res 26(5):1093–100.

Perrotte P, Matsumoto T, Inoue K, Kuniyasu H, Eve BY, Hicklin DJ, Radinsky R, Dinney CP (1999). Anti-epidermal growth factor receptor antibody C225 inhibits angiogenesis in human transitional cell carcinoma growing orthotopically in nude mice. Clin Cancer Res 5(2):257–65.

Petit AM, Rak J, Hung MC, Rockwell P, Goldstein N, Fendly B, Kerbel RS (1997). Neutralizing antibodies against epidermal growth factor and ErbB-2/neu receptor tyrosine kinases down-regulate vascular endothelial growth factor production by tumor cells in vitro and in vivo: angiogenic implications for signal transduction therapy of solid tumors. Am J Pathol 151(6):1523–30.

Plowman J, Narayanan VL, Dykes D, Szarvasi E, Briet P, Yoder OC, Paull KD (1986). Flavone acetic acid: a novel agent with preclinical tumor activity against colon adenocarcinoma 38 in mice. Cancer Treat Rep 70:631–5.

Prise VE, Honess DJ, Stratford MRL, Wilson J, Tozer GM (2002). The vascular response of tumor and normal tissues in the rat to the vascular targeting agent, combretastatin A-4-phosphate, at clinically relevant doses. Int J Oncol 21:717–26.

Raben D, Bianco C, Damiano V, Bianco R, Melisi D, Mignogna C, D'Armiento FP, Cionini L, Bianco AR, Tortora G, Ciardiello F, Bunn P (2004). Antitumor activity of ZD6126, a novel vascular-targeting agent, is enhanced when combined with ZD1839, an epidermal growth factor receptor tyrosine kinase inhibitor, and potentiates the effects of radiation in a human non-small cell lung cancer xenograft model. Mol Cancer Ther 3(8):977–83.

Seed L, Slaughter DP, Limarzi LR (1940). Effect of colchicine on human cancer. Surgery 7:696–709.

Siemann DW, Rojiani AM (2002). Enhancement of radiation therapy by the novel vascular targeting agent ZD6126. Int J Radiat Oncol Biol Phys 53(1):164–71.

Siemann DW, Rojiani AM (2005).The vascular disrupting agent ZD6126 shows increased antitumor efficacy and enhanced radiation response in large, advanced tumors. Int J Radiat Oncol Biol Phys 62(3):846–53.

Smith GP, Calveley SB, Smith MJ, Baguley BC (1987). Flavone acetic acid (NSC 347512) induces haemorrhagic necrosis of mouse colon 26 and 38 tumours. Eur J Cancer Clin Oncol 23:1209–11.

Steel GG (ed) (2002). Basic clinical radiobiology for radiation oncologists, 3rd edition. Edward Arnold, London.

Steel GG, Peckham MJ (1979). Exploitable mechanisms in combined radiotherapy-chemotherapy: the concept of additivity. Int J Radiat Oncol Biol Phys 5(1):85–91.

Tozer GM, Prise V E, Bell KM (1995). The influence of nitric oxide on tumour vascular tone. Acta Oncol 34(3):373–7.

Tozer GM, Prise VE, Chaplin DJ (1997). Inhibition of nitric oxide synthase induces a selective reduction in tumor blood flow that is reversible with L-arginine. Cancer Res 57(5):948–55.

Tozer GM, Prise VE, Wilson J, Locke R J, Vojnovic B, Stratford MR, Denis MF, Chaplin DJ (1999). Combretastatin A-4 phosphate as a tumor vascular-targeting agent: early effects in tumors and normal tissues. Cancer Res 59(7):1626–34.

Tozer GM, Prise VE, Wilson J, Cemazar M, Shan S, Dewhirst MW, Barber PR, Vojnovic B Chaplin DJ (2001). Mechanisms associated with tumor vascular shut-down induced by combretastatin A-4 phosphate: intravital microscopy and measurement of vascular permeability. Cancer Res 61(17):6413–22.

Tozer GM, Kanthou C, Lewis G, Prise VE, Vojnovic B, Hill SA (2008). Tumour vascular disrupting agents: combating treatment resistance. Br J Radiol 81 Spec No 1:S12–20.

Vincent L, Kermani P, Young LM, Cheng J, Zhang F, Shido K, Lam G, Bompais-Vincent H, Zhu Z, Hicklin D J, Bohlen P, Chaplin DJ, May C, Rafii S (2005). Combretastatin A4 phosphate induces rapid regression of tumor neovessels and growth through interference with vascular endothelial-cadherin signalling. J Clin Investigation 115:2992–3006.

Wachsberger PR, Burd R, Marero N, Daskalakis C, Ryan A, McCue P, Dicker AP (2005). Effect of the tumour vascular-damaging agent, ZD6126, on the radioresponse of U87 glioblastoma. Clin Cancer Res 11(2 Pt 1):835–42.

Walsh WH (1844). The anatomy, physiology, pathology and treatment of cancer. Boston: Ticknor and Co.

Wilson WR, Li AE, Cowan DS, Siim BG (1998). Enhancement of tumor radiation response by the antivascular agent 5,6-dimethylxanthenone-4-acetic acid. Int J Radiat Oncol Biol Phys 42(4):905–8.

Zwi LJ, Baguley BC, Gavin JB, Wilson WR (1989). Blood flow as a major determinant in the antitumor action of flavone acetic acid. J Natl Cancer Inst 81:1005–13.

Index

A

AIF. *See* Arterial input function
Animal models
  autochthonous tumour, 52
  bioluminescence/fluorescence imaging, 64–65
  hollow fibre assay, 69
  interstitial fluid pressure (IFP), 69
  isolated limb perfusion, 53
  MRS and MRI, 65–67
  orthotropic and metastatic, 51–52
  PET, 67–68
  scintigraphic imaging, tumour hypoxia, 68
  subcutaneous and ectopic, 50–51
  transgenic knockout mice, 53
  vascular function (*see* Vascular function)
  vascular morphology (*see* Vascular morphology)
  zebrafish, 54
Antiangiogenic drugs
  circulating endothelial progenitor cells (CEPs)
    anti-tumour effect assessment, 125–126
    anti-vascular effect, 122–123, 132
    bone marrow-derived cells (BMDCs), 119
    building blocks, 120
    colonization, bone marrow derived cells, 121–122
    growth factors, cytokines and chemokines, 124
    Lewis lung carcinoma, 121, 127
    maximum tolerated dose (MTD), 118, 125
    MeWo tumours, 122–126
    microscopy methods, 120–121
    relative tumour necrosis, 127
    tumour necrosis, 122–123
    VEGF pathway, 122
  clinical assessment, DCE-MRI
    conventional therapies, 146, 147
    monotherapy, 147
    phase I studies, 146–147
  clinical studies
    patient population, 129
    results, 129–132
    study design, 128–129
  flavone acetic acid (FAA), 118
Anti hypertensive therapy, 90
Arterial input function (AIF), 141, 142
ASA404 (5,6-dimethylxanthenone–4-acetic acid)
  biomarkers, 224–225
  chemical structure, 220–221
  clinical development, 218–219
  cytokine induction, 220–221
  cytotoxic drugs, 222, 226
  FAA, 220–221
  histological assay, 219
  in vivo assay, 218
  MTD, 222–223
  NSCLC, 223, 225
  preclinical development, 218–220
  treatment, 224
  tumour vasculature, 220–221
  XAA, 219

B

Bevacizumab
  biomarker effect, 148
  colorectal and NSCLC, 168
  DCE-MRI parameters, 147–148
  VEGF, 3–4
Bone marrow-derived cells (BMDCs), 119

C
Cancer research campaign (CRC), 189
Cardiac ischemia, 89
CECs. *See* Circulating endothelial cells
CEPs. *See* Circulating endothelial progenitors
Cetuximab, 244–245
Chemotherapy
  antiangiogenic agents, 84
  complementary targets, 78–83
  cytotoxic drug pharmacokinetics, 86–87
  endothelial cells and progenitors, 84, 91
  microenvironmental changes, 85
  non-steroidal anti-inflammatory drugs, 86
  pharmacodynamic biomarkers, 90
  preclinical studies, 78–84
  sequencing and timing
    chemotherapeutic agents, 79, 86
    Ewing's and Kaposi's sarcoma, 88
    toxicity, 89–90
    trapping effect, 86–87
    vascular disrupting agents and cytotoxic drugs, 90
  synergistic activity, 84
Circulating endothelial cells (CECs), 90
Circulating endothelial progenitor cells (CEPs)
  anti-tumour effect assessment, 125–126
  anti-vascular effect, 122–123, 132
  bone marrow-derived cells, 119
  building blocks, 120
  chemokines and cytokines, 126–127
  colonization, bone marrow derived cells, 122
  growth factors, 126–127
  Lewis lung carcinoma, 121, 127
  maximum tolerated dose, 118, 125
  MeWo tumours, 123–124
  microscopy methods, 120–121
  relative tumour necrosis, 127
  tumour necrosis, 122–123
  VEGF pathway, 122
Circulating endothelial progenitors (CEPs), 83
CLSM. *See* Confocal laser scanning microscopy
Colchicine, 235
Coley's toxins
  Corynebacterium parvum, 7
  Haemophilus somnus, 8
  Streptococcus pyogenes, 7
Combretastatin A4 phosphate (CA4P)
  combined activity, 186–187
  cytotoxic agents, 195–198
  DCE-MRI, 100, 157–160
  magnetic resonance imaging (MRI),98
  pharmacodynamics, 201–202
  pharmacokinetics, 199–201
  plasma profile, 201–202
  positron emission tomography (PET), 157–158
  radiotherapy/antibodies, 200–201, 238–240
  single-agent activity, 185
  structure and mechanism, 184–185
  toxicity, 198–199
  VEGF, 16–18
Combretum caffrum, 14, 236
Computed tomography (CT), 158
Confocal laser scanning microscopy (CLSM), 63
CRC. *See* Cancer research campaign

D
DCE-MRI. *See* Dynamic contrast enhanced magnetic resonance imaging
Diazonamide A, 211
5,6-Dimethylxanthenone 4-acetic acid (DMXAA)
  apoptosis, 240
  biomarkers, 99
  blood volume and vessel size, 103
  colon cancer xenograft models, 149
  complex nature, 102
  DCE-MRI, 100
  fibrosarcomas, 102
  KHT sarcoma, 88
  K^{trans} and IAUGC, 98
  mechanisms, 157
  β-NTP/Pi ratio, 108
  post radiation,241
  potentiating effect, melphalan, 85
  tumour-associated inflammatory cells, 85
  tumour blood flow, 111
  vessel shut down,86
Docetaxel, 88
Doppler optical coherence tomography (DOCT), 57–58
Dose-limiting toxicity (DLT)
  acute coronary syndrome, 194
  atrial fibrillation, 205
  bevacizumab, 128
  coronary ischemia, 208
  coronary syndrome, 194
  cytotoxic drugs, 201
  intravenous infusion, 208
  MTD, 201
  neutropenia, 201, 208
  vascular disruptive activity, 138
  Vinca alkaloids, 207

Dynamic contrast enhanced magnetic resonance imaging (DCE-MRI)
  antiangiogenic agents assessment, 145–146
  CA1P (OXi–4503), 156
  CA4P, 100, 154–156
  colon cancer xenograft models, 149
  DMXAA assessment
    IAUGC, 98
    macromolecular contrast medium (MMCM), 96
  P22 carcinosarcoma model, 149
  quantification, 142–144
  vascular biomarker, 144–145
  ZD6126
    DCE-MRI, 98–99
    GH3 prolactinoma model, 98–99
    necrosis, 99
Dynamic susceptibility enhanced magnetic resonance imaging (DSC-MRI), 137, 141, 145

E
Endothelial cell apoptosis, 235–236, 241
Ewing's sarcoma, 88
Extravascular–extracellular space (EES)
  macromolecular contrast medium, 96
  tissue perfusion and permeability, 142–143
  vascular shutdown, 149

F
Flavone acetic acid (FAA), 118, 220–222
Flavonoids, 14–15
  vascular disruptive agents
    5,6-dimethylxanthenone–4-acetic acid, 240–241
    flavone acetic acid, 240
Fluorine–18 fluorodeoxyglucose-positron emission tomography ([18F]-FDG-PET), 110–111
FOLFOX chemotherapy, 4
Folkman hypothesis, 166

G
Gastrointestinal stromal tumours (GIST), 143
Gene therapy
  Pseudomonas exotoxin, 10
  viral and non-viral vectors, 10
Genetically engineered mouse models (GEMMs), 52

H
Haemophilus somnus, 8
Hollow fibre assay, 69
5-Hydroxyindole–3-acetic acid (5-HIAA), 219, 221, 223, 225
Hyperthermia, 243–244

I
Integrated area under gadolinium-time curve (IAUGC)
  gadolinium concentration curve, 97–98
  MRI measurements, 98
  prolactinoma tumour model, 101
  semi-quantitative analysis, 98
Interstitial fluid pressure (IFP), 69
Intravital video microscopy (IVM), 61
^{125}Iodoantipyrine (IAP), 149

K
Kaposi's sarcoma, 88
Kety's dynamic model, 142

L
Laser Doppler flowmetry (LDF), 58
Lewis lung carcinoma, 122, 127

M
Macromolecular contrast medium (MMCM)
  administration, 102
  fibrosarcomas, 101
  intrinsic susceptibility MRI, 104
  permeability, 101–102
  PET, 112
  tumour tissue selection, 101
Magnetic resonance imaging (MRI)
  biomarkers, oncology drug development, 97
  CA4P assessment, 100
  contrast agents/medium, 96
  DCE-MRI
    antiangiogenic agents, 145–148
    CA1P (OXi–4503), 156
    CA4P, 154–156
    colon cancer xenograft models, 149
    DMXAA and tumour tissue, 102–103
    EES, 96
    IAUGC, 96–97
    K^{trans} measurement, 96–97, 102
    non-enhancing (NE) pixels, 143
    P22 carcinosarcoma model, 149

Magnetic resonance imaging (MRI) (*cont.*)
quantification, 142–144
semi-quantitative analysis, 98
vascular biomarker, 144–145
ZD6126, 153
diffusion-weighted MRI, 106–107
DMXAA assessment
IAUGC, 101
MMCM, 101–102
dynamic MRI, 141–142
extravascular–extracellular space (EES), 96
hypoxia and necrosis, 96
non-MR imaging modalities, 110–111
susceptibility contrast MRI, 103
VDA therapy, 96–97
ZD6126 assessment
DCE-MRI, 98–99
GH3 prolactinoma model, 98–99
necrosis, 99
treatment, 105–106
Magnetic resonance spectroscopy (MRS), 67–69, 107–109
Matrigel plug assay, 60
Maximum tolerated dose (MTD), 137, 138, 224–225, 237, 240
MMCM. *See* Macromolecular contrast medium
MRI. *See* Magnetic resonance imaging
Multi-photon fluorescence microscopy (MPFM), 63
Multitarget tyrosine kinase inhibitors (MTKIs), 146

N
Near infrared spectroscopy (NIRS), 58
N(omega)-nitro-L-arginine (L-NNA), 52, 85, 243–244
Non-enhancing (NE) pixels, 143
Non-small cell lung cancer (NSCLC), 223, 243, 245
Non-steroidal anti-inflammatory drugs (NSAIDs), 51, 85

O
Orthotropic and metastatic models, 51–52

P
PET. *See* Positron emission tomography
Pharmacodynamics
CA4P infusion, 202
MTD, 201
Pharmacokinetics
AVE8062, 204–205
BNC–105, 209
CA4P, 199–201
Positron emission tomography (PET)
blood flow, 195
CA4P administration, 154
external imaging system, 55
fluorine–18 fluorodeoxyglucose (18F-FDG), 67–68
tumour angiogenesis, 169
tumour perfusion measurements, 157–158

R
Radiotherapy
clinical trials, 245
combretastatin A4 phosphate (CA4P), 236–239
cytotoxic chemotherapy, 233
flavonoid VDAs
DMXAA, 240–241
flavone acetic acid, 240
hyperthermia, 241–242
MTD, 235, 238
novel agents
bioreductive agents, 243
nitric oxide synthase inhibition, 243–244
OXi4503 (CA1P), 238–239
targeted therapies, 244–245
TCD50 value, 236–238, 242
timing, sequence and schedule, 234
tubulin-binding VDAs
actin cytoskeleton, 236
colchicine, 235
vascular disruptive agents (VDAs)
advantages and disadvantages, 233–234
non-interactive mechanisms, 233
therapeutic modalities, 235
tumour oxygenation,234
vascular effects, 233–234
Response evaluation criteria in solid tumours (RECIST), 166

S
Serratia marcescens, 7
Small immune protein (SIP), 35–36, 40–41
Small molecule vascular disrupting agents
colchicine, 13–14
flavonoids/xanthenones, 12–13
metals and metalloids, 12
N-cadherin antagonists, 13

Sorafenib, 147
Stanniocalcin (STC1), 34
Streptococcus pyogenes, 7
Subcutaneous and ectopic model, 50–51

T

TEMs. *See* Tumour endothelial markers
Tirapazamine, 245
TNF. *See* Tumour necrosis factor
Tofts' two-compartment kinetic model, 142
Tubulin binding vascular disrupting agents
- ABT–751, 208–209
- actin cytoskeleton, 236
- animal toxicity, 188
- AVE8062, 204–206
- BNC–105P, 209
- cemadotin (LU103793, NSC D–669356), 206
- clinical development
  - phase Ib and II trials, 192–193
  - phase I trials, 189–193
- colchicine, 235
- combretastatin A4 phosphate (CA4P)
  - combined activity, 186–187
  - cytotoxic agents, 195–198
  - pharmacodynamics, 201–202
  - pharmacokinetics, 199–201
  - plasma profile, 201–202
  - radiotherapy/antibodies, 200–201
  - single-agent activity, 185
  - structure and mechanism, 184–185
  - toxicity, 198–199
- CRC, 189
- CYT–997, 210
- diazonamide A, 211
- DLT, 195
- dolastatin–10 (NSC–376128), 206
- ILX651, 207
- infusion frequency and duration, 187–188
- LP–261, 210
- MN–029, 208
- NPI–2358, 208
- OXi4503, 205
- radiotherapy
  - actin cytoskeleton, 236
  - colchicine, 235
- symplostatin and malevamide, 211
- TZT–1027, 206–207
- ZD6126 (ANG453), 203–204

Tubulin depolymerizing agents
- anti-mitotic activity, 15
- combretastatin A4 phosphate (CA4P), 14–16
- *Combretum caffrum,* 14
- cytotoxic agents, 16

Tumour angiogenesis
- anti-angiogenic therapies, 172
- bevacizumab, 166
- contrast ultrasound, 168–169
- Folkman hypothesis, 166
- imaging, 167–168
- immunohistochemical staining, 170
- MiaPaCa–2 tumours, 172, 173
- microbubbles (MB), 168–169
- non-invasive imaging, 172–173
- normalization process, 167
- PET-based imaging techniques, 168
- potential markers, 171, 172
- response evaluation criteria in solid tumours, 166
- targeted MB and ultrasound
  - VEGF receptor 2 (VEGFR2), 170–171
  - *in vitro* conditions, 172
- VEGF, 166–167

Tumour endothelial markers (TEMs)
- bioactive molecules, 31
- combretastatins, 32
- ligand-based pharmacodelivery, 35–36
- vascular tumour targets
  - annexin A1, 38
  - EDA and EDB, fibronectin, 36–37
  - endoglin, 37–38
  - endosialin/TEM1 and TEM7, 40
  - fibronectin, 33
  - phosphatidylserine phospholipids, 38–39
  - prostate-specific membrane antigen, 38
  - proteins labeling, 34–35
  - radioimmunotherapy, 40
  - robo4, 39–40
  - SIP (L19), 40–42
  - stanniocalcin (STC1), 34
  - tenascin-C, 37
  - transcriptomes, 33
  - tumour angiogenesis, 32
  - VEGF-a and VEGF receptors, 39

Tumour hypoxia, 68
Tumour necrosis factor (TNF), 53

U

U87 glioblastoma model, 239, 244

V

Vascular endothelial growth factor (VEGF)
- angiogenesis promoting factor, 122
- angiogenic factors, 2
- anti-angiogenic therapies, 2, 3, 16–17
- antibody-based approaches, 9–10
- anti-tumour activity, 7, 11, 15, 19
- anti-VEGF therapy, 170–172
- apocryphal reports, 6
- bevacizumab (avastin), 3–5, 17
- chemotherapeutic agents, 4
- clinical status, 17
- Coley's toxins
  - *Corynebacterium parvum,* 7
  - *Haemophilus somnus,* 8
  - *Streptococcus pyogenes,* 7
- colorectal cancer, 3
- elevated levels, 132
- engineered ligands, 8–9
- FOLFOX chemotherapy, 4
- gene therapy
  - *Pseudomonas* exotoxin, 10
  - viral and non-viral vectors, 10
- genetically modified tumours, 61
- neutralizing antibody, 127
- pericyte recruitment, 167
- plasma levels, 126
- protein synthesis, 8
- receptors, 37
- signal transduction, 3–5
- small molecule vascular disrupting agents
  - colchicine, 13–14
  - flavonoids/xanthenones, 12–13
  - metals and metalloids, 12
  - N-cadherin antagonists, 13
- testicular torsion, 5–6
- therapies, 16–17
- tubulin depolymerizing agents
  - anti-mitotic activity, 15
  - combretastatin A4 phosphate (CA4P), 14–16
  - *Combretum caffrum,* 14
  - cytotoxic agents, 16
  - intravascular coagulation, 15
- tumour clamping studies, 6–7

Vascular function
- blood flow rate, 54–55
- Doppler optical coherence tomography (DOCT), 57–58
- high frequency micro-ultrasound, 57
- intravital video microscopy (IVM), 61
- LDF and NIRS, 58
- matrigel plug assay, 60
- multifluorescence microscopy, 58–60

Vascular morphology
- CLSM and MPFM, 63
- microvascular corrosion casting, 61–62
- transmission electron microscopy (TEM), 62–63

VEGF. *See* Vascular endothelial growth factor

X

Xanthenone acetic acid (XAA), 219

Xanthenones, 12–13

Z

ZD6126 drug
- DCE-MRI, 98, 157
- endothelial cell apoptosis,84
- GH3 prolactinoma model, 98–99
- induced necrosis, 99
- N-acetylcolchinol, 88
- paclitaxel, 87–88
- tubulin binding vascular disrupting agents, 203–211
- tumour model, 67
- tumour necrosis, 244
- vascular disruption, 64
- vessels shut down, 60

Lightning Source UK Ltd.
Milton Keynes UK
UKOW06n0005120617
303078UK00001B/8/P

9 781441 966087